ATLAS OF PHLEBOGRAPHY OF THE LOWER LIMBS

INCLUDING THE ILIAC VEINS

SERIES IN RADIOLOGY 6

Series ISBN: 90-247-2427-9

ATLAS OF PHLEBOGRAPHY OF THE LOWER LIMBS

INCLUDING THE ILIAC VEINS

JACQUES CHERMET

Associate Professor of Radiology,
Department of Cardiovascular Radiology,
St. Antoine School of Medicine,
6th University, Paris

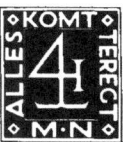

1982

Springer-Science+Business Media, B.V.

Distributors:

for the United States and Canada

Kluwer Boston, Inc.
190 Old Derby Street
Hingham, MA 02043
USA

for all other countries

Kluwer Academic Publishers Group
Distribution Center
P.O. Box 322
3300 AH Dordrecht
The Netherlands

Library of Congress Cataloging in Publication Data

Chermet, J., 1941-
    Atlas of phlebography of the lower limbs.

    (Series in radiology ; v. 6)
    1. Extremities, Lower--Blood-vessels--Diseases--
Diagnosis--Atlases. 2. Extremities, Lower--Blood-
vessels--Radiography--Atlases. 3. Veins--Radiog-
raphy--Atlases. 4. Iliac vein--Radiography--
Atlases. I. Title. II. Series.
RC951.C43   616.1'4075   81-18989
                               AACR2

ISBN 978-94-009-7463-0   ISBN 978-94-009-7461-6 (eBook)
DOI 10.1007/978-94-009-7461-6

Photography: C.T. Ruygrok, Leiden
Figures 39, 40, 41, 225, 226, 284a, b, 354, 355 and 356 have been redrawn from H. Dodd and F.B. Cockett, The Pathology and Surgery of the Veins of the Lower Limb (2nd edition), published by Churchill Livingstone, Edinburgh, 1976.

CONTENTS

FOREWORD

This book is not meant to be a textbook or a handbook of phlebography of the lower limbs. It is an atlas aimed only at teaching one how to read an interpret phlebograms, and is of considerable importance as it represents the standard investigatory method used to check the reliability of other diagnostic methods concerning venous circulation.

Regarding diagnosis, nothing is more certain than the phlebographic demonstration of a thrombus; moreover, even if the thrombus is not demonstrable, as in certain phlebites. it is still possible to establish the diagnosis with adequate knowledge of the radioanatomy of the non-opacified veins and the demonstration of marked collateral circulation. Therefore this investigation must be carried out very carefully with particular attention to interpretation.

The technique was first used in man in 1923 and is now employed world wide; better tolerated contrast materials render it almost innocuous; the occurrence of very few incidences of non-tolerance does not diminish the value of this method. We have purposely reduced the text to legends of the illustration and withheld the bibliography in so far as it is meant to be a teaching program by way of pictures without any reference to past or present publications.

In all the chapters the reader will learn to recognize normal phlebograms and attention is drawn to possible pitfalls present in the phlebographic technique. The pathology mainly concerns the phlebitic involvements of the lower limbs and of the iliocaval system; it is widely illustrated with figures and the related text allows the reader to use his own knowledge of diagnosis to interpret the figures.

Finally, some chapters are devoted to post-operative pathology, varicose veins and dysplasiae, as well as some rare causes such as traumatisms and certain extrinsic compressions. The author's purpose will have been achieved if the reader, whether he is a radiologist, a physician or a surgeon, is able to interpret, and eventually to criticize, the data provided by this investigation, which remains the reference examination for the entire pathology of the veins of the lower limbs, of the iliac veins, and often of the inferior vena cava.

The collaboration of drs. C. Bourde, J.P. Cécile, J.F. Huguet, and E. Kieffer is gratefully acknowledged. Dr. Aslam R. Siddiqui was kind enough to write the chapter on Radioisotope Phlebography.

Chapter 1

RADIOANATOMY AND VENOGRAPHIC ILLUSTRATION OF THE TECHNIQUES

Figures 1–62

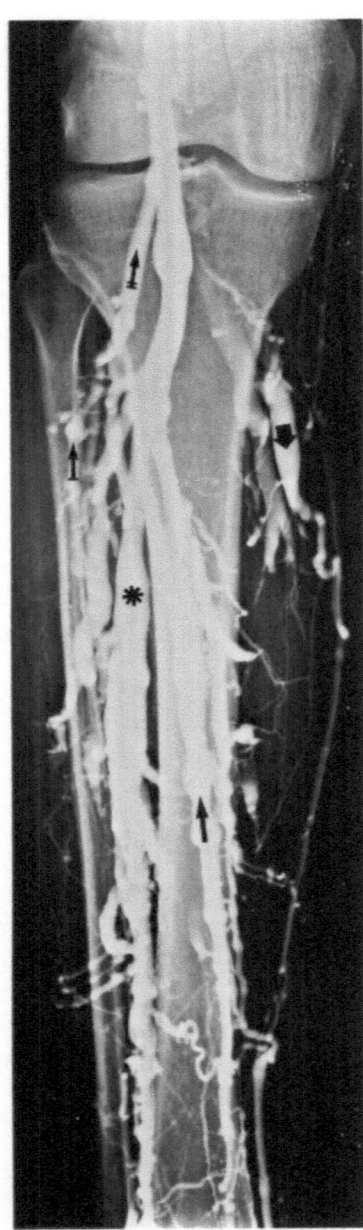

Fig. 1: Phlebography of the right lower limb. Vertical position, frontal projection. Injection into a vein of the medial part of the dorsum of the foot. The tourniquet is not utilized. Opacification of the deep veins: posterior tibial veins ⵏ anterior tibial veins ⵏ and peroneal veins ✳. The peroneal veins are always the largest and often have a "blasted" appearance at their termination. Note that the anterior tibial veins join separately via a common trunk ⵏ at the level of the knee-joint line. Note also that with this technique, the valves are clearly shown and the reflux in the initial segment of the perforating veins of the leg. Note also the opacification of the internal gastrocnemial veins ♠. On this projection the median and lower part of the anterior peroneal and tibial veins are superimposed and are not dissociable.

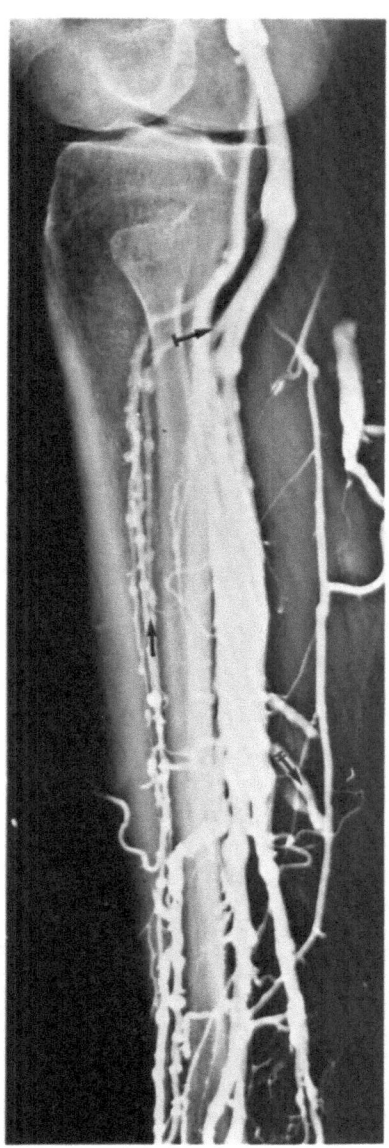

Fig. 2: Same patient as in Fig. 1. Lateral projection. This projection is easily performed with a remote controlled table in the vertical position or tilted by 60°, with the patient rotated by 90°. The orthogonal representation can thus be obtained with a single injection of contrast medium. The lateral projection displays entirely the anterior tibial veins which are small and perfectly valved ↑; it also shows that one ↟ of the anterior tibial veins is anastomosed with a peroneal vein to form a common trunk which joins the middle portion of the popliteal vein. Unfortunately, on this projection, the posterior peroneal and tibial veins are superimposed at the level of the superior and middle third of the leg, and thus ill-dissociable. There is also reflux in some perforating veins of the leg ↕ but this is a rather common finding with this technique and has no pathologic value as the perforating veins of the leg do not seem to be dilated.

4

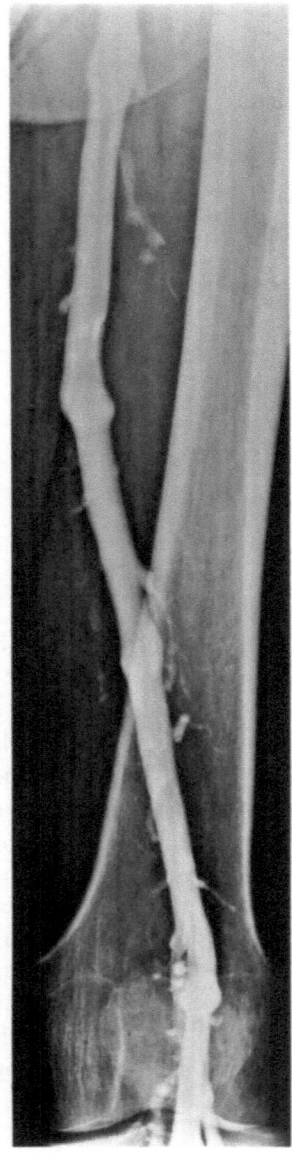

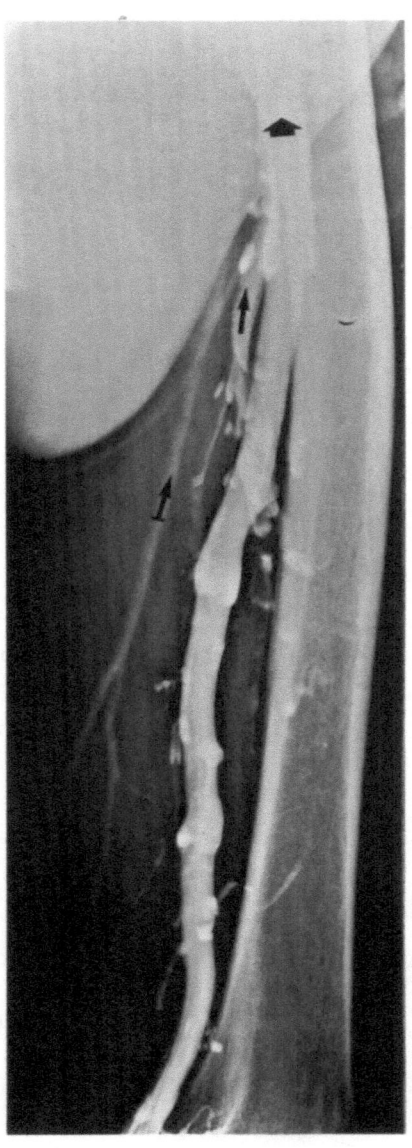

Fig. 3: Phlebography in the vertical position. Frontal projection centered on the thigh. Normal appearance of the perfectly valvulated femoro-popliteal axis. Note that the technique in the vertical position provides excellent distension of the valves.

Fig. 4: Same patient as in Fig. 3. False lateral projection (3/4 projection) centered on the thigh. The venogram has been taken at a slightly later phase and shows faint opacification of the deep femoral vein ↑ as well as a saphenous branch posterior to the thigh ↥. Superficial femoral vein crosses the femur from posterior to anterior at the upper portion of the thigh (this is not a true lateral projection) ◄.

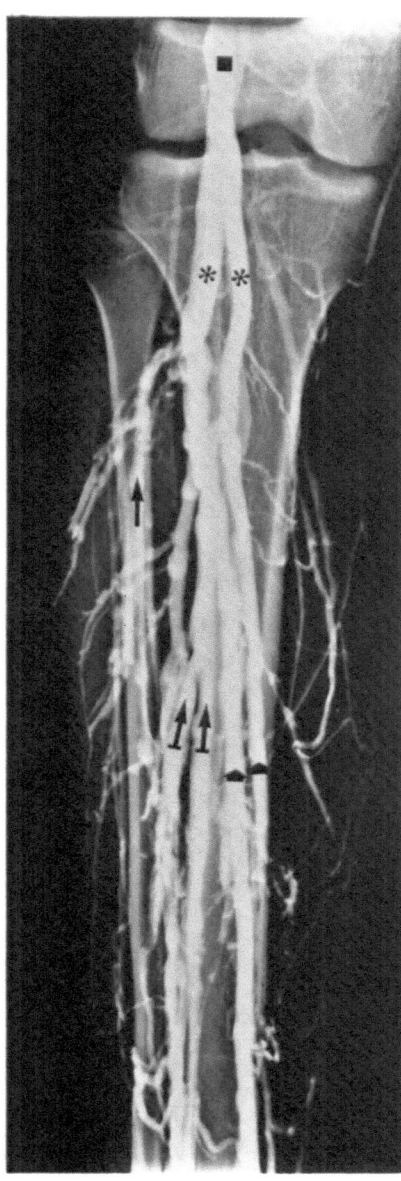

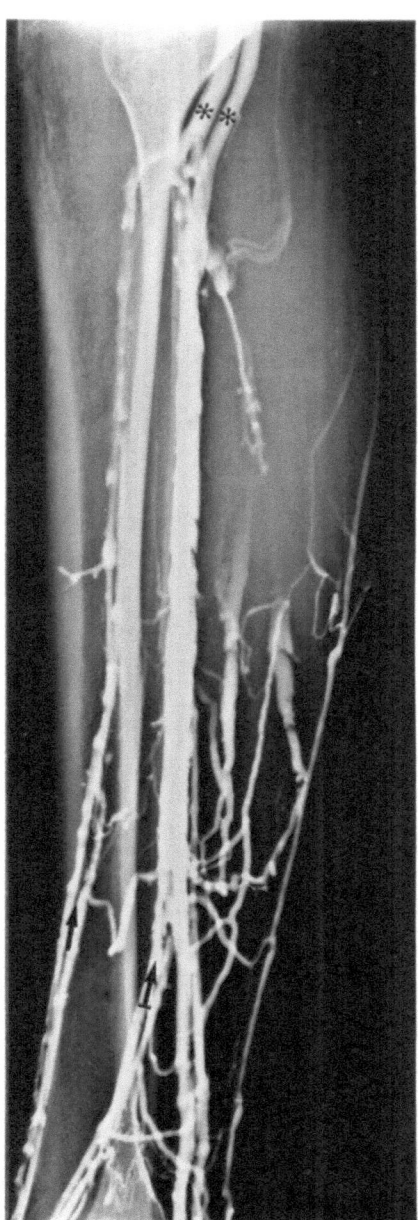

Fig. 5: Phlebogram in the vertical position. Projection frontal to the leg. Opacification of three deep venous groups: anterior tibial ↑, peroneal ↟ and posterior tibial ◣. The deep veins of the leg are always duplicated. The tibioperoneal venous trunk is double ∗ ∗ and forms the popliteal vein ▪ at the level of the knee-joint line. Note the marked reflux occurring in the perforators with the technique in the vertical position.

Fig. 6: Same patient as Fig. 5. Lateral projection. This incidence shows clearly the anterior tibial veins which are of small caliber ↑. Note at the ankle the classical disposition of the deep veins of the lower limb (lateral projection), i.e. from posterior to anterior: the posterior tibial, the peroneal ↟ and the anterior tibial veins ↑. Note also on this projection the important reflux in the perforating veins as well as in the muscular venous plexus of the calf.

6

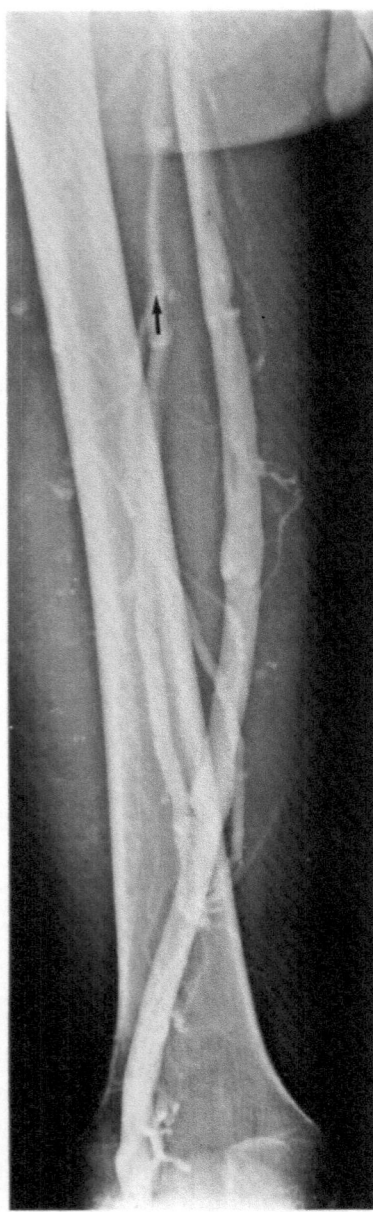

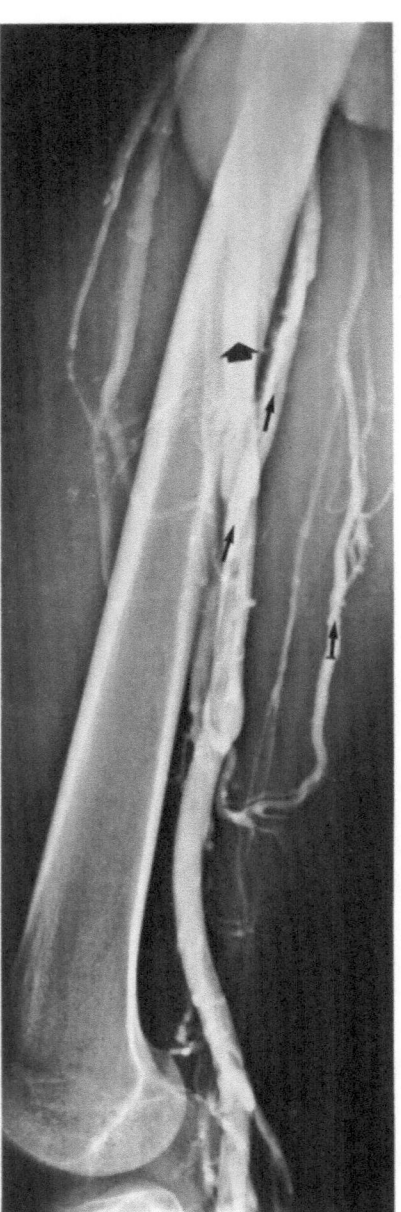

Fig. 7: Venography in the vertical position. Centering on the thigh. Hand injection at low rate. The opacification of the femoro-popliteal axis is faint but demonstrates the patency of the axis and clearly outlined valves. Opacification of the profunda femoris vein ↑.

Fig. 8: Same patient as in Fig. 7. Note the usual topography of the superficial femoral ● vein which crosses the femur from posterior to anterior, and of the profunda femoris vein which remains longer behind the femoral diaphysis ↑. Note the posterior opacification of a vein of the sciatic nerve (↕). It is not a superficial vein insofar as it branches from the popliteal vein.

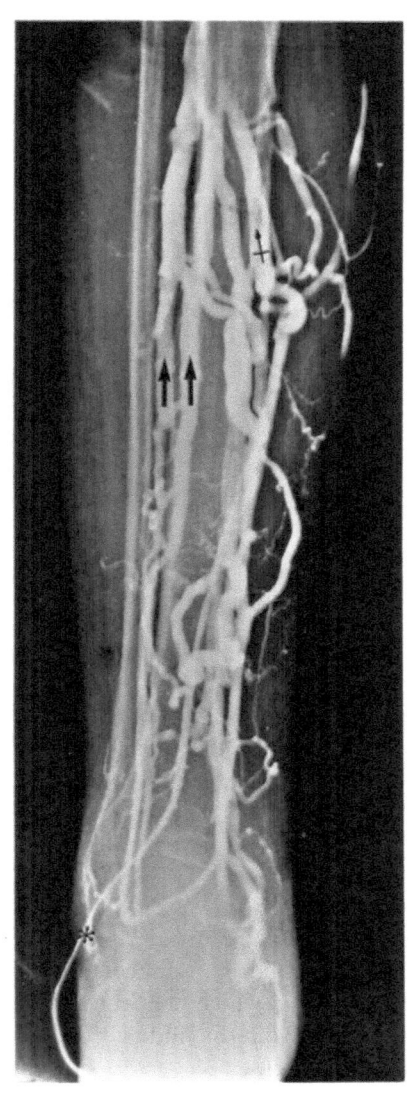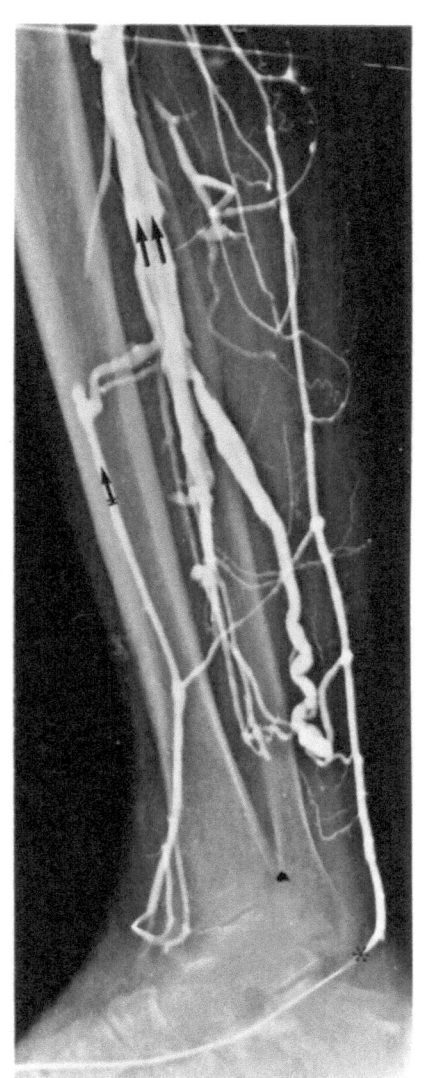

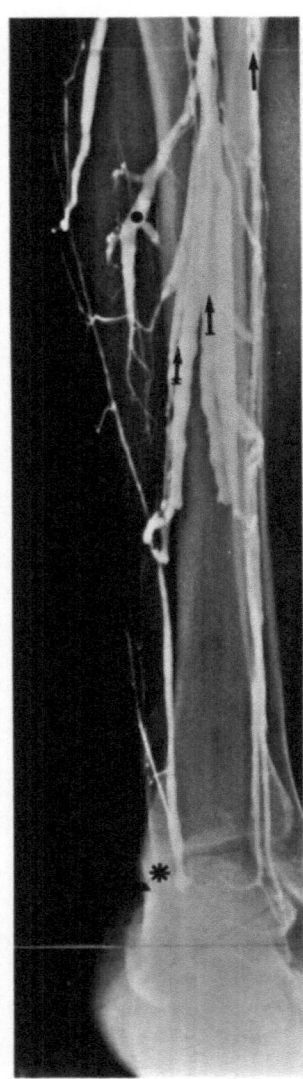

Fig. 11: Phlebogram in the dorsal decubitus. Upstream injection into the internal saphenous vein at the level of the malleolus ✳. Film centered onto the leg. Opacification of the anterior tibial veins ↑ which are thin. Filling of the peroneal ↕ and posterior tibial veins ↨ only from the middle third of the leg on. Reflux into the internal veins ● of muscles.

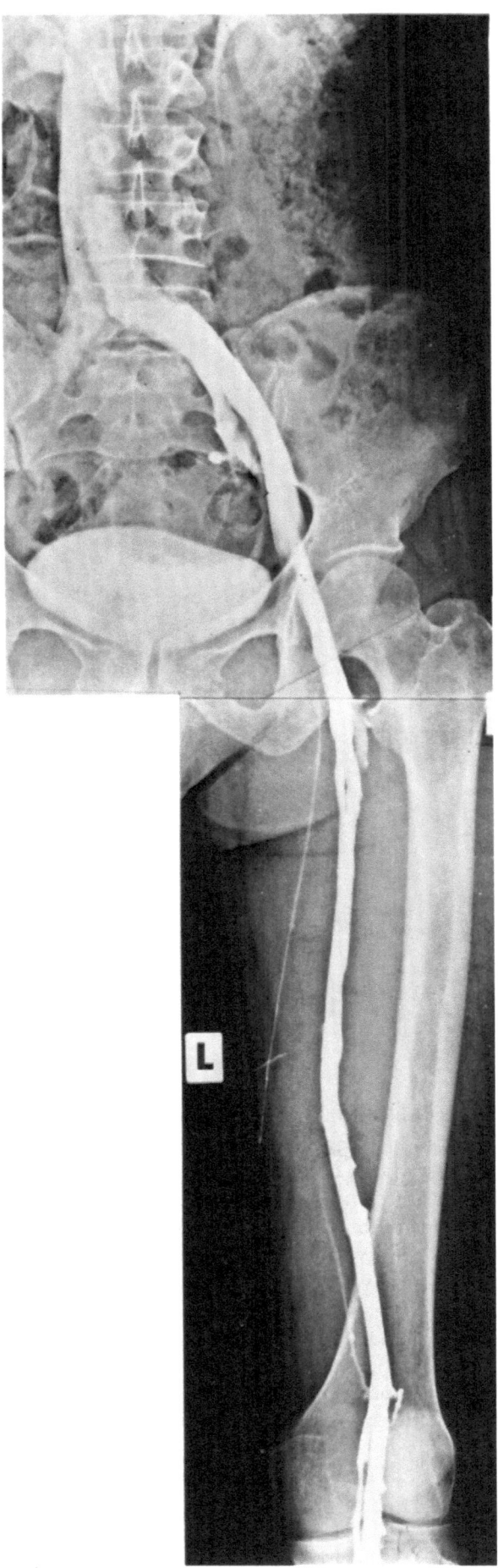

Fig. 12: Phlebogram in the dorsal decubitus. Excellent opacification of the deep femoro-popliteal venous axis, of the ilio-femoral venous system and of the infrarenal inferior vena cava. A large amount of contrast medium is necessary: 100 ml of a material containing 380 mg/ml iod, injected at a rate of 6 ml/s. Retrograde injection into a large superficial vein (the internal saphenous vein at the ankle) provides excellent filling of the veins.

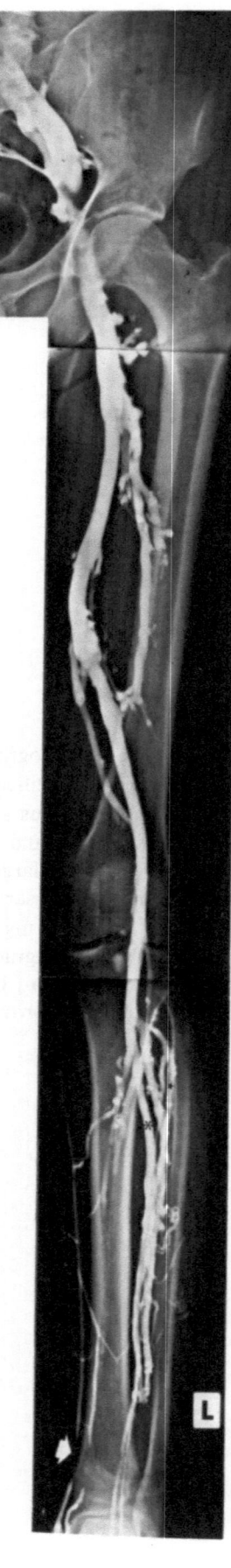

Fig. 13: Phlebography performed in the dorsal decubitus. Upstream injection into the superficial dorsal venous arch (medial portion). Large dose of contrast medium: 100 ml. Six films in large 30 × 120 cm cassettes. Very good opacification of the peroneal veins *. The posterior tibial veins are squeezed by a very tight tourniquet above the ankle ♦. The anterior tibial veins ★ are opacified from the middle third of the leg. Very good opacification of the femoro-popliteal axis, of the profunda femoris vein (from below upward, which is quite normal), and finally, of the ilio-fermoral venous axis. This technique with large cassettes provides complete visualization of the morphology of the venous system of the lower limb.

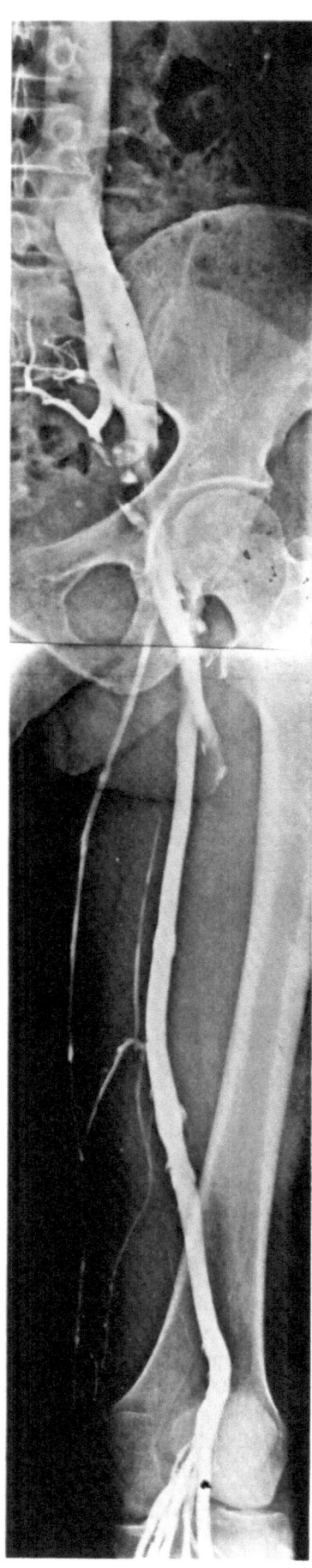

Fig. 14: Phlebography performed in the dorsal decubitus. Large dose of contrast medium: 100 ml. Film centered onto the pelvis and the thigh. Note the excellent opacification of the femoro-popliteal axis, then of the ilio-femoral, and finally of the inferior vena cava. The latter is very well opacified without using abdominal compression maneuvers.

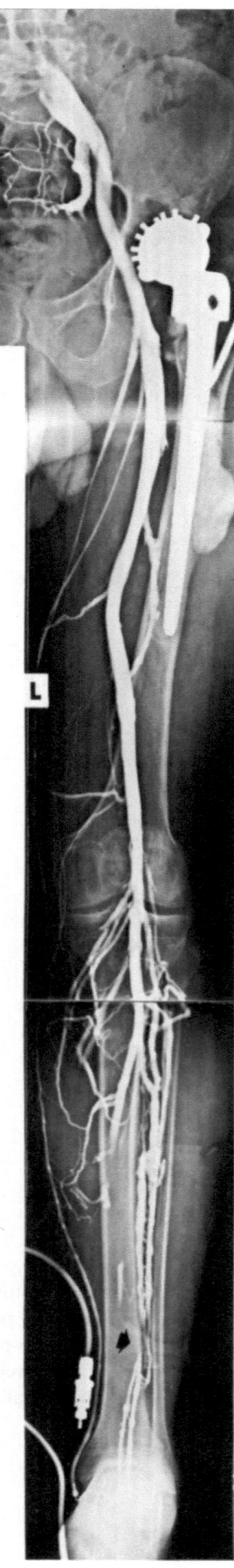

Fig. 15: Phlebography of the left lower limb. Upstream injection into the internal saphenous vein at the ankle. Large volume of contrast: 100 ml. Large cassette. Correct opacification of all peroneal veins. A tourniquet ← applied very tightly around the leg prevents correct opacification of the posterior tibial veins. The anterior tibial veins are opacified in the upper part of the leg and are superimposed onto the peroneal veins. Excellent opacification of the femoro-popliteal axis, of the ilio-femoral route and of the inferior vena caval origin.

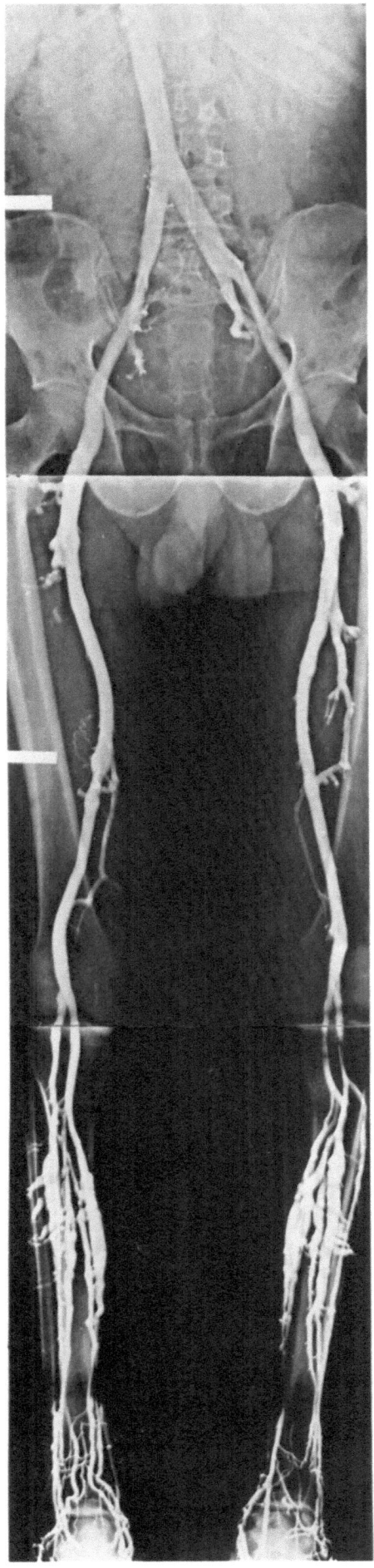

Fig. 16: Phlebography with the patient in the supine position. Large cassettes. Large volume of contrast: 200 ml, as both legs are examined. Excellent opacification of the right and of the left venous system as well as of the inferior vena cava.

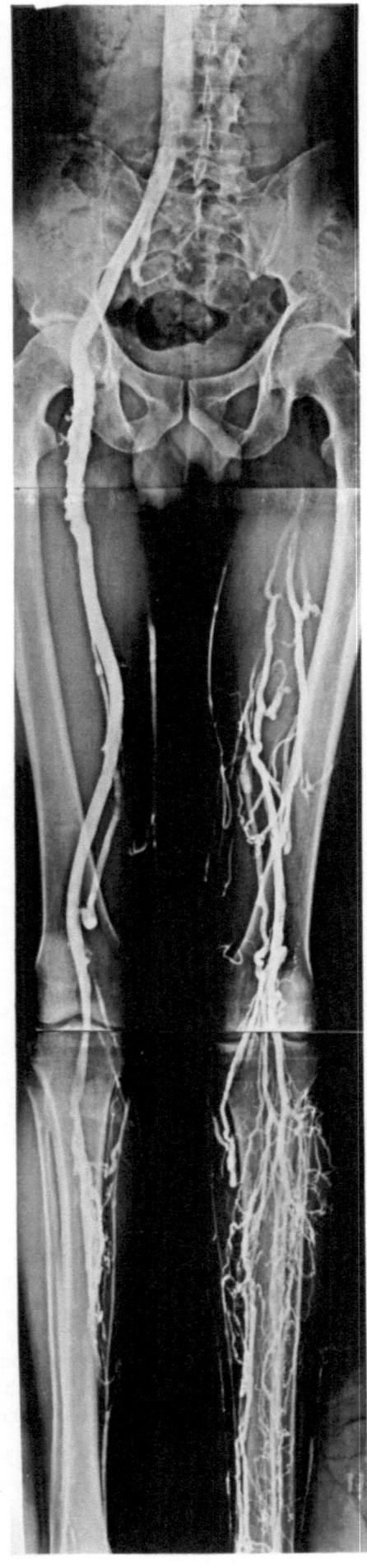

Fig. 17: Phlebography with the patient lying supine. Bilateral injection of 100 ml of contrast into a dorsal vein of the foot on the right and on the left. This volume is notoriously insufficient for a correct opacification of the venous system of the right and left lower limbs. The left venous system, which shows signs of chronic phlebitis with recanalization changes on the leg as well as on the femoro-popliteal system, presents retarded progression of the contrast; there is no iliofemoral opacification so that it is impossible to make the diagnosis of occlusion or of patency of the left iliac system. In the absence of a 100 ml double syringe, phlebography with entirely free circulation is performed separately, first on the right, then on the left side.

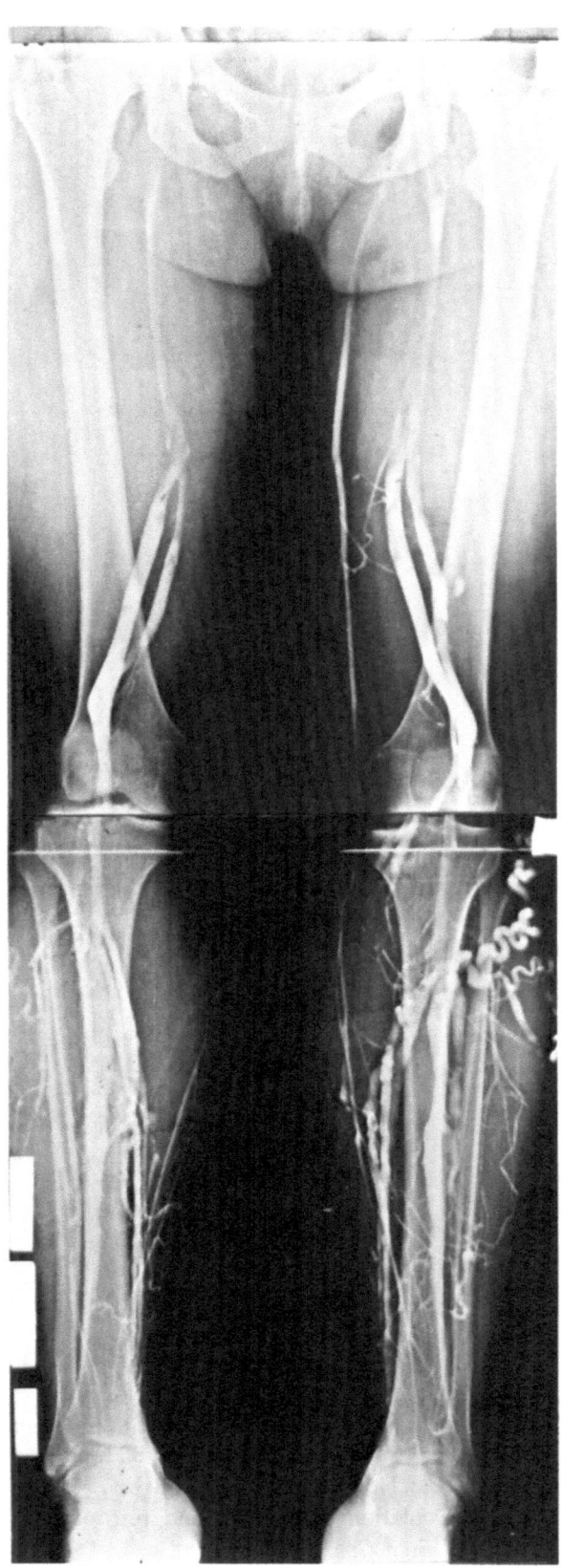

Fig. 18: Another case. Phlebography in the supine position. Bilateral hand injection of 100 ml contrast medium. Varicose veins of the left leg. Because of the hand injection (though it is a later phase, it is here an X-ray film with a 40 s exposure time), there is no opacification of the upper part of the superficial femoral system. The use of a small amount of contrast medium combined with hand injection render this technique inadequate. Preferably venography of the lower limbs should be carried out with an automatic injector with constant delivery rate, and with a large volume of contrast medium (80 to 100 ml for each side).

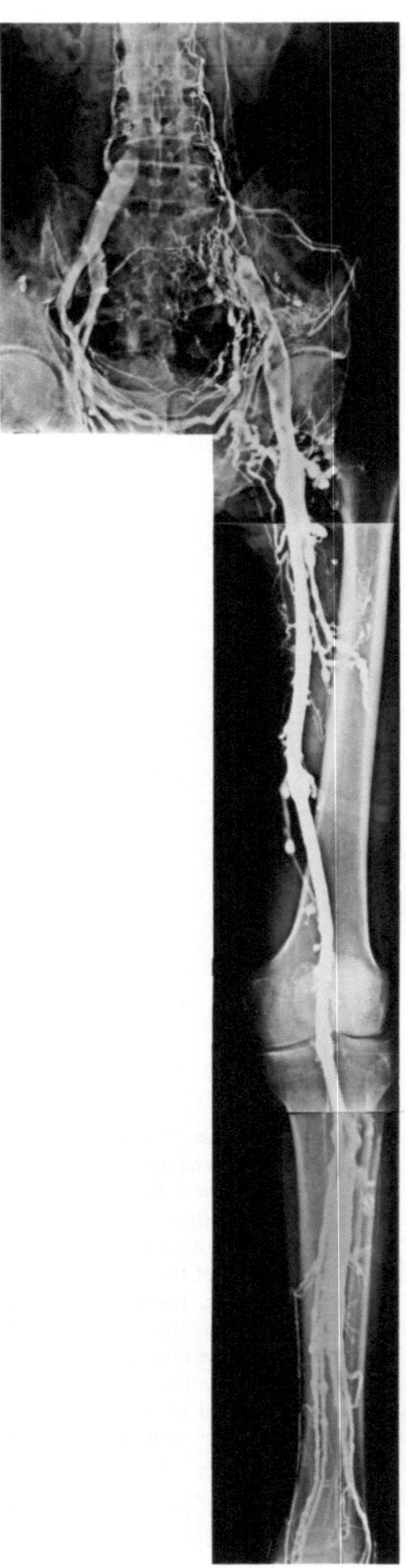

Fig. 19: Phlebography in the supine position. Injection of a large volume: 100 ml. Demonstration of a left iliofemoral free thrombus. Note the opacification of the left-to-right collateral circulation via supra- and retropubic plexuses. Compare to Fig. 17.

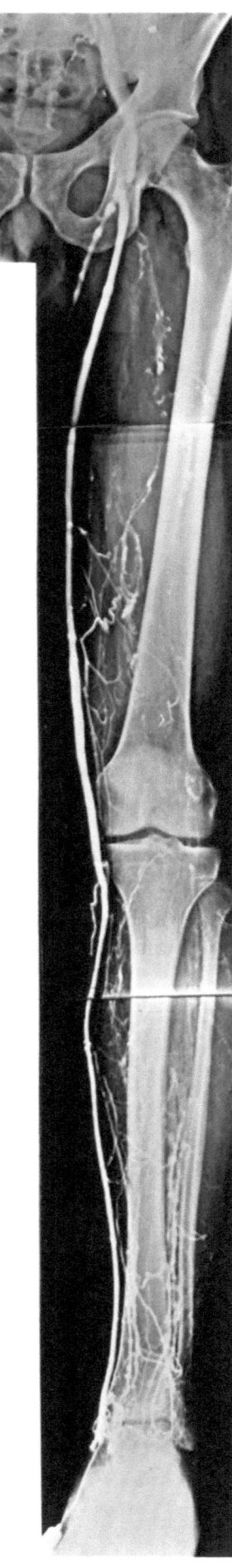

Fig. 20: Free circulation phlebography of the left lower limb. Downstream injection into the internal saphenous vein at the level of the ankle. Example of a technique not to be used: this demonstrates nothing but the internal saphenous vein on the medial aspect of the left leg, and some fragmentary opacifications of the deep system. When the injection into the internal saphenous vein is performed at the ankle, it should be done in the upstream direction to opacify the deep veins (the perforating veins of the ankle and of the foot are mostly valveless and permit filling of the deep venous system).

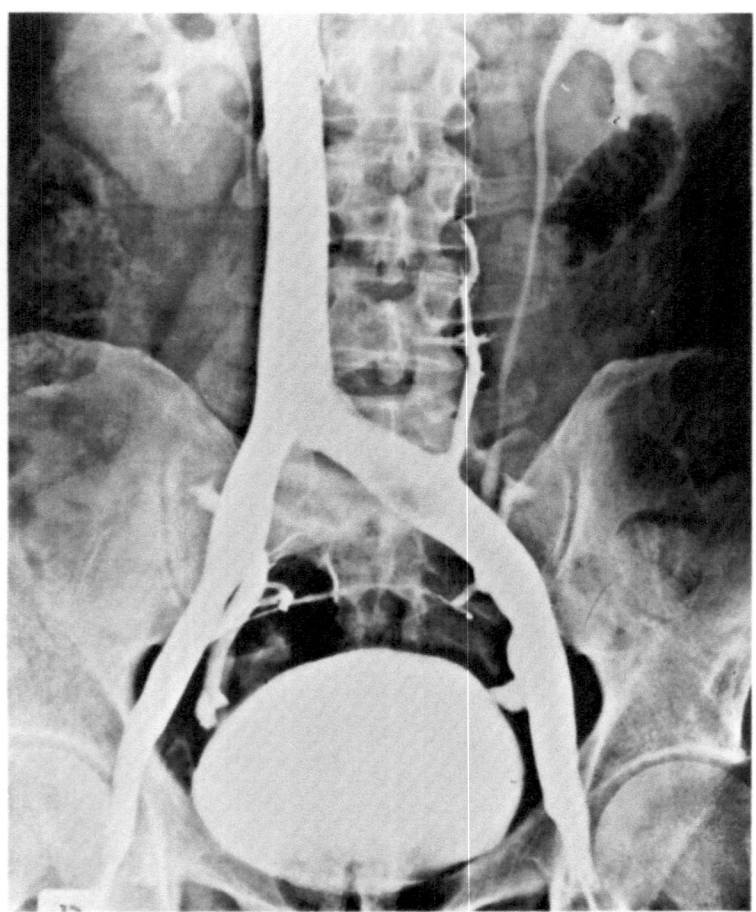

Fig. 21: Bifemoral percutaneous inferior vena cavography performed with two small needle-catheters introduced into the common femoral vein on the right and on the left side. Normal radiologic appearance. Normal slight opacification of the left ascending lumbar vein.

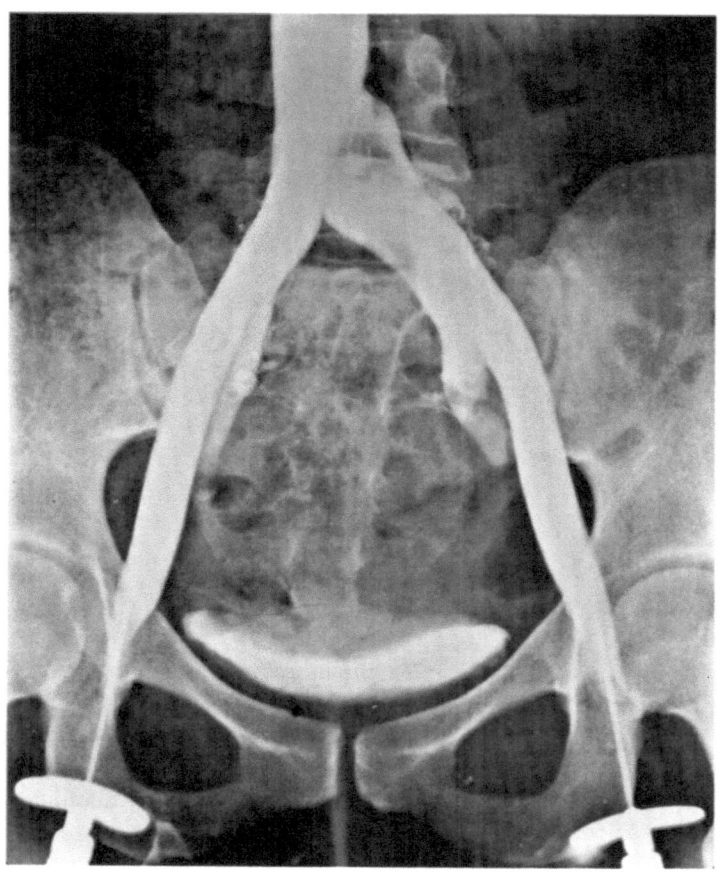

Fig. 22: Another case. Bifemoral percutaneous inferior vena cavography performed with two metal Seldinger-type trocars. Normal reflux, up to the first valve, in the right and left hypogastric system.

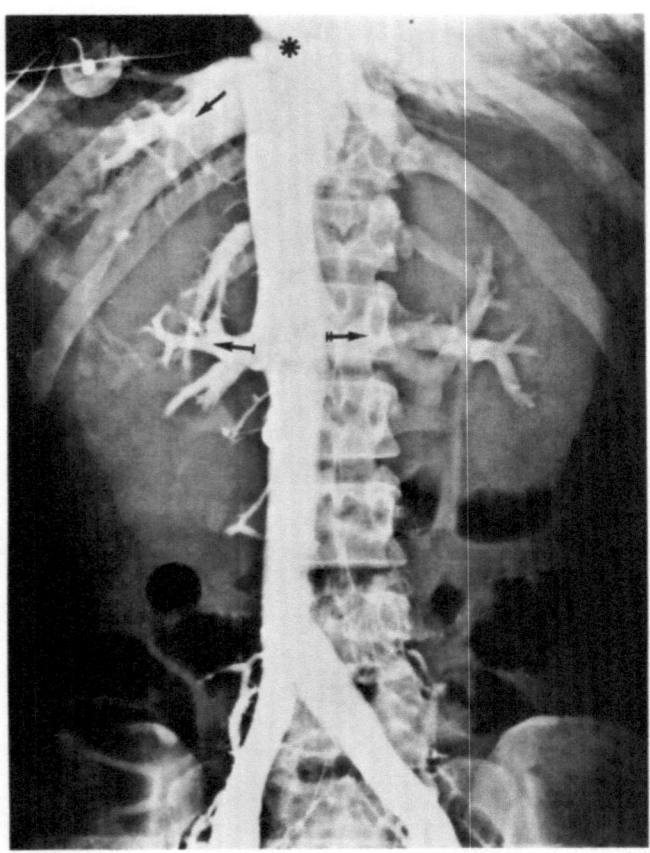

Fig. 23: Bifemoral percutaneous iliocavography. Centering onto the upper abdomen up to the floor of the right atrium ✳. Valsalva maneuver with sus-hepatic ↑ and left ↓ and right ↑ renal reflux. Normal radiologic appearance.

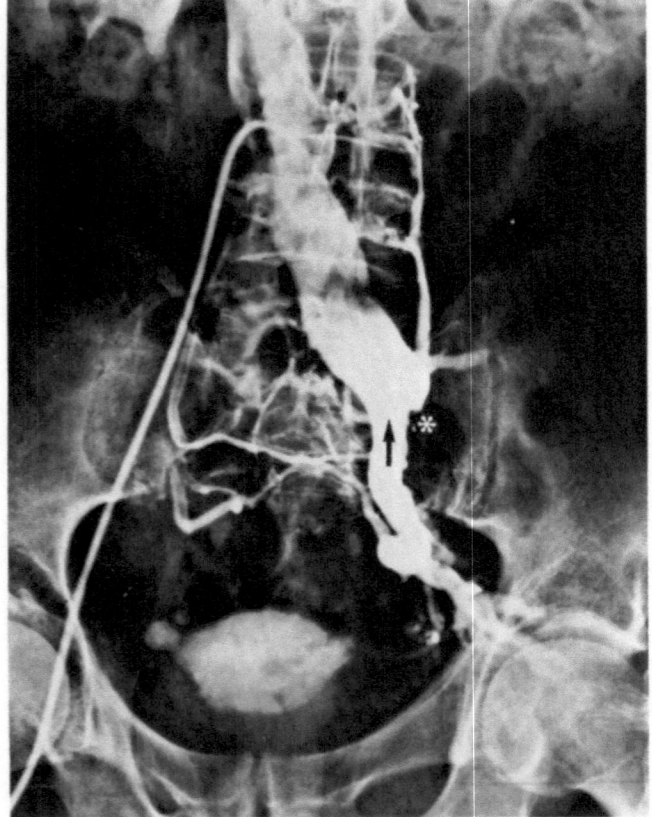

Fig. 24

Figs. 24 and 25: Retrograde iliac venography.

24: The contrast medium moulds the head of a thrombus in the left iliofemoral system. Note the upwardly concave stop * . Reflux into the left internal iliac vein ↑. Catheterization of the right femoral vein according to the Seldinger technique.

25: Later phase of the same injection show stagnation above the head of the left iliofem thrombus ●. This latter image rules out the p ence of a valve in the external iliac vein, w would have the same morphology but would produce stagnation of the contrast medium.

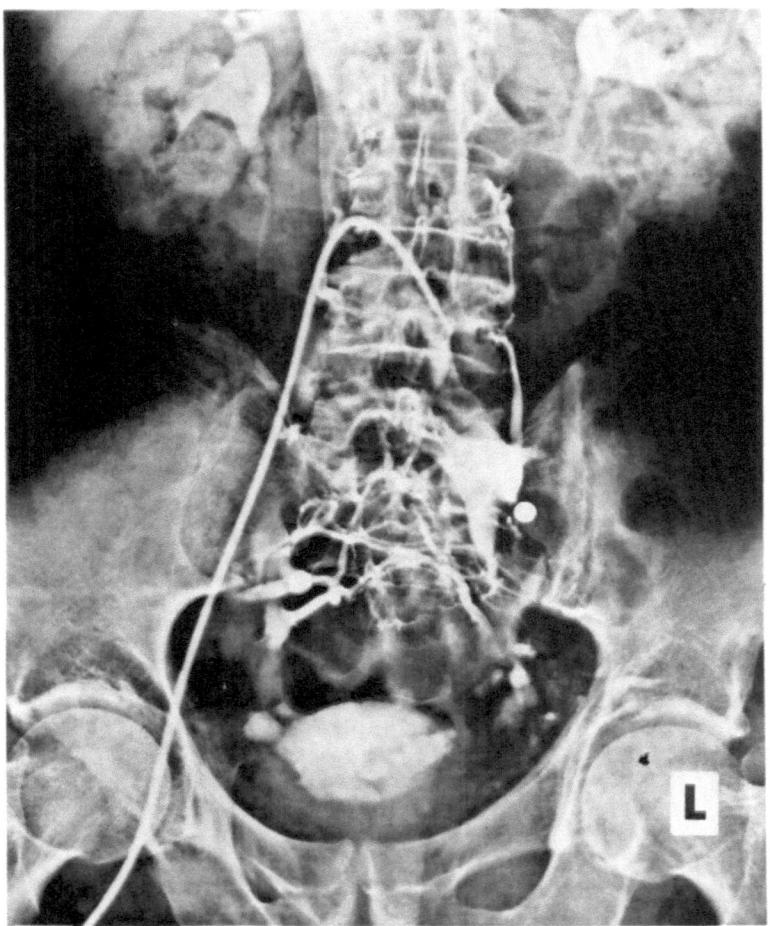

Fig. 25

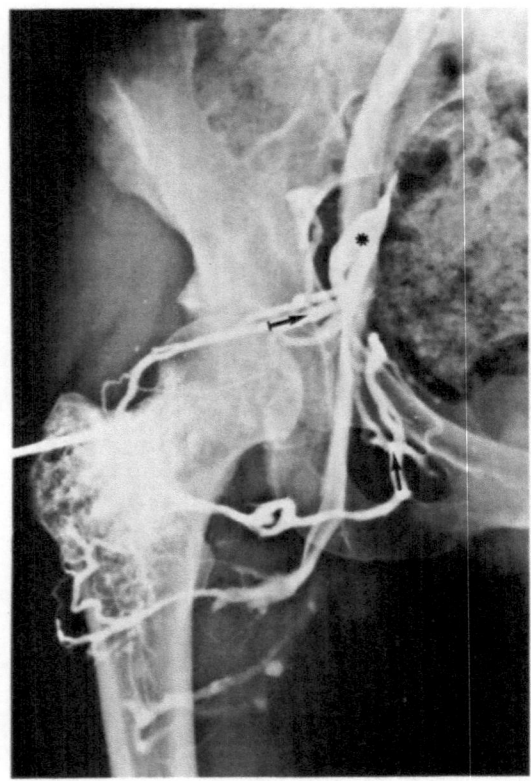

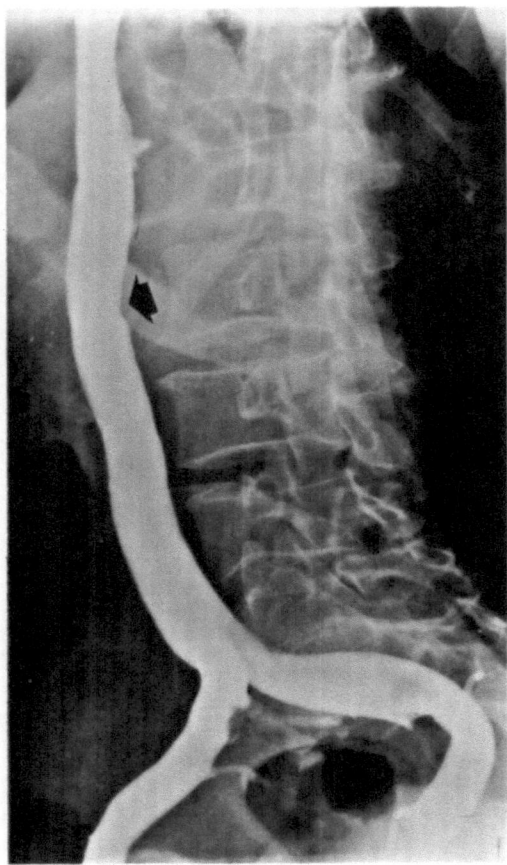

Fig. 26: Transosseous right pertrochanteric venography. Opacification of the circumflex veins connected with the obturator ⭡ and inferior gluteal ⭡ venous system draining toward the right internal iliac vein ✳. This technique is dangerous and entails the risk of fat embolism; moreover it requires general anesthetic. It is no longer used.

Fig. 27: Percutaneous bifemoral cavography. Left anterior oblique projection separating perfectly the image of the posterior aspect of the cava and the image of the spine. Note the arciform imprint of the right renal artery on the posterior aspect of the interrenal segment of the inferior vena cava ◄.

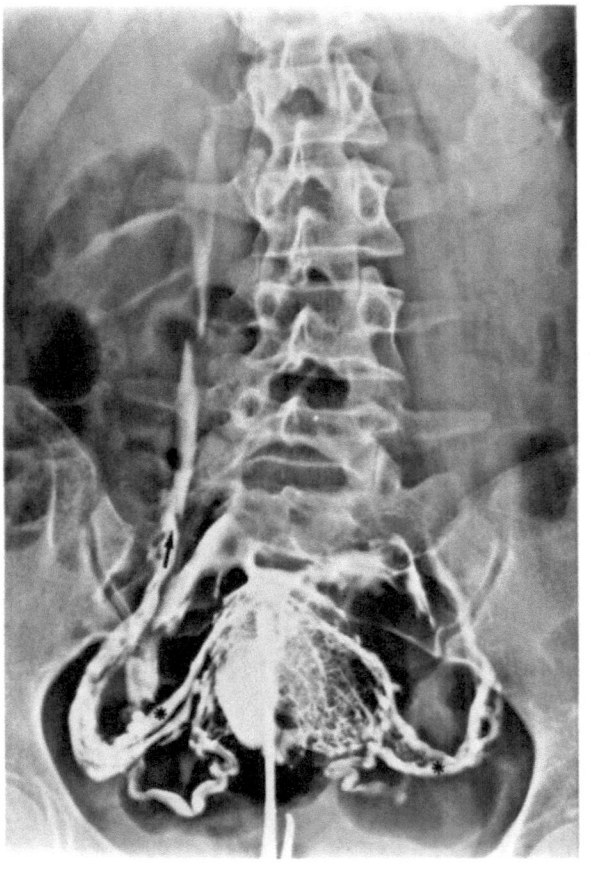

Fig. 28

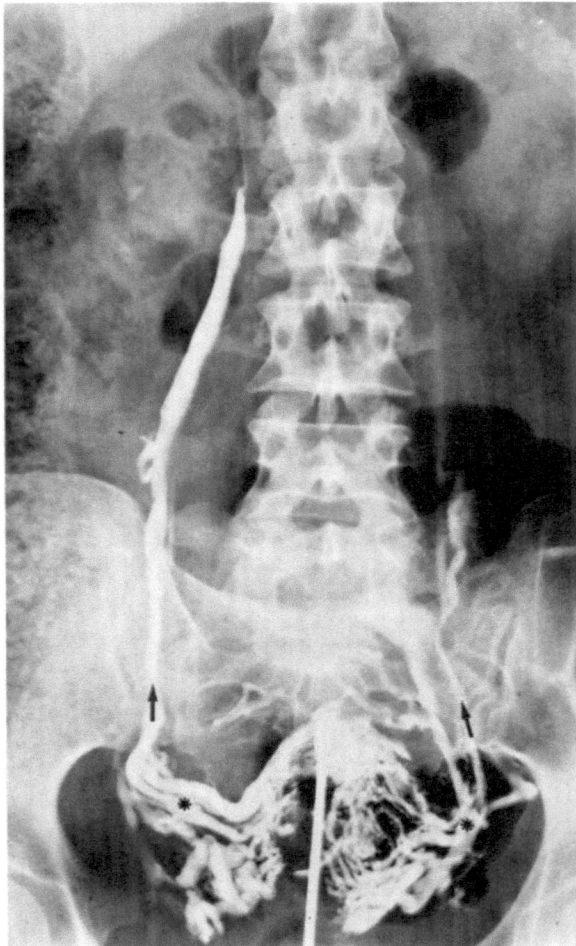

Fig. 29

Figs. 28 and 29: Hysterophlebography by puncture of the fundus of the uterus. This technique (Pr. Tavernier) opacifies only the hypogastric ✳ and ovarian venous systems ↑.

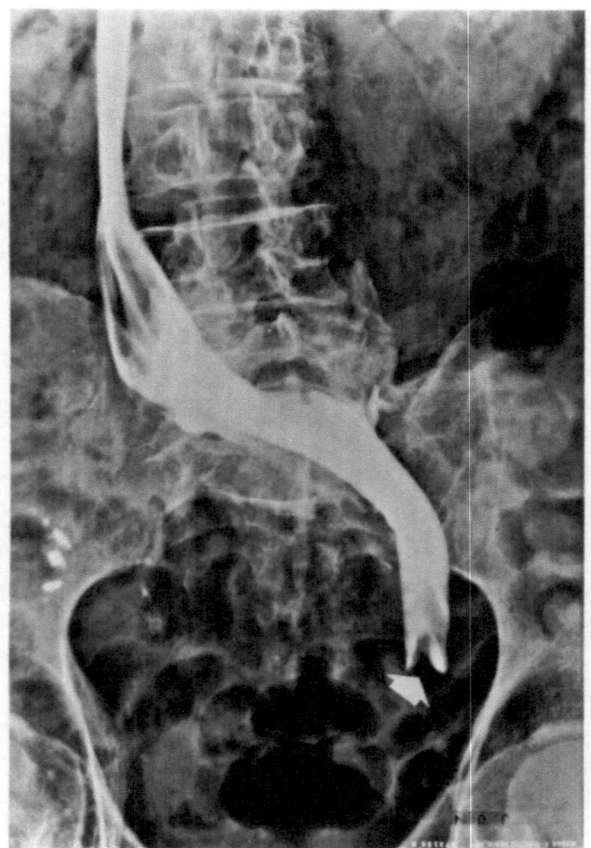 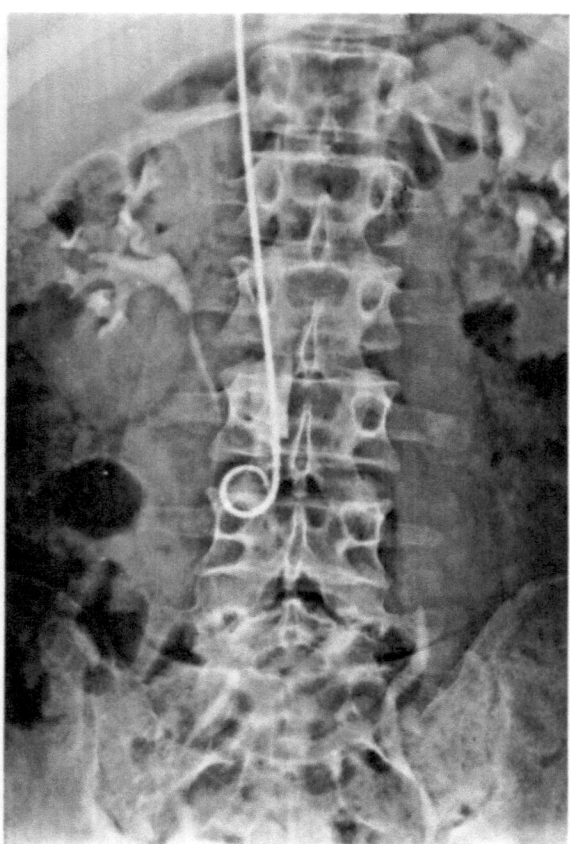

Fig. 31

Fig. 30: Descending cavography. The catheter is in the left common iliac vein. Opacification by reflux as far as the first valve, which corresponds to the external iliac valve, shows clearly on this film ◄.

Figs. 31 and 32: Descending cavography by percutaneous brachial approach (a pigtail-shaped catheter is introduced at the bend of the right elbow by means of a Desilets).

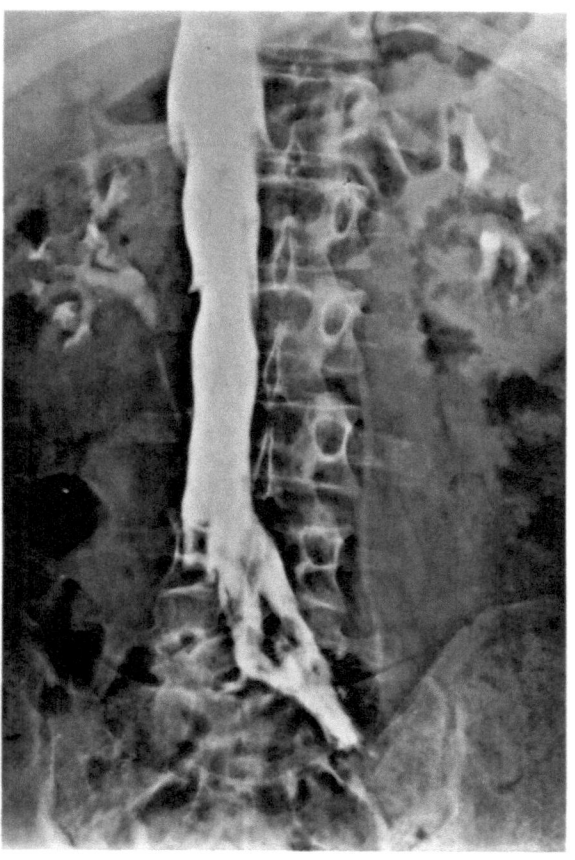

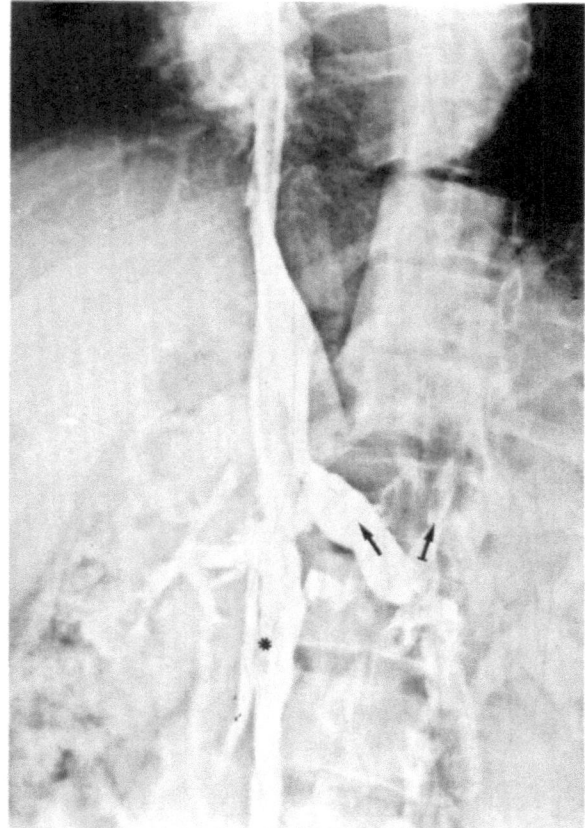

Fig. 32

Fig. 33: Descending cavography by brachial injection. This investigation was carried out after a venogram of the lower limbs had shown obstruction of both iliac veins. The technique is performed to show the upper level of the obstruction in the event of an involvement of the inter- and suprarenal portion of the inferior vena cava. The suprarenal and the interrenal portion of the inferior vena cava is patent. The infrarenal inferior vena cava ✱ has a narrow and straticulate appearance, a sign of chronic thrombosis. The left anterior oblique projection shows a reflux into the left renal vein ↑ which opacifies the onset of a renoazygos collateral circulation ↥.

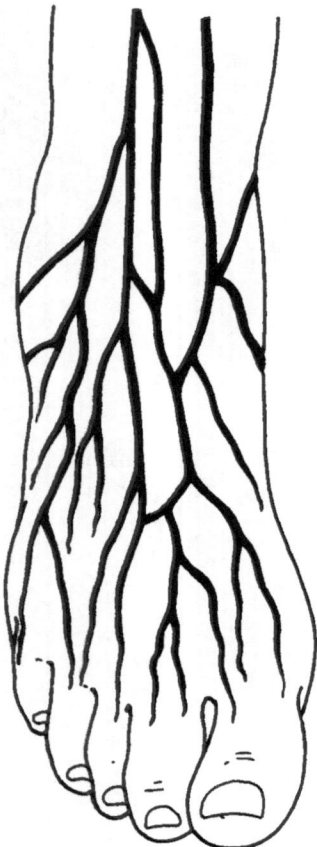 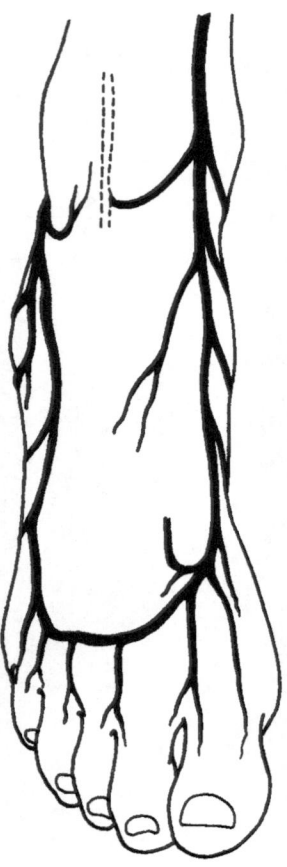

Fig. 34: Superficial dorsal venous system of the foot.

Fig. 35: Dorsal venous arch and superficial system of both saphenous veins.

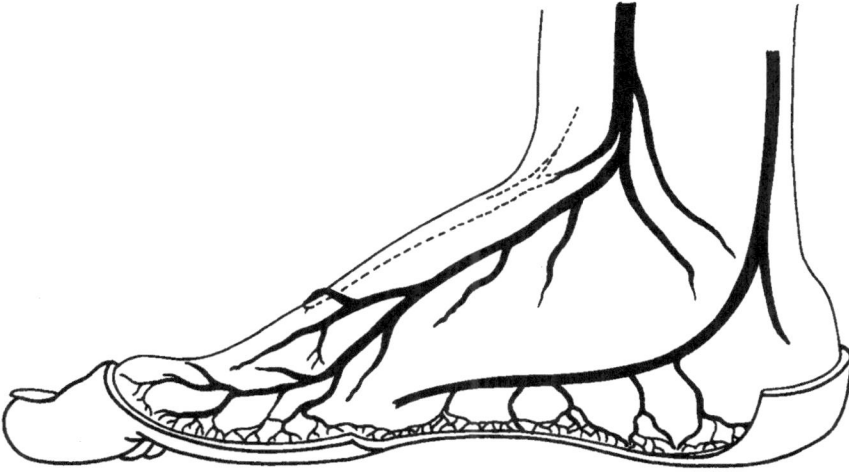

Fig. 36: Superficial plantar venous network. This plexus drains into the plantar veins but also into the dorsal veins of the foot (superficial veins and saphenous system).

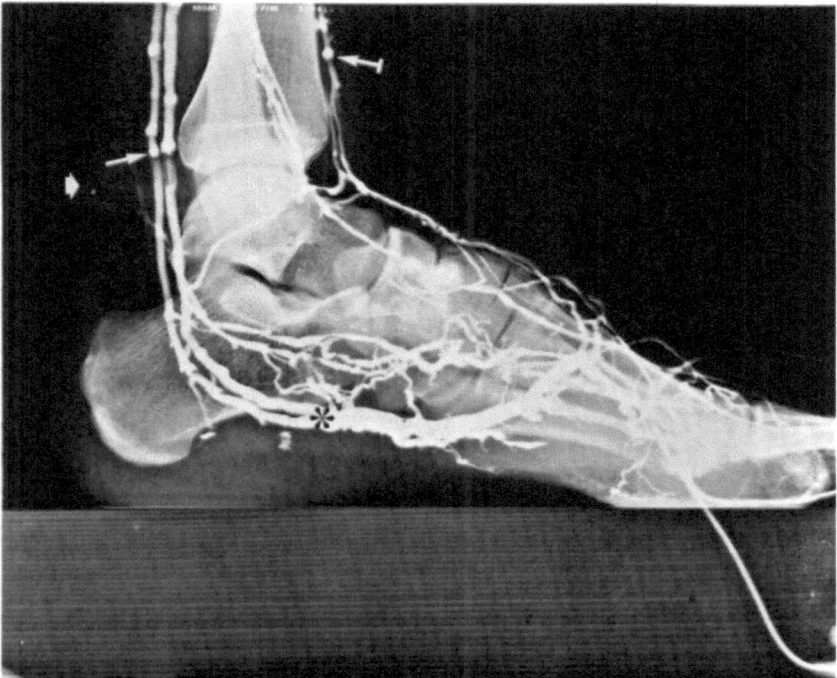

Fig. 37: **Lateral venogram of the foot. Injection into a vein of the superficial dorsal system** (tourniquet applied close to the malleoli ✦). Opacification of the deep veins of the foot and of the lower third of the leg. The large veins are lateral plantar veins ✻ . Note the presence of well-delineated valves in the posterior tibial ↑ and anterior tibial veins ↿.

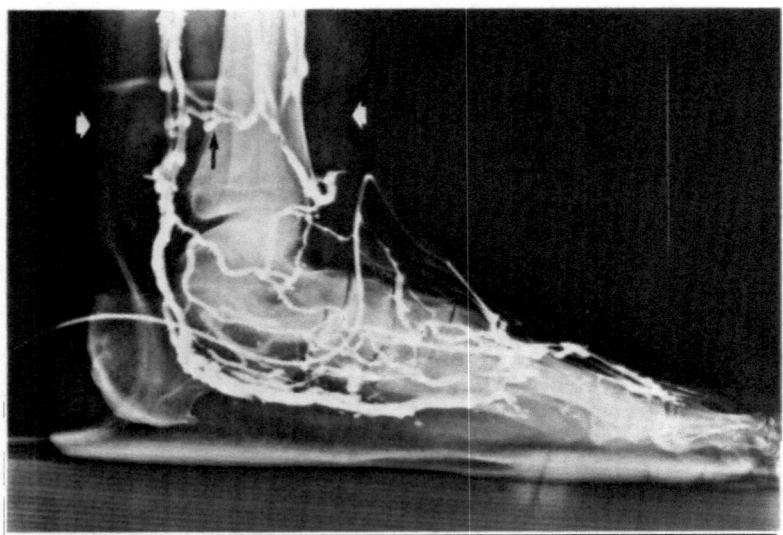

Fig. 38: Lateral venogram of the foot. Upstream injection at the medial part of the dorsal venous arch. Opacification through perforating veins of the lateral plantar veins, and to a lesser degree of the medial plantar veins. The anterior peroneal and tibial veins are opacified only through perforating veins ↑ situated above the ankle. Thus, there is only incomplete opacification of the deep veins of the foot. Note the elective site of the tourniquet ◄ which must be applied at the level of the malleoli and not the lower third of the leg: this latter location would impede the mechanism of the perforating veins which are sometimes very useful for opacifying the deep venous system of the leg.

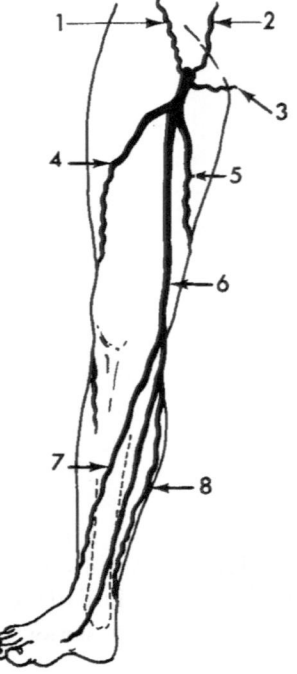

Fig. 39: Diagram showing the internal saphenous venous system with its tributaries. Note that it consists of several veins and not of a single vein. (Redraw from H. Dodd and F.B. Cockett, fig. 3.3)

The internal saphenous vein with its tributaries.
1. S.C.I.V. = Superficial circumflex iliac vein.
2. S.E.V. = Superficial epigastric vein.
3. S.E.P.V. = Superficial external pudic vein.
5. P.M.V. = Postero-medial vein.
6. L.S.V. = Long saphenous vein.
8. P.A.V. = Posterior arch vein.
7. A.V.L. = Anterior vein of leg.
4. A.L.V. = Antero-lateral vein of thigh.

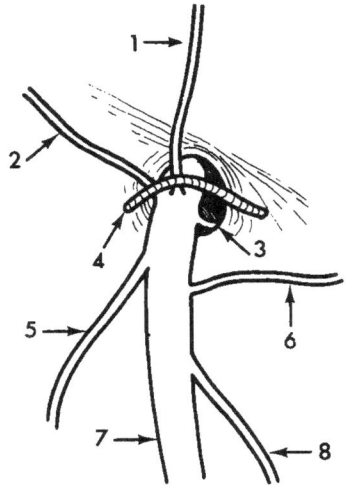 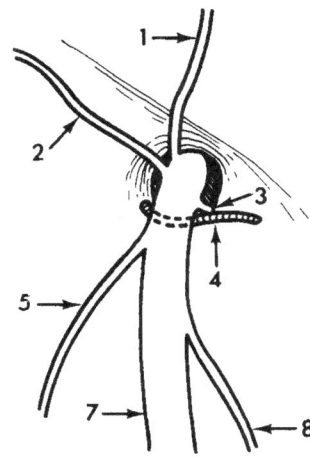

Fig. 40: Diagram showing the termination of the internal saphenous vein and its collateral branches. These two diagrams depict two possible relationships of the superficial external pudic artery (4) to the termination of the internal saphenous vein. (Redrawn from H. Dodd and F.B. Cockett, fig. 3.5.)

1. SEV = Superficial epigastric vein.
2. SCIV = Superficial circumflex iliac vein.
3. DEPV = Deep external pudendal vein.
4. SEPA = Superficial external pudic artery.

5. ALV = Antero-lateral vein of thigh.
6. SEPV = Superficial external pudic vein.
7. ISV = Internal saphenous vein
       (long saphenous vein).
8. PMV = Postero-medial vein.

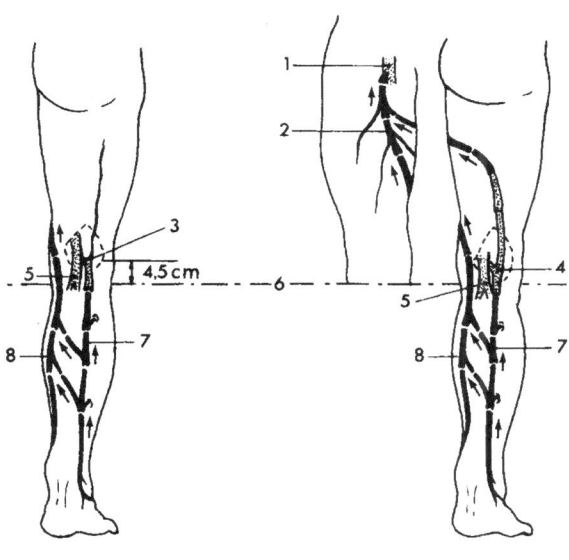

Fig. 41: The external saphenous vein at the posterior aspect of the lower limb. The left diagram depicts the most frequent disposition. The right one shows a variation with an anastomosis of large caliber between the internal and the external saphenous system at the posterior aspect of the thigh (Giacomini vein). (Redrawn from H. Dodd and F.B. Cockett).

1. Common femoral vein.
2. Internal saphenous vein.
3. Sapheno-popliteal union.
4. Division of external saphenous vein.
5. Popliteal vein.
6. Knee-joint line.
7. External saphenous vein.
8. Internal saphenous vein.

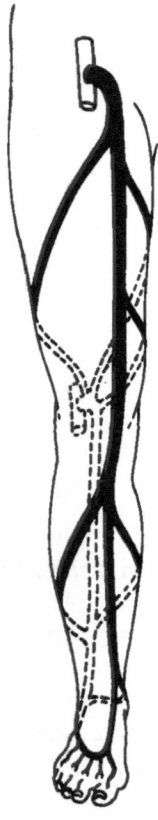

Fig. 42: Drawing presenting the sapheno-saphenous anastomoses. Black: Internal saphenous vein. White: External saphenous vein.

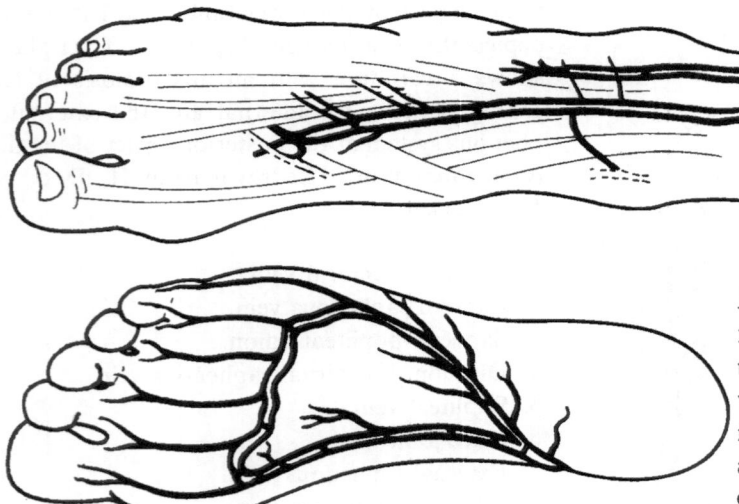

Fig. 43: Deep venous system of the foot. The dorsal veins of the foot and the perforating veins of the peroneal veins are on the dorsal aspect. The internal and the external plantar veins as well as the plantar venous arch are depicted on the sole of the foot.

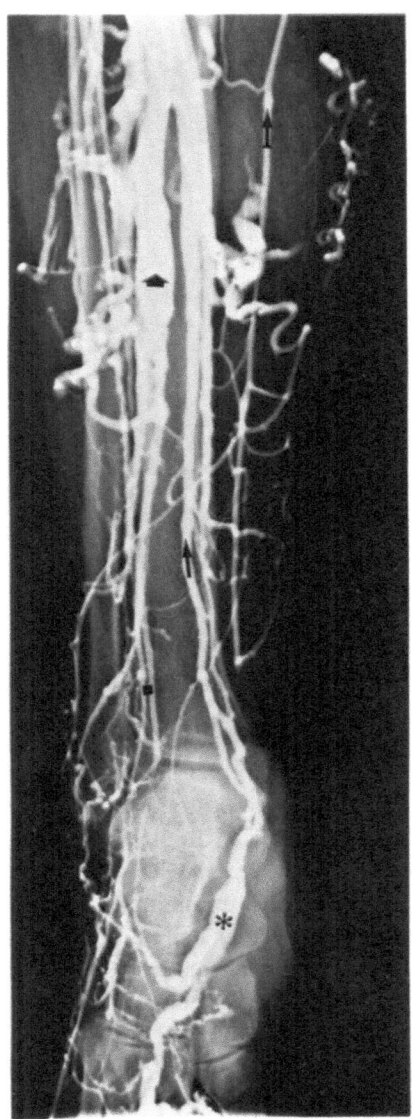

Fig. 44: Injection into a vein of the big toe. Venography of the deep veins of the right leg. Note the opacification of the large plantar veins ✳ drained by the posterior tibial veins ↑ which are related to the medial malleolus. The peroneal veins have a large caliber ◄ and are seen in the intertibio-peroneal space. The anterior tibial veins ■ are opacified, they are very thin and, on this frontal projection, they are superimposed onto the peroneal veins at the level of the middle and upper third of the leg. Reflux into some perforating veins opacifies the internal saphenous system which is thin ↥.

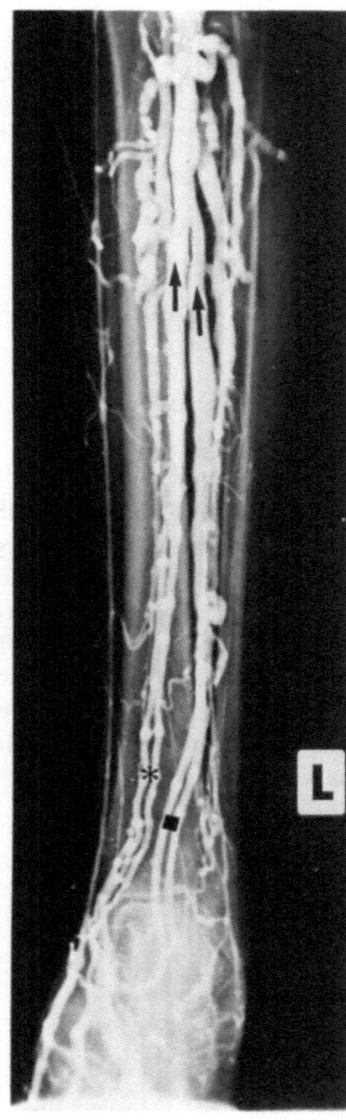

Fig. 45: Phlebogram of the left lower limb from an injection into the vein of the big toe. Frontal projection centered onto the leg. The three groups of deep veins are opacified. The posterior tibial veins ∗ ascend from the medial malleolus onwards. The peroneal veins in the intertibioperoneal space have a spindle-shaped termination, which is a normal appearance ↑↑. The anterior tibial veins ▪ are almost always the thinnest of the deep veins; they are superimposed onto the peroneal veins in the upper part of the leg. Note the presence of valves on all these deep veins. The fusiform appearance of the peroneal veins termination must not be misinterpreted as an ectasia of the deep veins; it is a normal feature.

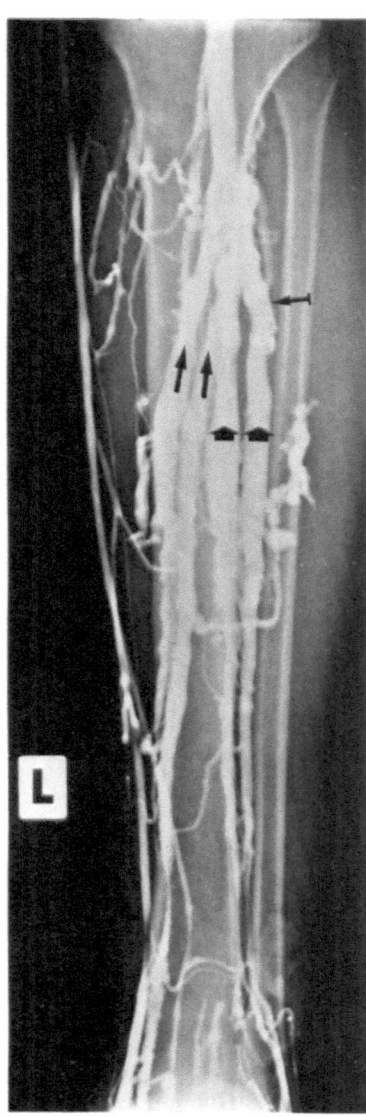

Fig. 46: Venogram of the left lower limb from an injection of a superficial dorsal vein. Frontal projection of the leg. On this film, only the peroneal ◄ and posterior tibial ↑ veins are well demonstrated. Both (in fact there are four of them) are pseudo-ectatic at their termination. However, they still have valves ↿.

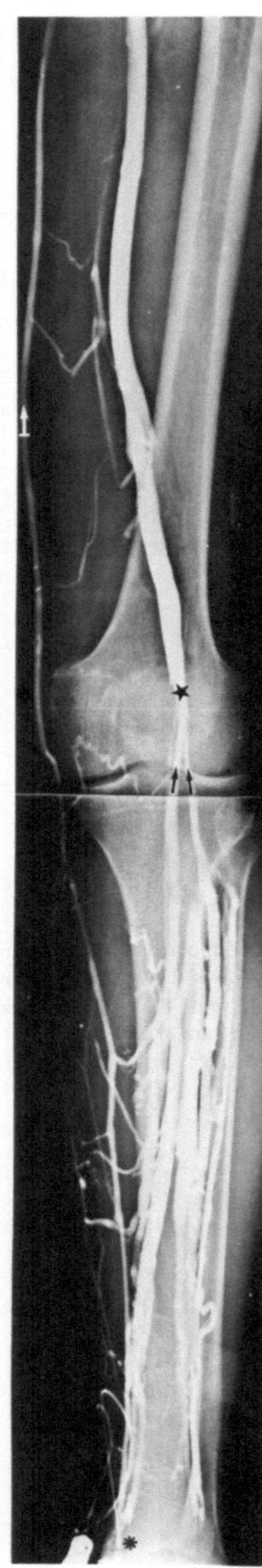

Fig. 47: Venogram of the left lower limb. Large cassette. Upstream injection into the internal saphenous vein at the ankle ❋. The deep leg veins are all opacified and perfectly patent. Duplication of the tibioperoneal trunk ↑. There is also a false appearance of duplication of the lower popliteal vein which resumes a normal caliber ★ above the condyles. The hyperextension of the knee accounts for pseudo-stenosis at this level (see chapter 2). Opacification of the internal saphenous vein on the medial aspect of the leg ↑.

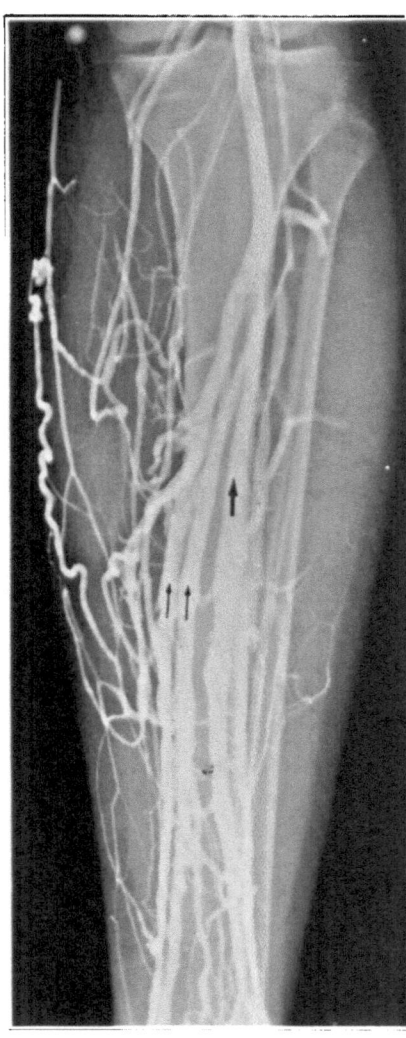

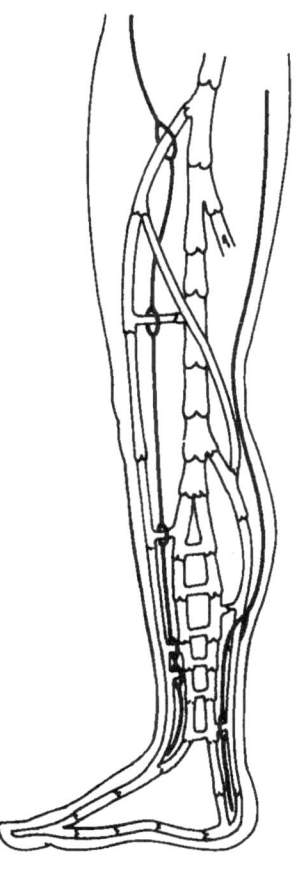

Fig. 48: Venography of the left lower limb. Projection frontal to the leg. Opacification of the posterior tibial veins ↑↑ and of the peroneal veins ↑. Faint and ill-defined opacification of the anterior tibial vein shown on this single frontal projection.

Fig. 49: Representation of the superficial and deep veins of the lower limb, as seen on a lateral film. Relations of these veins with the aponeuroses.

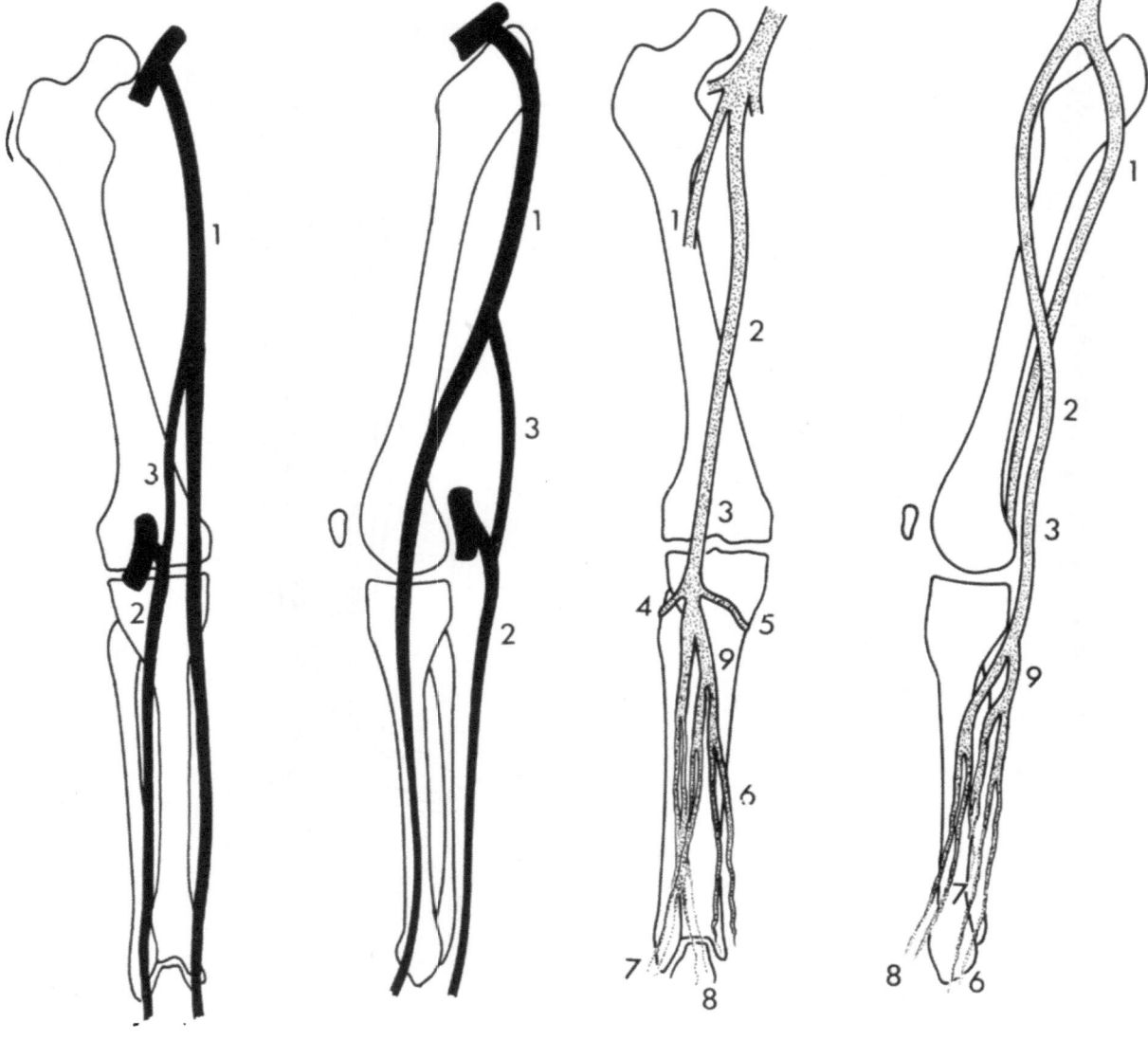

Fig. 50: Diagram showing the relation of the superficial and deep veins, as seen on a lateral and on a frontal film, with the bone structures.

A. Superficial saphenous system
   1. Internal saphenous vein
   2. External saphenous vein
   3. Vein of Giacomini

B. Deep venous system
   1. Profunda femoris vein
   2. Superficial femoral vein
   3. Popliteal vein
   4. External gastrocnemial vein
   5. Internal gastrocnemial vein
   6. Posterior tibial veins
   7. Peroneal veins
   8. Anterior tibial veins
   9. Tibioperoneal trunk.

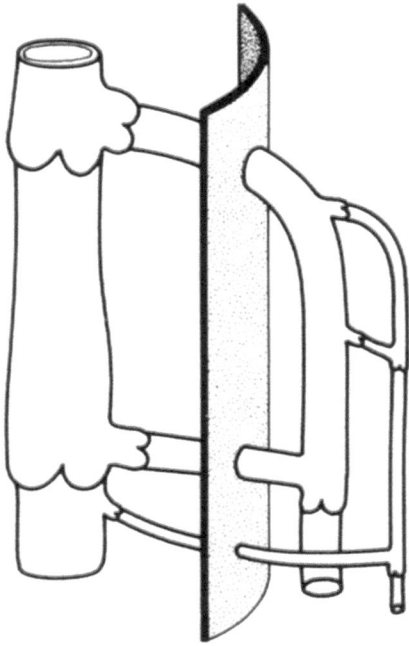

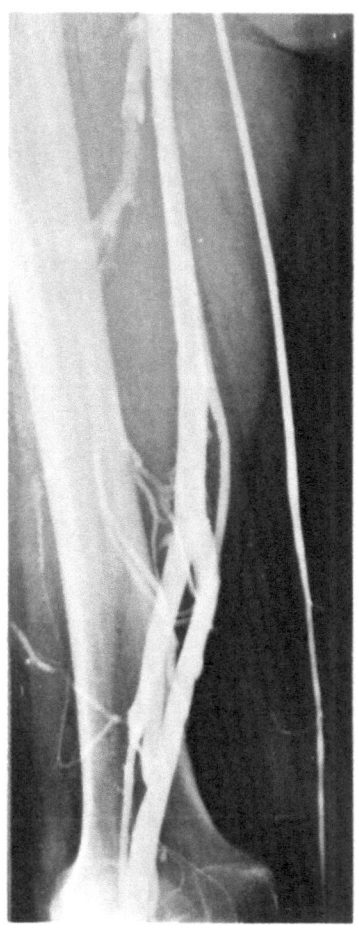

Fig. 51: Diagram showing the connections of the superficial venous system with the saphenous veins and with the deep veins. The perforating veins connect the superficial with the deep veins. They are of two types, viz. (i) the direct perforating veins which connect the deep system with the saphenous system (large veins), and (ii) the indirect perforating veins (small veins) which are certainly the most common, connecting the subcutaneous veins (collateral branches of the saphenous veins) with the deep venous system. All perforating veins are valved, so that in a normal person, the blood can only pass from the superficial to the deep veins.

Fig. 52

Figs. 52, 53, 54 and 55: Congenital variation showing duplications of different shape and extent, at the level of the femoropopliteal venous axis. Figure 54 (see p. 38) shows a venogram in a 5-year-old child.

38

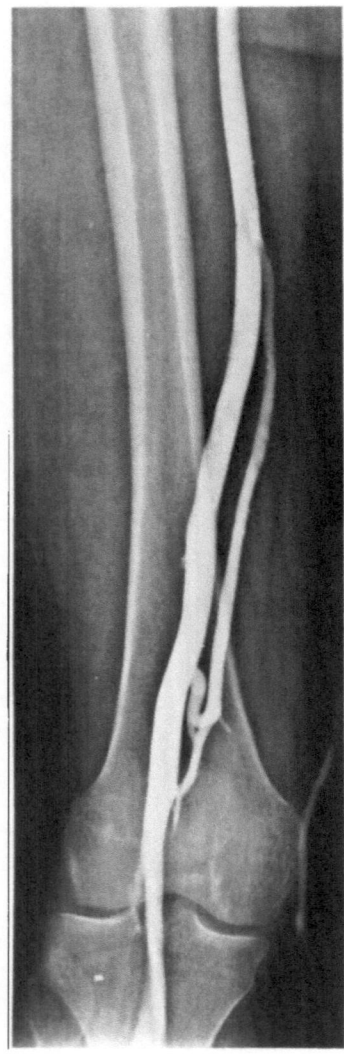

Fig. 53

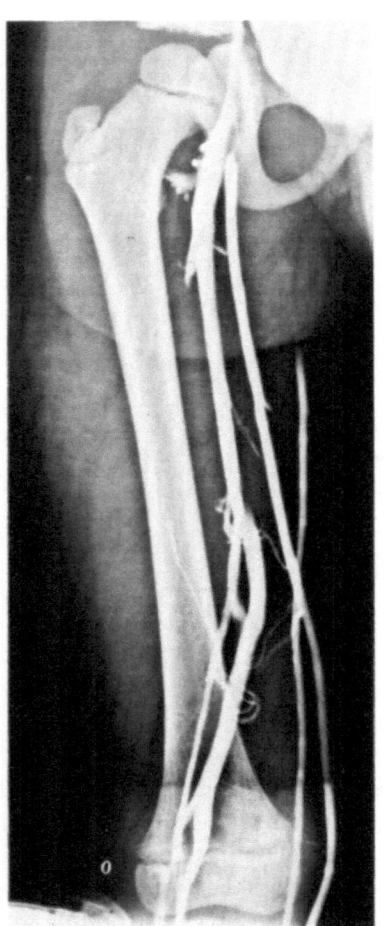

Fig. 54

Figs. 52 (see p. 37), *53, 54 and 55:* Congenital variation showing duplications of different shape and extent, at the level of the femoropopliteal venous axis. Figure 54 shows a venogram in a 5-year-old child.

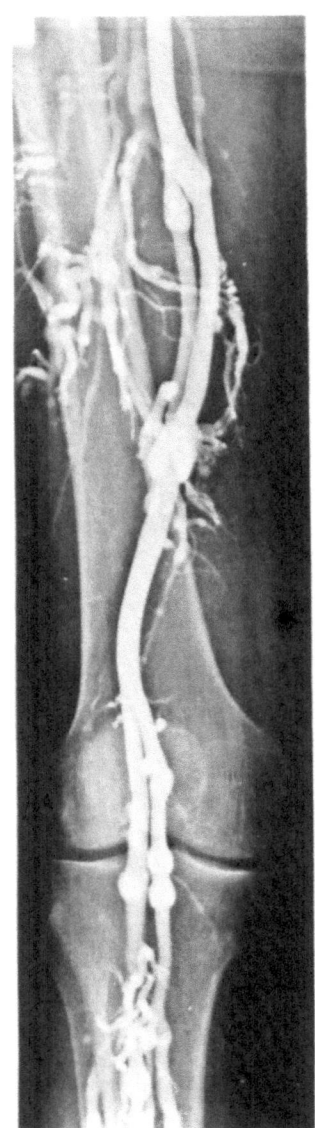

Fig. 55

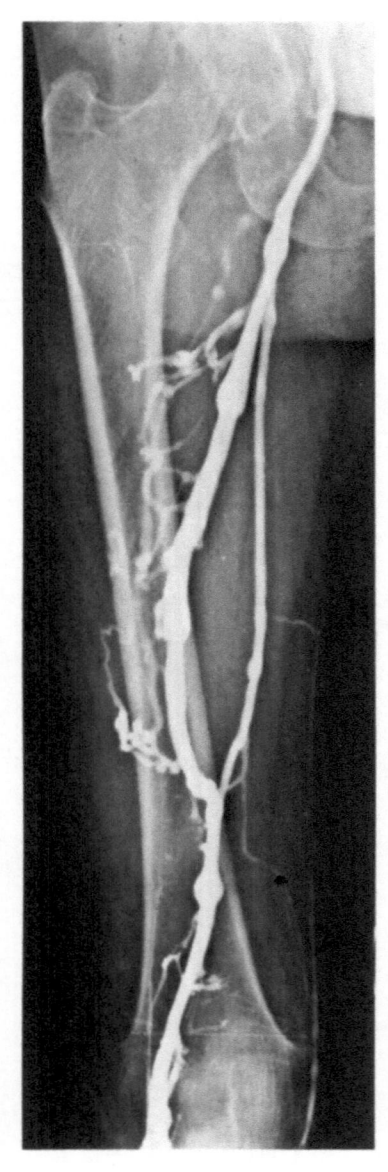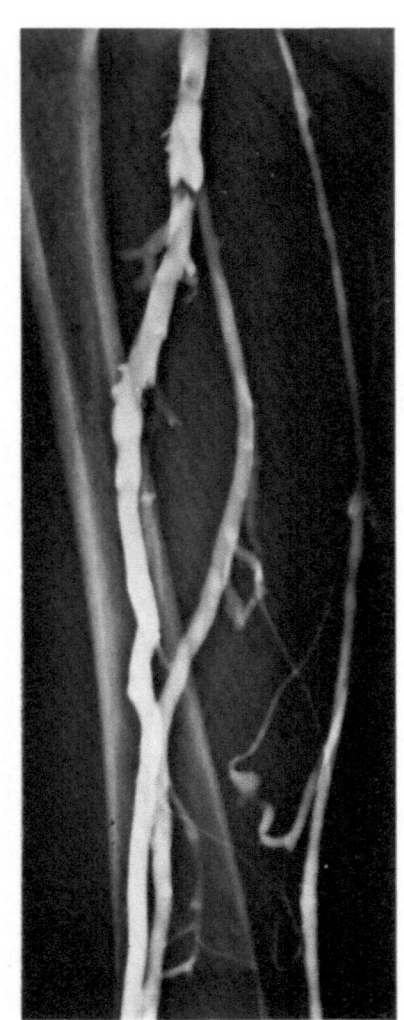

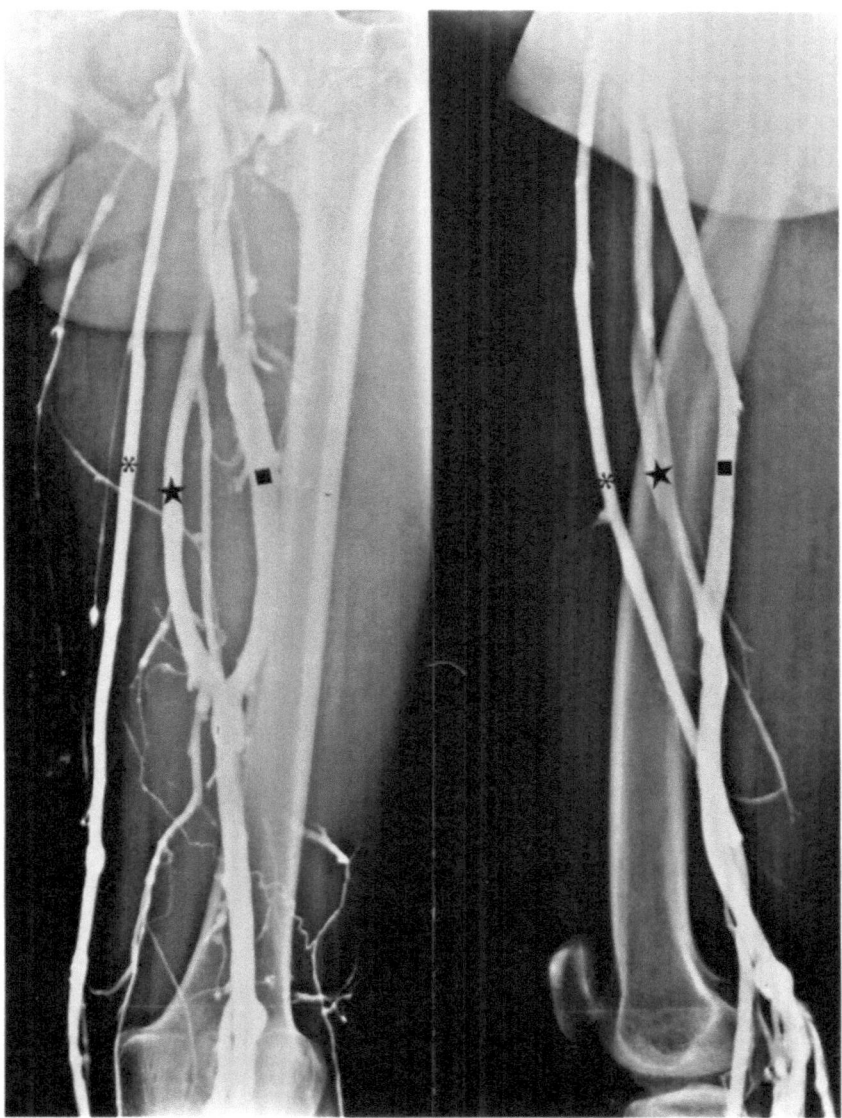

Fig. 58   Fig. 59

Figs. 58 and 59: Frontal and lateral film in the same patient, showing a congenital anomaly with duplication of the superficial femoral vein at the middle third of the thigh. The lateral projection (Fig. 59) confirms that it is merely a duplication of the superficial femoral vein and not the opacification of the superficial and of the deep femoral vein. Indeed, on the latter projection (Fig. 59) there is an opacification, from anterior to posterior, of the internal saphenous vein ✳ and then of the two branches of the superficial femoral channel (★ and ■). A profunda femoris vein would be parallel to the posterior aspect of the femoral shaft over a longer distance. Note also on the lateral projection (Fig. 59) the fainter opacification of the anterior part of the superficial femoral collateral channel, due to a change in the patient's position ★.

42

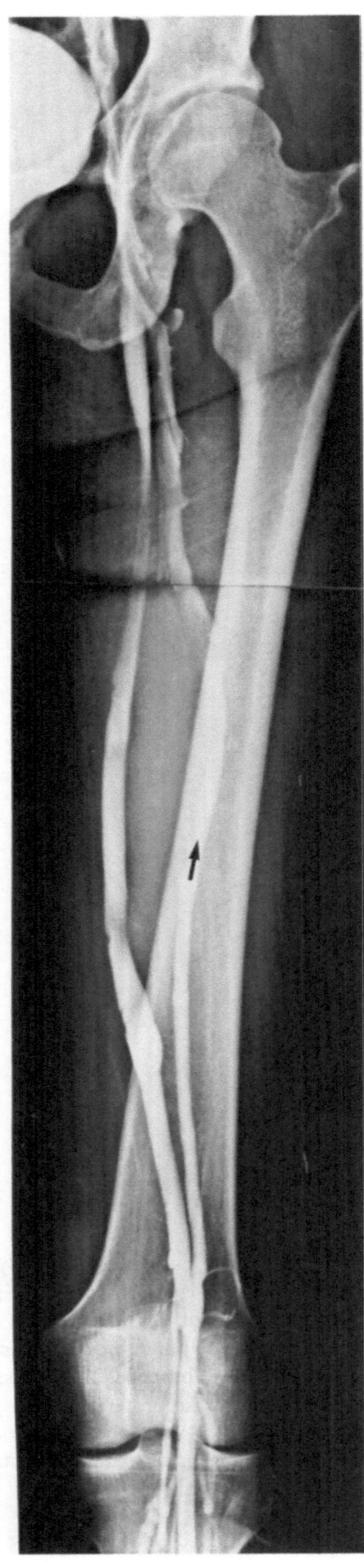

Fig. 60

Figs. 60 and 61: Venogram of the left lower limb and then of the right in a patient demonstrating a certain symmetry in the duplication of the femoropopliteal venous route. The venogram of the left lower limb (Fig. 60) corresponds very probably to drainage by a retro-adducting vein ↑ which is prolonged by the profunda femoris vein. Figure 61 shows the venogram of the left lower limb which is consistent with real duplication with a collateral channel. In both cases it is difficult to diagnose positively on the basis of the sole frontal view.

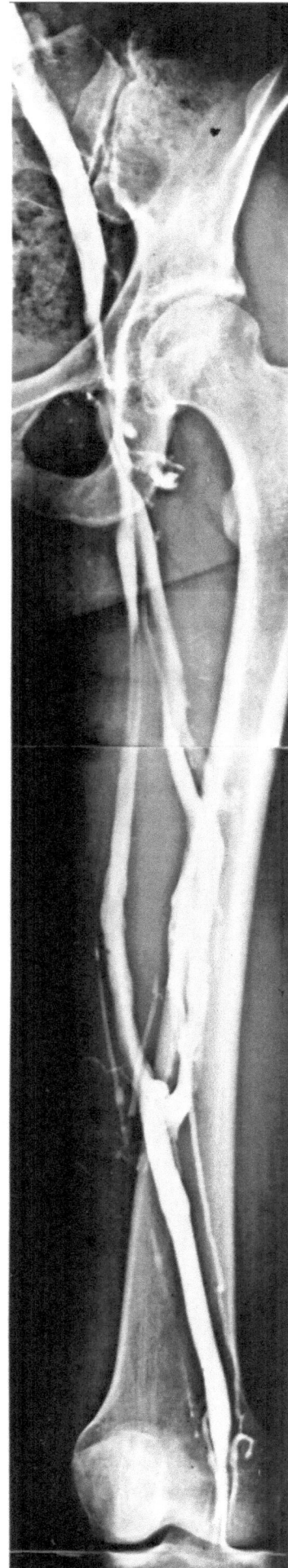

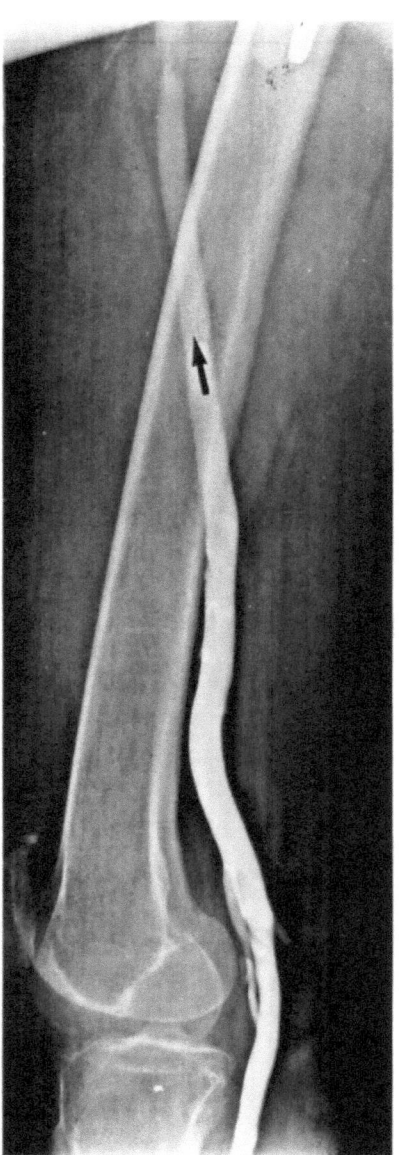

Fig. 62: Venogram of the right lower limb. Lateral projection of the thigh. Isolated opacification of the femoral vein showing clearly its topography with regard to the femoral shaft. This vein crosses the shaft posteriorly to anteriorly at the level of its middle third ⬆.

Fig. 61

Chapter 2

ARTEFACTS AND INCIDENTS

Figures 63–100

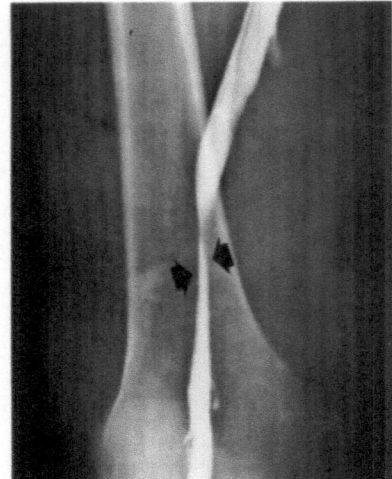

Fig. 63

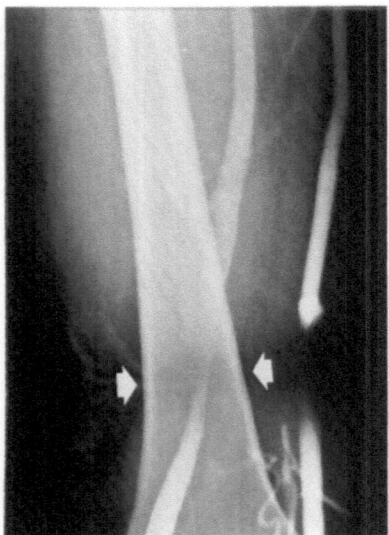

Fig. 64

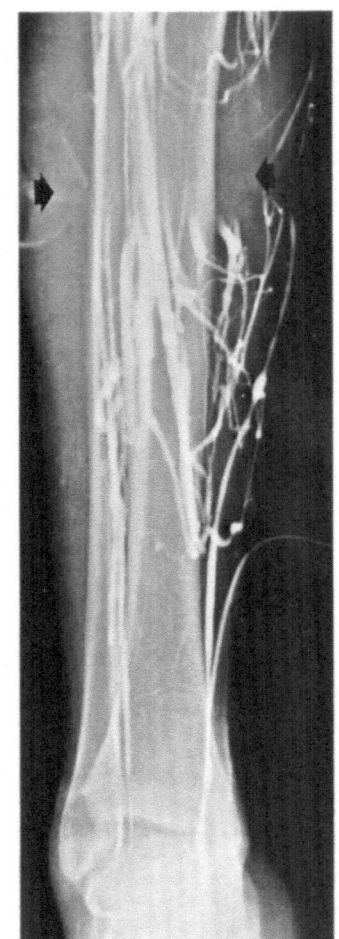

Fig. 65

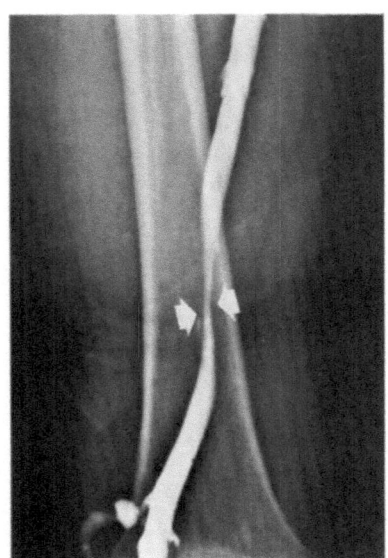

Figs. 63, 64, 65, 66, 67 and 68: Artefact due to a too tight tourniquet ▲ which compresses the deep venous system

Fig. 66

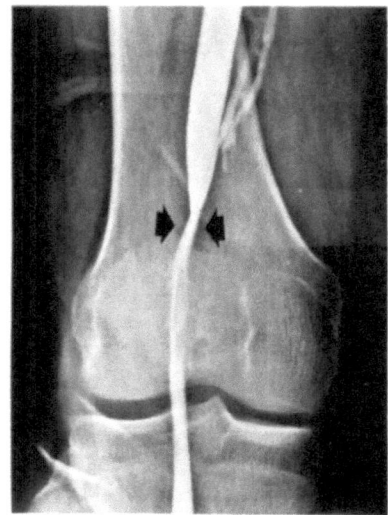

Fig. 67

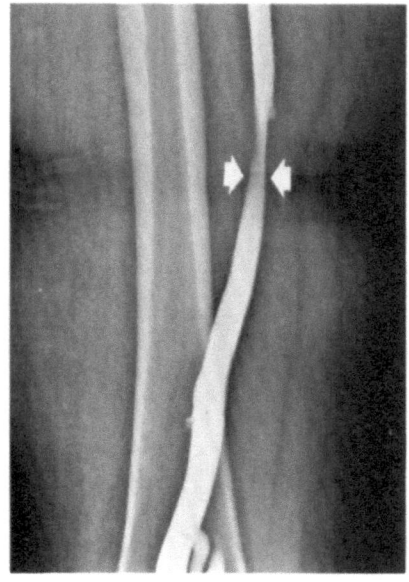

Fig. 68

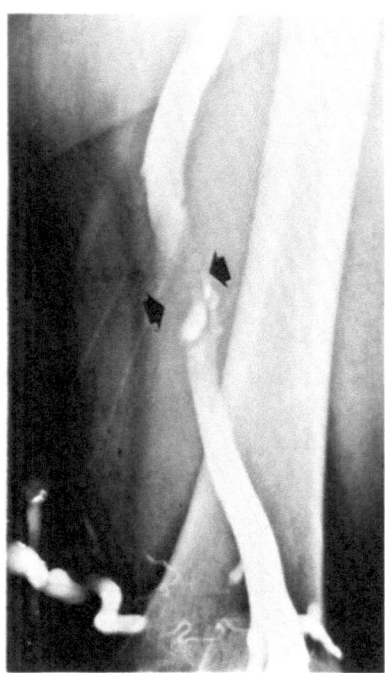

Fig. 69

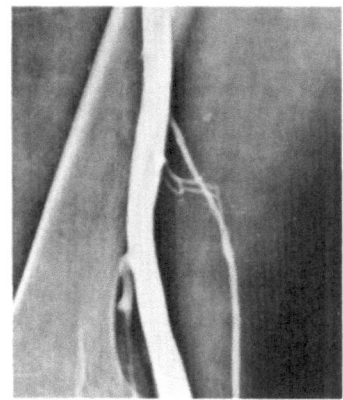

Fig. 70

Figs. 69 and 70: Artefact due to a too tight tourniquet ◄. The artefact is no longer seen on the lateral projection after the tourniquet has been withdrawn.

48

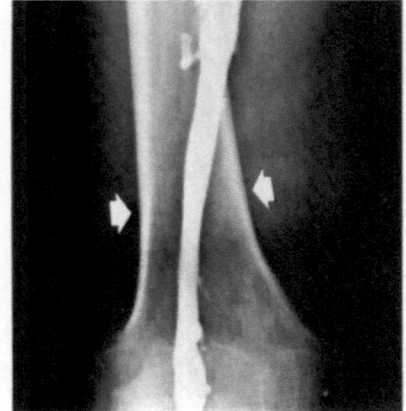

Fig. 71

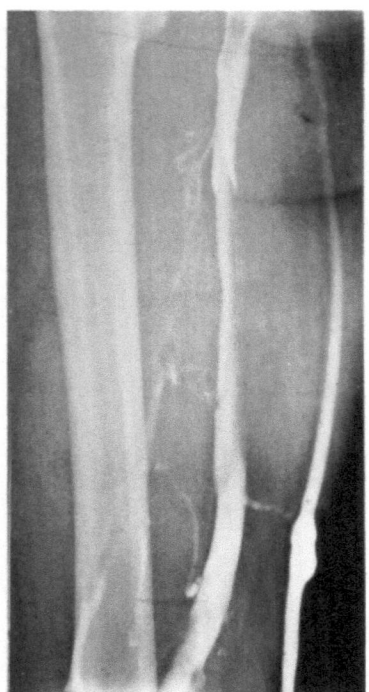

Fig. 73

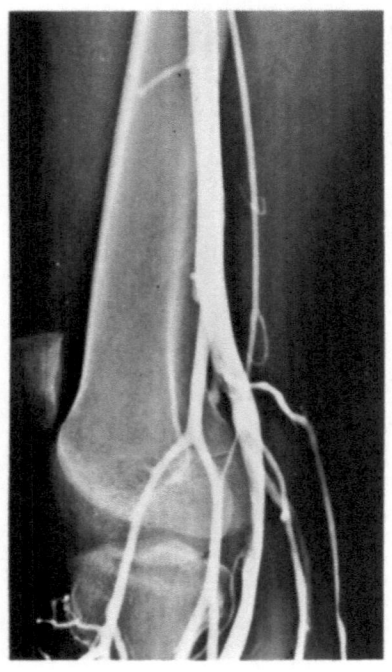

Fig. 72

Figs. 71 and 72: Same caption as for Figs. 69 and 70.

Figs. 73, 74, 75, 76 and 77: Venograms performed with the patient supine, showing layering effect due to low-rate hand injection. This artefact is mainly seen on the middle portion on the superficial femoral vein. It is sometimes increased by the arrival on non-opacified blood in a large perforating vein of the thigh, as is clearly shown in Fig. 74.

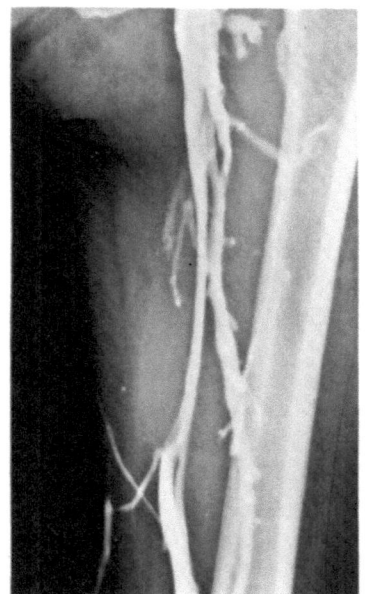

Fig. 74

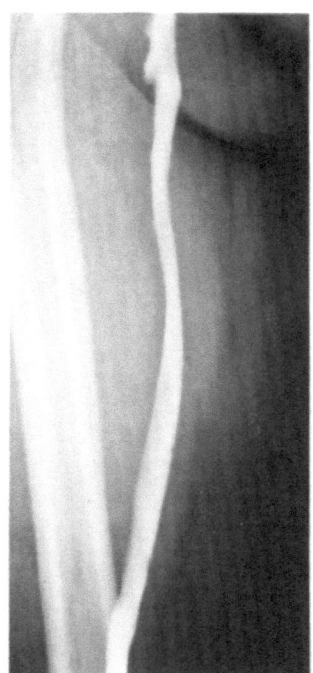

Fig. 76

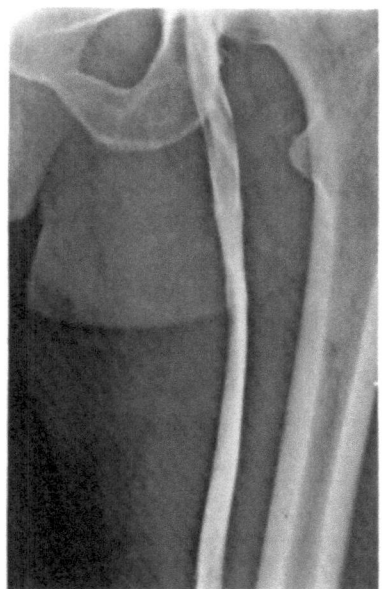

Fig. 75

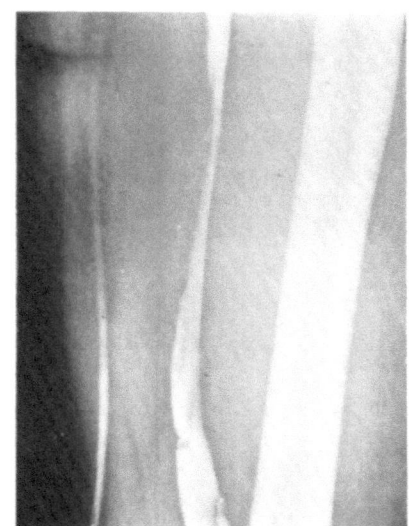

Fig. 77

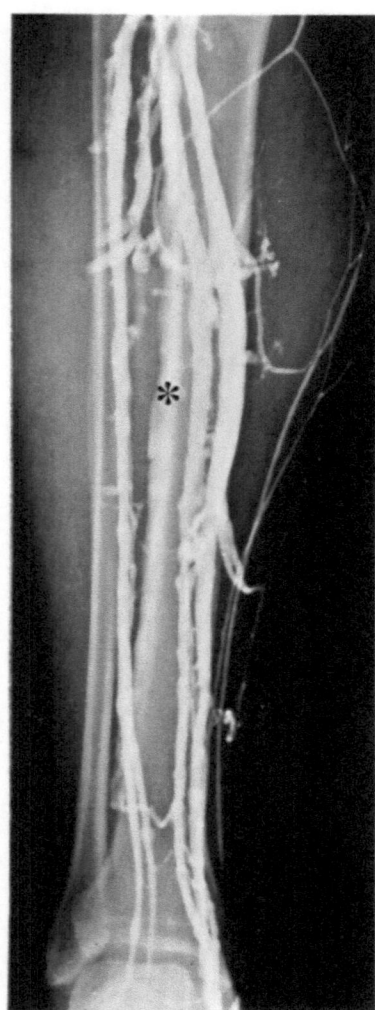

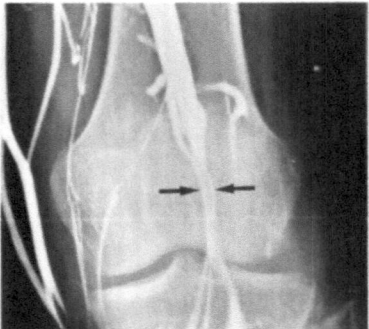

Fig. 79

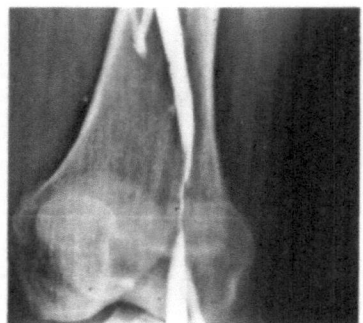

Fig. 80

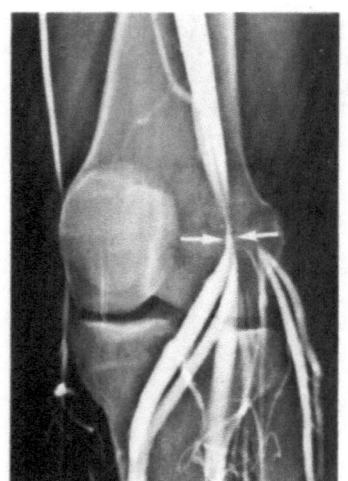

Fig. 78: Non-filling of part of the deep veins of the leg. The peroneal veins ∗ are, as it were, not opacified. This artefact is related, on the one hand, with the site of the injection on the dorsum of the foot, and no the other with a certain degree of compression of the calf muscles on the investigation table (patient in the supine position).

Fig. 81

Figs. 79, 80 and 81: Narrowing of the popliteal vein ↑ due to hyperextension of the knee. Hyperextension of the knee can produce an apparent obstruction of the vein in the popliteal space.

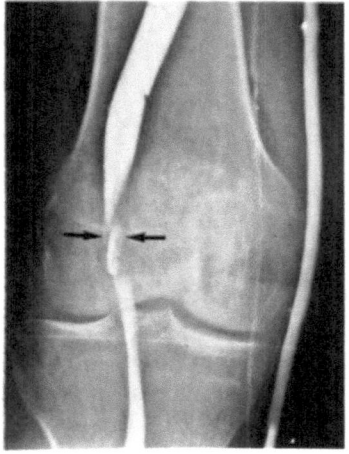

Fig. 82

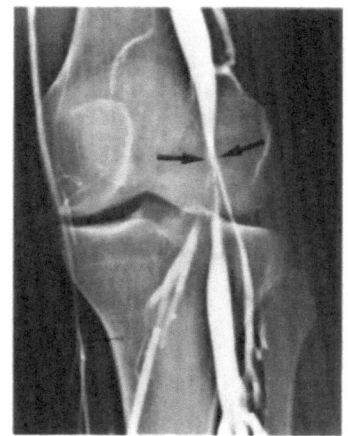

Fig. 84

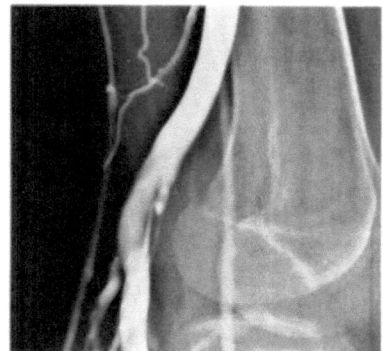

Fig. 83

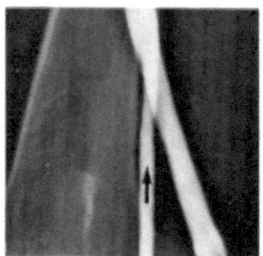

Fig. 85

Figs. 82 and 83: Stenosis of the middle popliteal vein due to hyperextension of the knee. Figure 83 corresponds to a lateral venogram (same patient as in Fig. 82) which shows that the stenosis disappears when the knee is slightly flexed. One can see, moreover, that this popliteal stenosis is largely due to compression against the femoral condyles.

Figs. 84 and 85: Stenosis of the middle popliteal vein by hyperextension of the knee. Figure 85 shows a lateral venogram (same patient as in Fig. 84) demonstrating that a slight flexion of the knee releases the stenosis. The lateral view (85) also shows the opacification of the internal saphenous vein ↑.

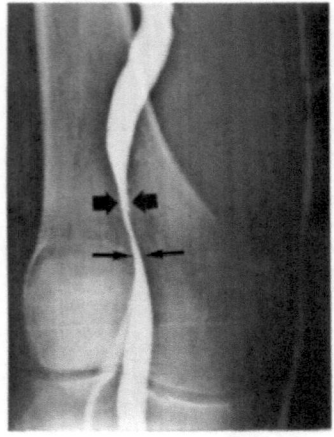

Fig. 86: Stenosis of the middle and upper portion of the popliteal vein. There is a triple artefact: i) narrowing of the popliteal vein due to hyperextension of the knee ↑; ii) too tight rubber tourniquet ♦; iii) compression of the muscles against the hard surface of the phlebography table when the patient is supine.

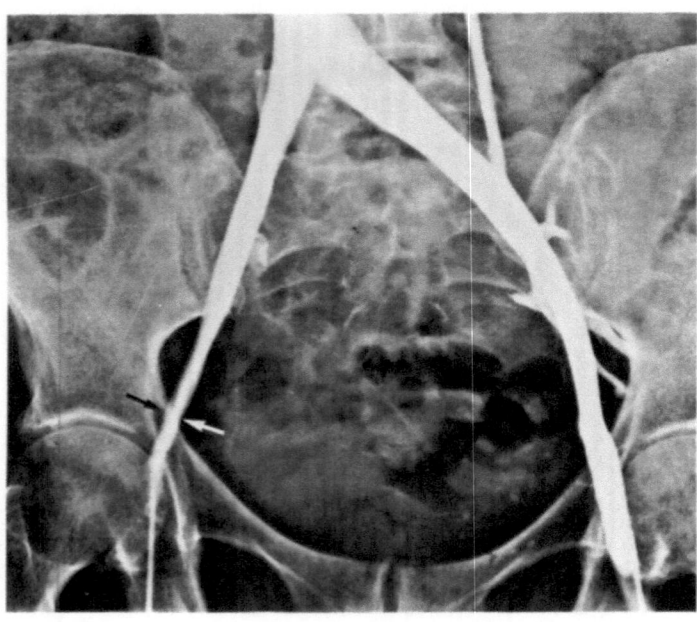

Fig. 87: Bifemoral percutaneous inferior vena cavography. Venturi effect ↑ in a right ilio-femoral vein. Under certain conditions the vein may have a tapered appearance: Venturi effect due to a too rapid injection of contrast medium into a large vein on hand with a cathether without side holes.

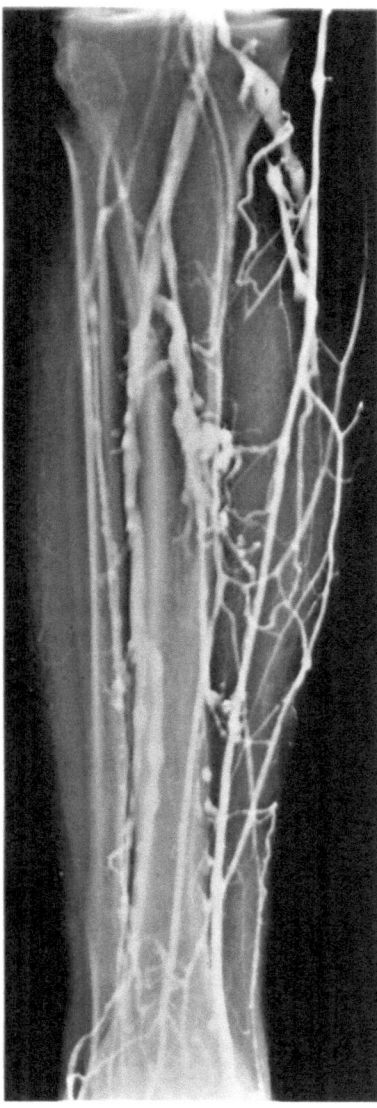

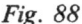

Fig. 88

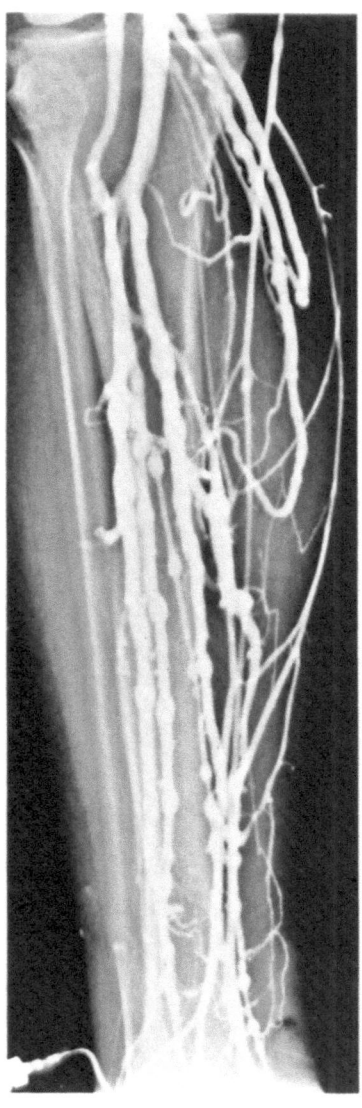

Fig. 89

Figs. 88 and 89: Frontal and lateral venogram of the right lower limb. The frontal projection (88) shows partial and poor opacification of the deep veins of the leg. This non-filling of the veins is mainly due to compression of the calf-muscles resulting from the supine position on the hard surface of the phlebography table. The lateral projection (89) suppresses the compression of the muscles and shows correct filling of the anterior and posterior tibial peroneal veins. Note the congenital variation with duplication of the lower popliteal vein and separate junction of the anterior tibial veins. This artefact, caused by the muscular compression on the examining plane, is often increased by contraction of the muscles.

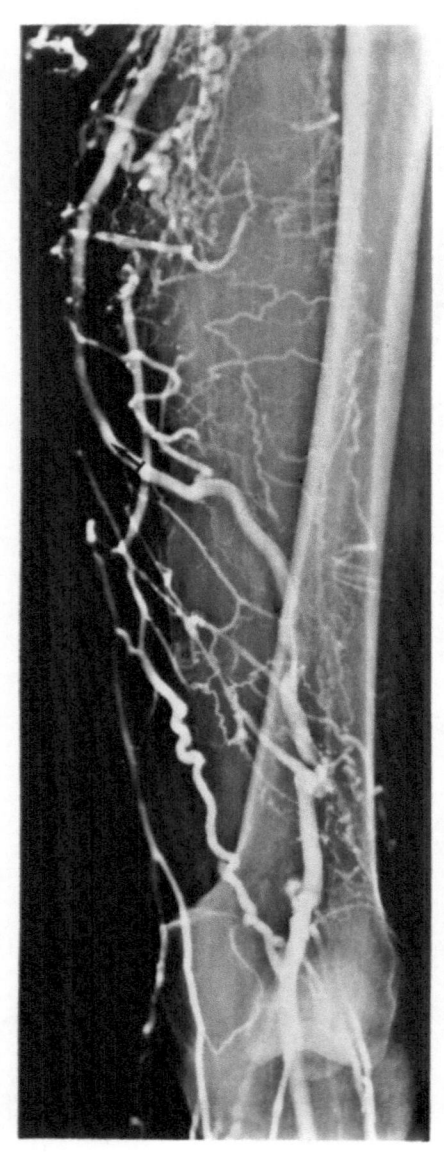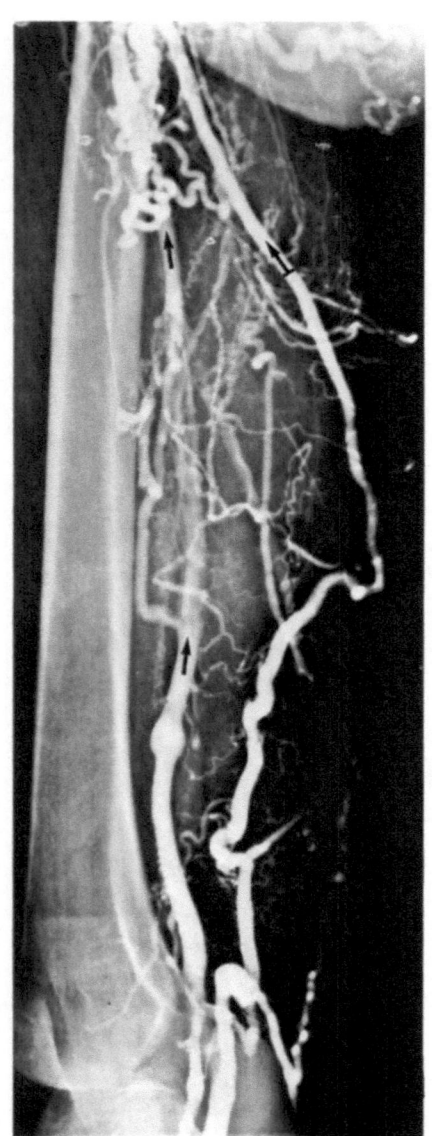

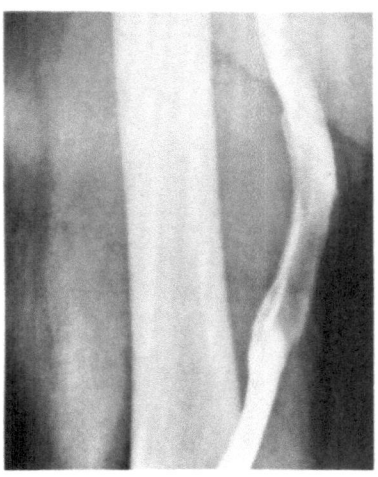

Fig. 92: False defect on the middle portion of the superficial femoral vein due firstly to a low rate hand injection, and secondly to a too tight rubber tourniquet which was withdrawn just before this film was taken. This feature is strikingly like phlebothrombosis (free thrombus). A second seriography with a constant delivery rate injection (not shown here) rules out thrombosis at this level.

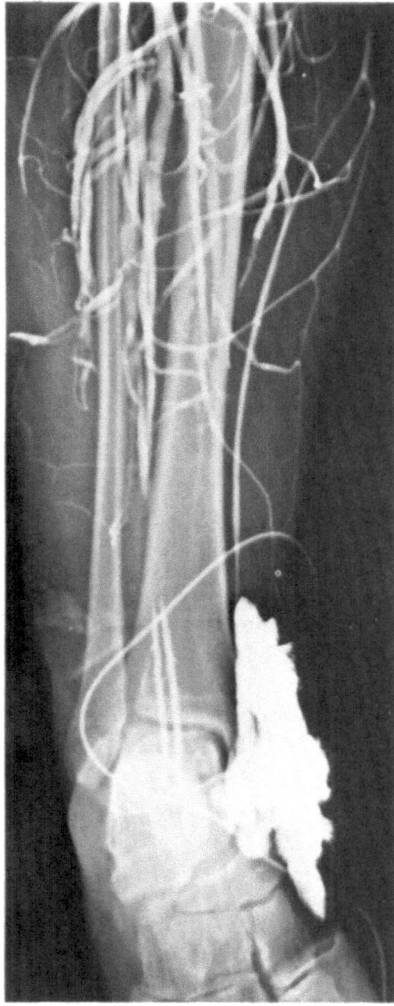

Fig. 93

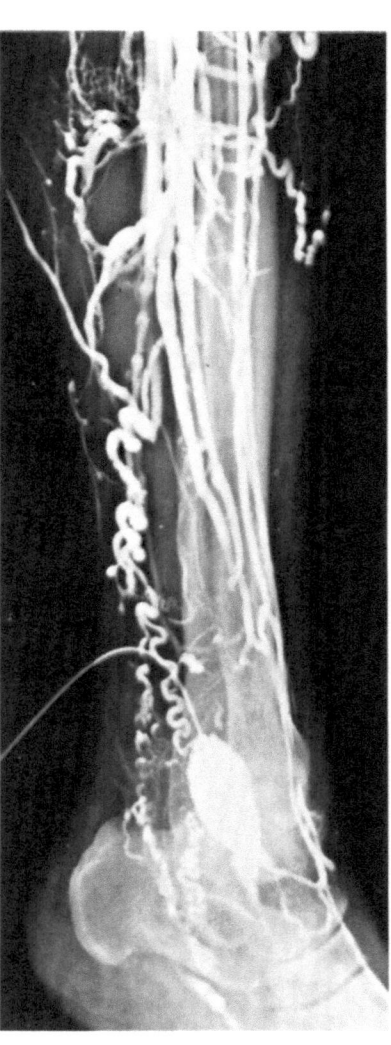

Fig. 94

Figs. 93 and 94: Extravasation and perivenous injection of contrast medium at the ankle.

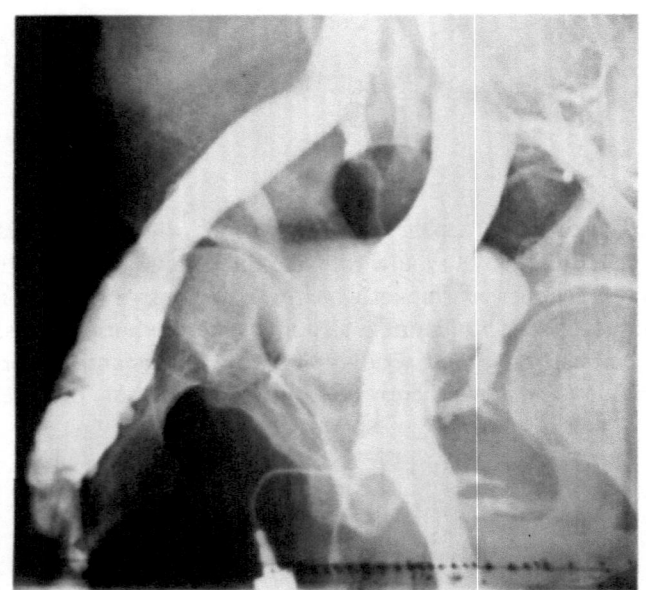

Fig. 95

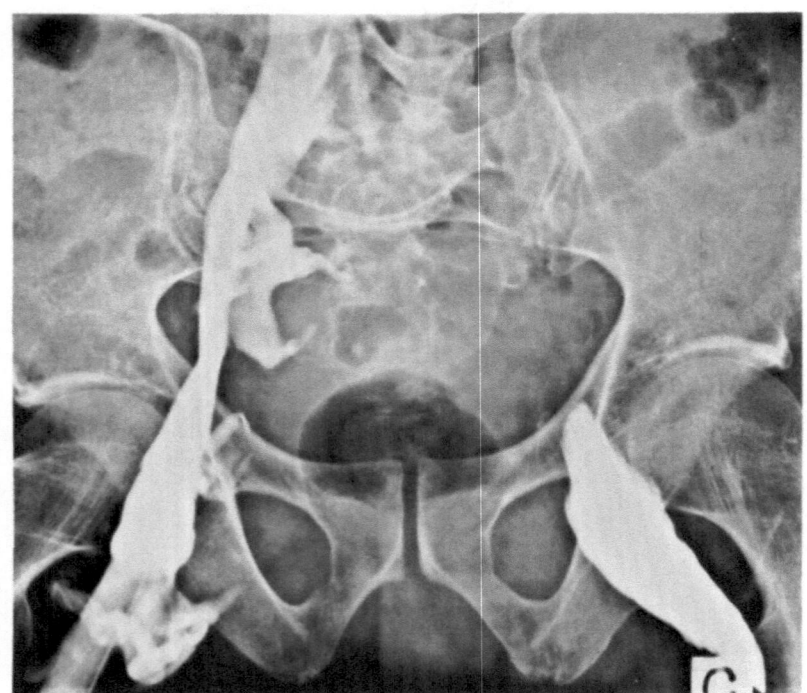

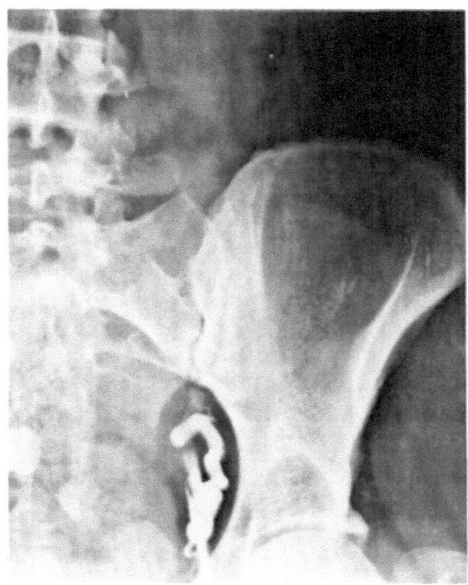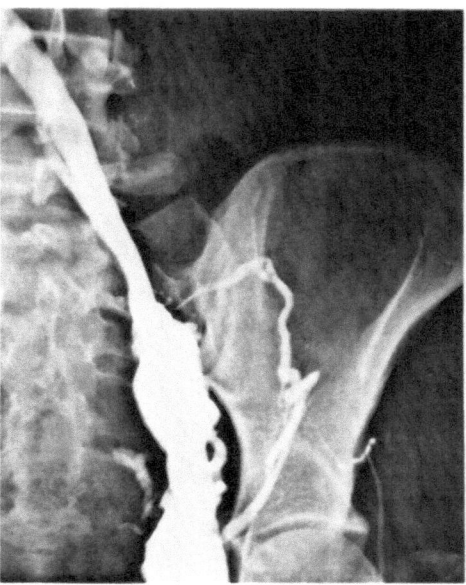

Fig. 98

Figs. 97 and 98: Left unilateral ilio-cavography. Too deep, intrapelvic catheterization. It corresponds in fact to injection into a vein of the hypogastric system, for which the high injection rate is not adequate; the left iliofemoral perivenous injection is well demonstrated in Fig. 98.

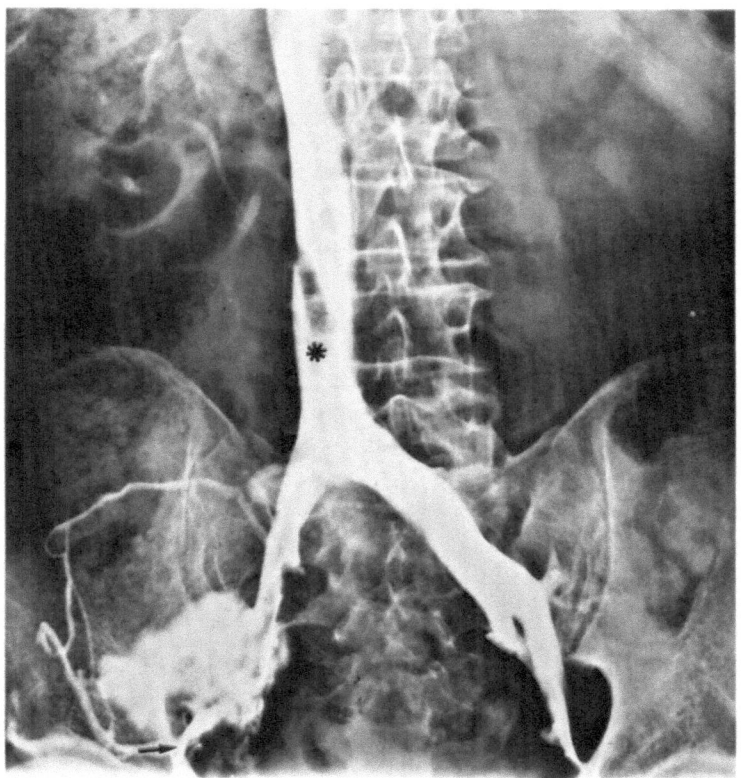

Fig. 99: Bifemoral percutaneous inferior vena cavography. On the right, catheterization is too deep and becomes intrapelvic. The catheterized vein is, in fact, the right gluteal vein ↑ which cannot stand the high injection rate. Note, moreover, the intracaval loose thrombus ✳.

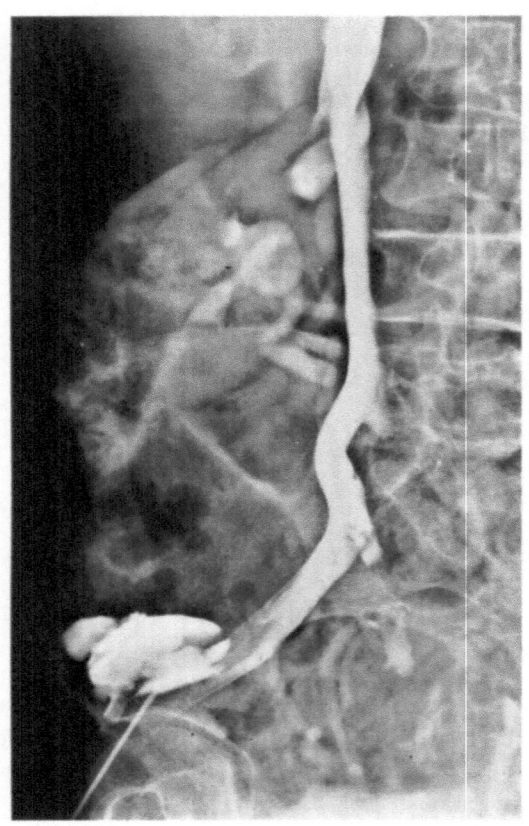

Fig. 100: Unilateral right iliocavography. Left anterior oblique projection. Perivenous injection with well-visible pooling of contrast medium.

Chapter 3

ACUTE THROMBOPHLEBITIS OF
THE VEINS OF THE LOWER LIMB

Figures 101–127

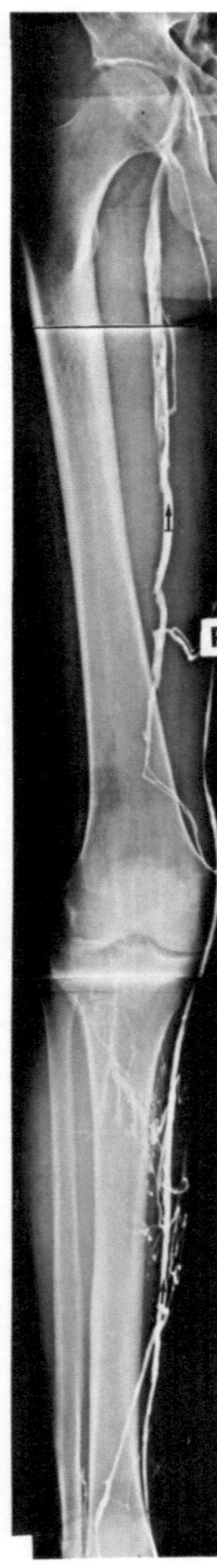

Fig. 101: Clinically typical phlebitis of the calf. Non-pressurized venography of the right lower limb. Complete obliteration of the deep veins of the leg. Collateral circulation via the internal saphenous vein ↑. Opacification of the superficial femoral vein ↕ through a perforating vein above the knee shows it to be occluded by a loose thrombus of the phlebothrombotic type. Venography is indicated for demonstrating that phlebitis of the calf may in fact be diffuse phlebitis of all veins of the leg.

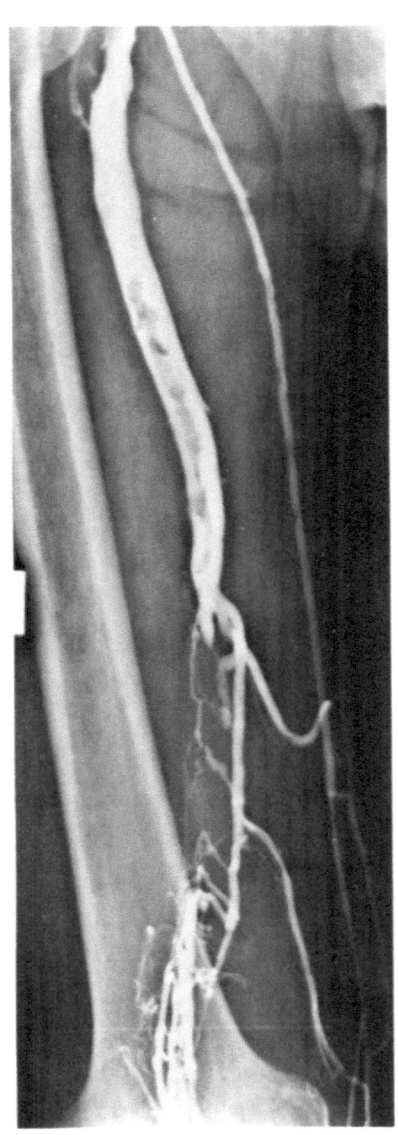

Fig. 102: Ancient popliteal obliteration with fenestration of the popliteal vein. Reopacification of the superficial femoral vein at the upper thigh showing a recent loose thrombus, type phlebo-thrombosis, in the femoral vein above the chronic obliteration. Example of recent acute phlebitis occurring on underlying chronic obstruction.

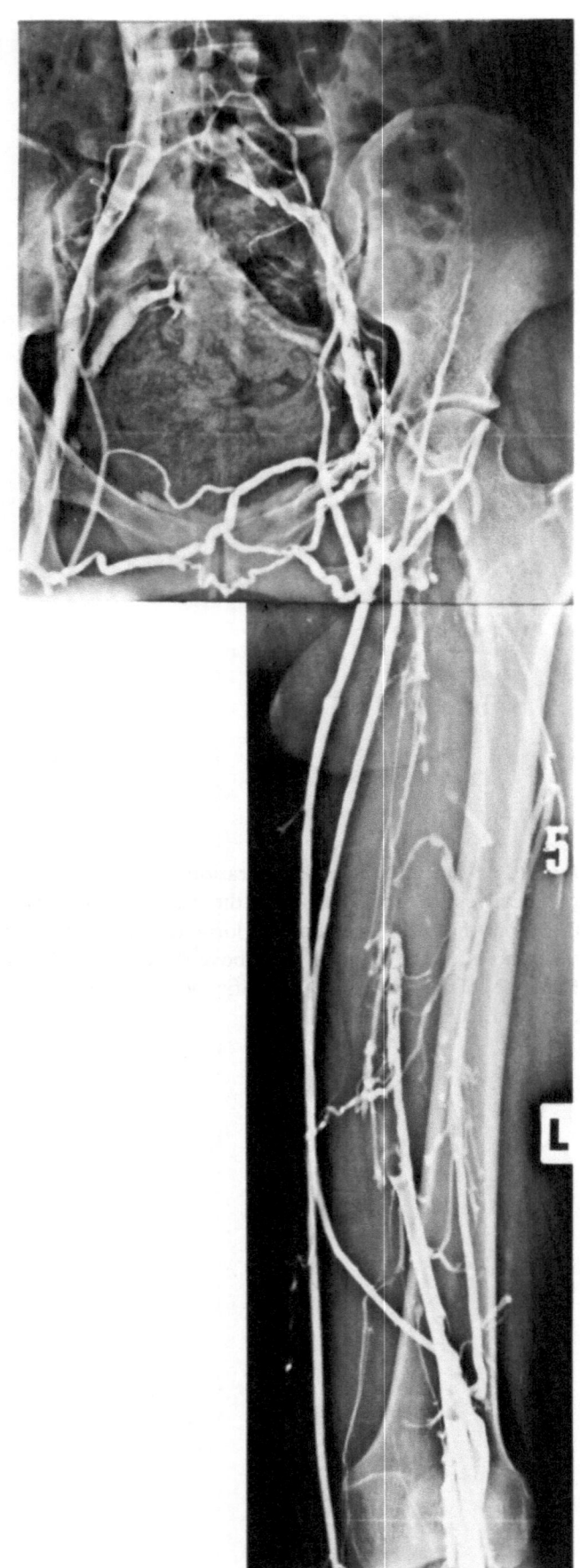

Fig. 103: Free flow venogram of the lower limb (100 ml contrast). Recent left iliofemoral phlebitis.

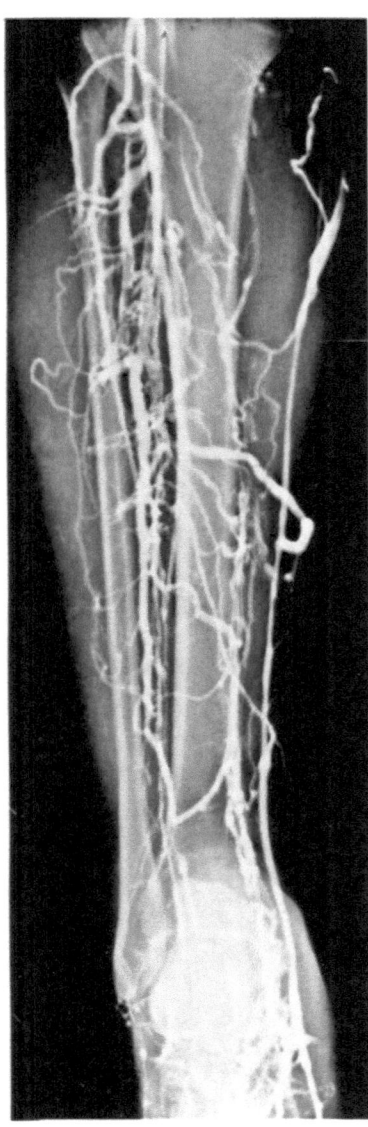

Fig. 104: Free flow venogram
of the left lower limb. Phlebitis
of the calf. Filling defects in the
deep veins of the leg as well as
in some perforating veins.

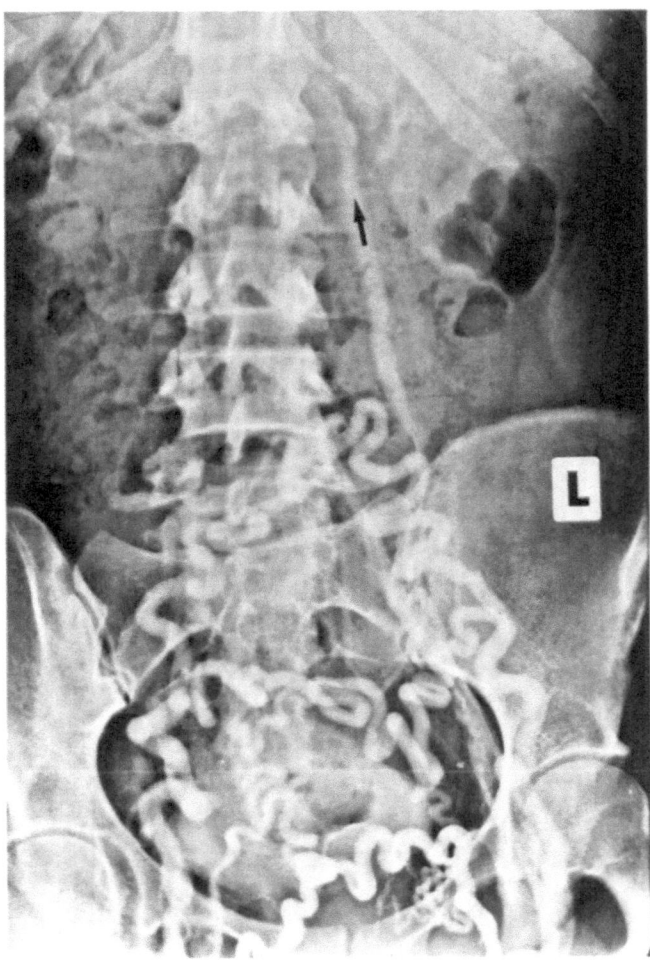

Fig. 105: Free flow venogram of the left lower limb.
Recent left iliofemoral phlebitis and subjacent obstruction of all veins of the left leg. Very marked superficial
collateral circulation and opacification ↑ of a left ovarian
vein bearing witness to inferior caval obstruction associated with the diffuse acute phlebitis of the entire left leg.
This shows the necessity for using large volumes of
contrast medium which produces opacification of the
upper parts and allows the accurate diagnosis of iliocaval
obstructions associated with acute phlebitis of the lower
limbs.

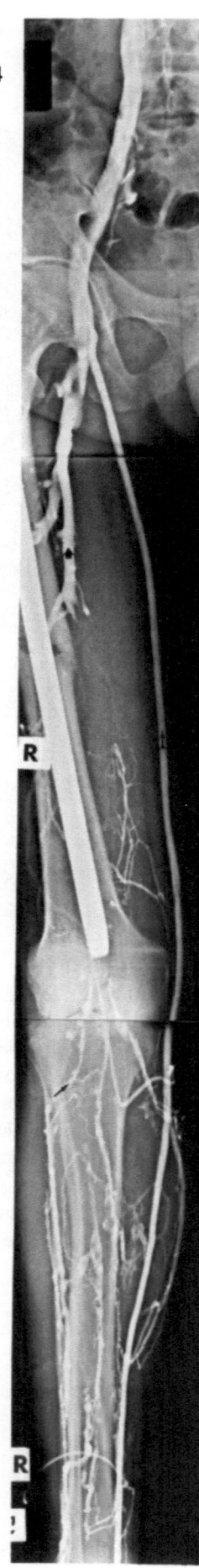

Fig. 106: Post-traumatic acute phlebitis of the right lower limb. Fracture of the femoral shaft treated by nailing. Filling defects in the deep leg veins. Only the anterior tibial veins ↑ are partly patent. Collateral circulation through the internal saphenous vein ↕. Complete femoropopliteal obstruction. Collateral circulation is via the profunda femoris vein ♠ which is perfectly patent, as is the iliac system and the inferior vena cava.

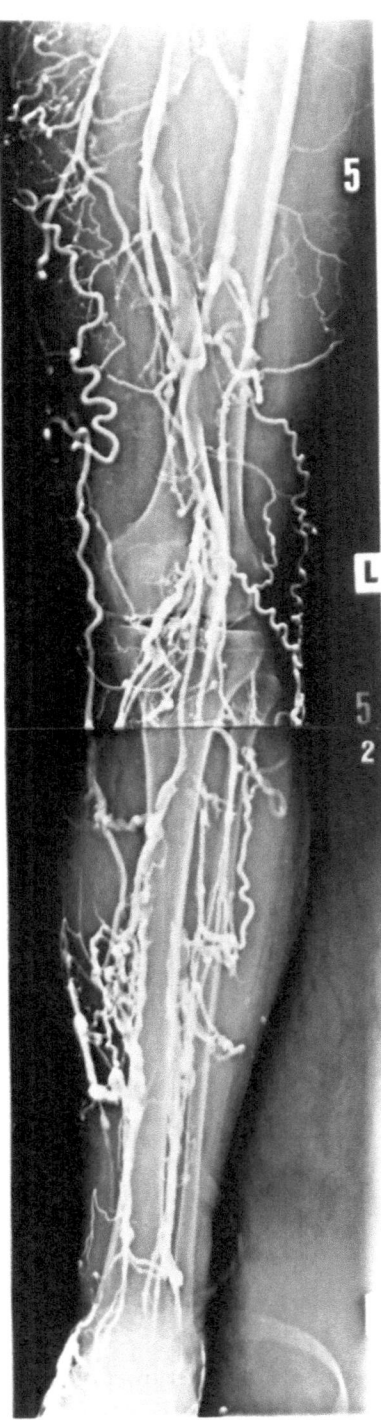

Fig. 107: Venogram of the left lower limb. Diffuse filling defects in the deep veins of the leg and in the femoro-popliteal axis. Acute phlebitis of the phlebothrombotic type.

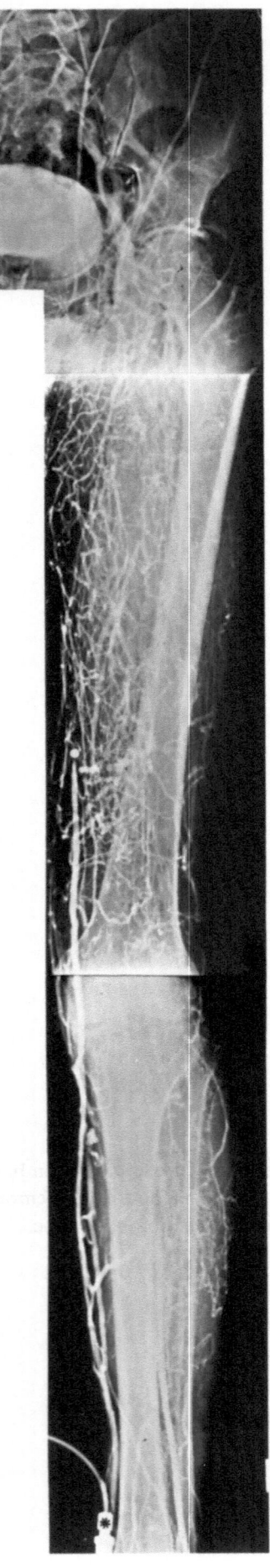

Fig. 108: Phlebogram of the left lower limb, through upstream injection into the internal saphenous vein at the dorsum pedis ✳. Acute phlebitis. No deep vein is opacified. Collateral circulation is via the superficial and the muscle veins. The three collateral pathways, internal saphenous, profunda femoris vein and the venae comitantes of the femoropopliteal axis are obstructed. The internal saphenous vein is obstructed at the lower third of the thigh ●. The injection is very painful, because of the filling of these superficial veins.

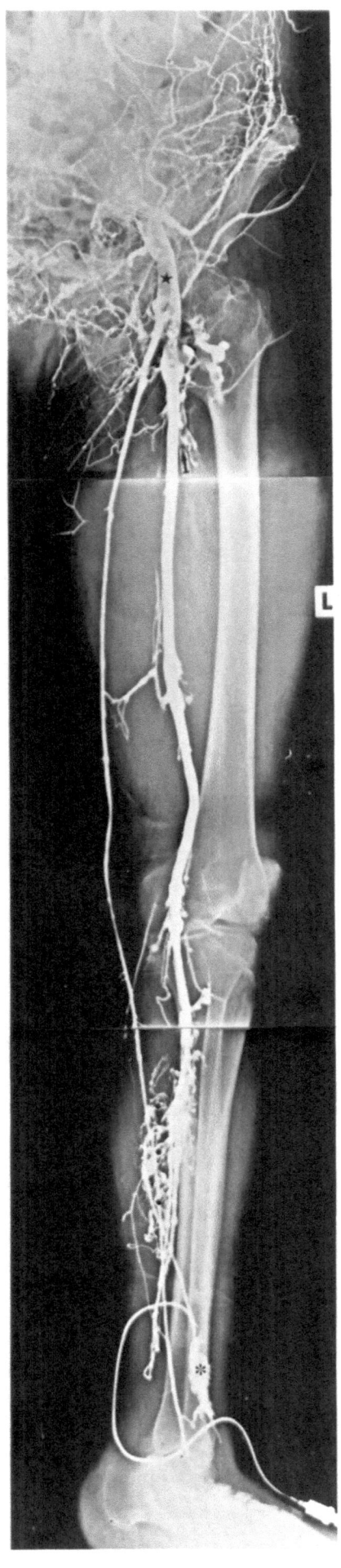

Fig. 109: Venogram of the left lower limb. Upstream injection into the internal saphenous vein at the ankle. Extravasation of contrast medium around the vein ∗. Filling of the posterior tibial veins with reflux into the calf-muscle veins, connected with the posterior tibial veins; There are numerous thromboses in the muscle veins ● ● ● . The femoropopliteal axis above is patent. But there is a suprajacent phlebitic obstruction in the common femoral vein ⋆ and the entire iliac axis is obstructed. Note also the reflux into the profunda femoris vein ⥮ which is thrombosed and contains a free thrombus. Backflow opacification of some veins of the femoral neck. Abdominal and suprapubic collateral circulation. Conclusion: left iliofemoral phlebitis associated with sural phlebitis with thrombi in numerous veins of the calf muscle. Two-leveled phlebitis.

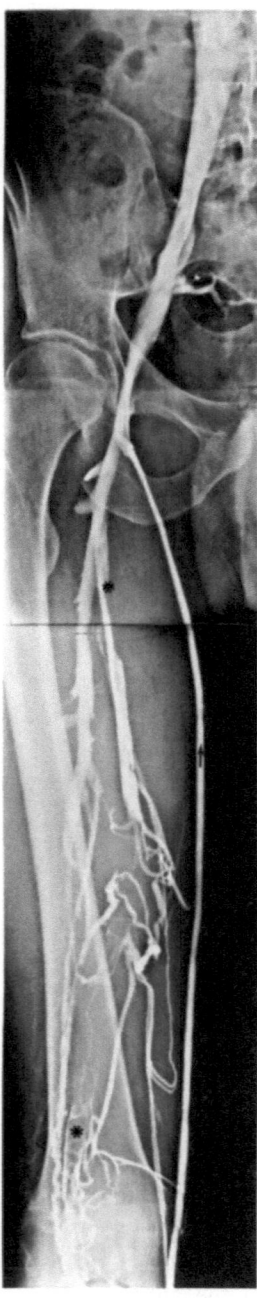

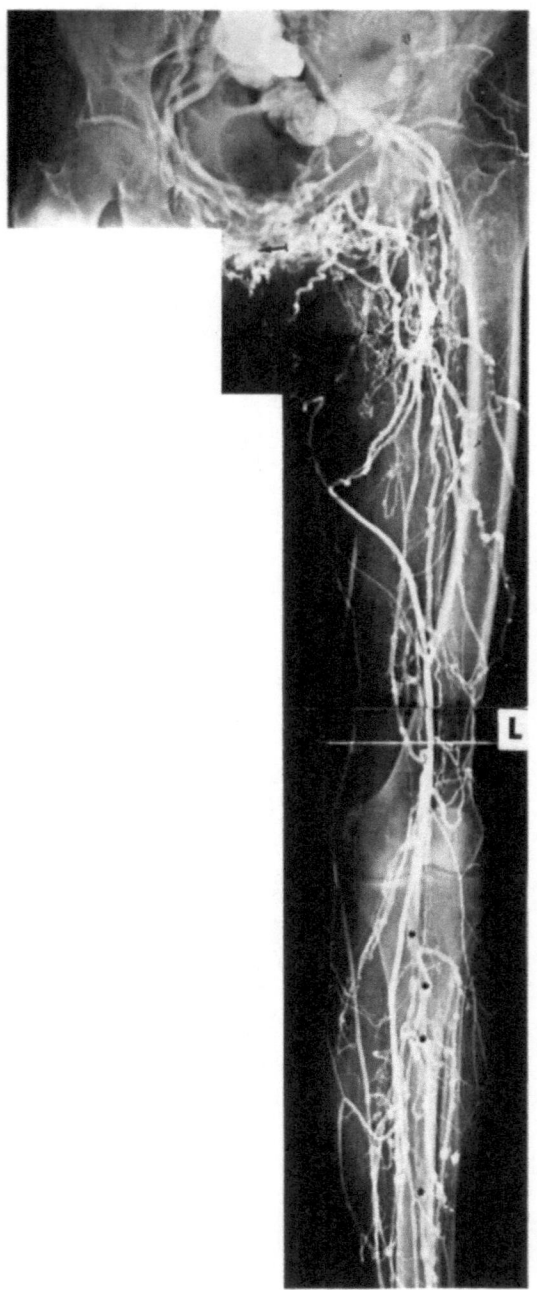

Fig. 110: Acute phlebitis of the right lower limb. Complete obstruction of the deep leg veins. Marked internal saphenous collateral circulation ↑. Numerous filling defects in the popliteal vein and in the upper superficial femoral vein ✳ which is reopacified via collateral veins. Competent iliocaval segment. Note the importance of injecting a large volume of contrast medium in order to demonstrate the patency of the ilio-inferior caval segment.

Fig. 111: Acute phlebitis of the left lower limb. The lower part of the deep veins of the leg remains patent with well-visible valves ◂. Multiple filling defects in the upper part of the leg veins ✳. Complete obstruction of the femoropopliteal system with collateral circulation through multiple superficial veins. The internal saphenous vein has undergone stripping. Iliac obliteration very probably due to supra-pubic left-to-right collateral circulation ↑. Large volumes of contrast medium allow demonstration of iliac obstruction.

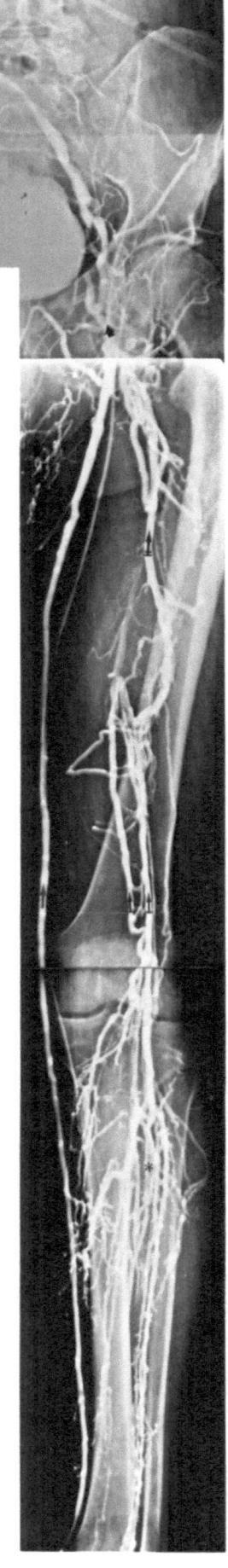

Fig. 112: Diffuse ilio-femoro-popliteal phlebitis associated with phlebitis of the calf veins. Partial obstruction of the deep veins of the leg with filling defects ∗ in veins which remain opacified. Femoropopliteal obstruction. Triple collateral circulation: internal saphenous vein ↑, venae comitantes of the thigh with their very characteristic "ladder" pattern ↑, and profunda femoris vein ↕. The common femoral vein is occluded, the iliac vein partially occluded. Collateral circulation is via the obturator veins ♠ which partly reopacify the left hypogastric system. Clinically: isolated sural phlebitis.

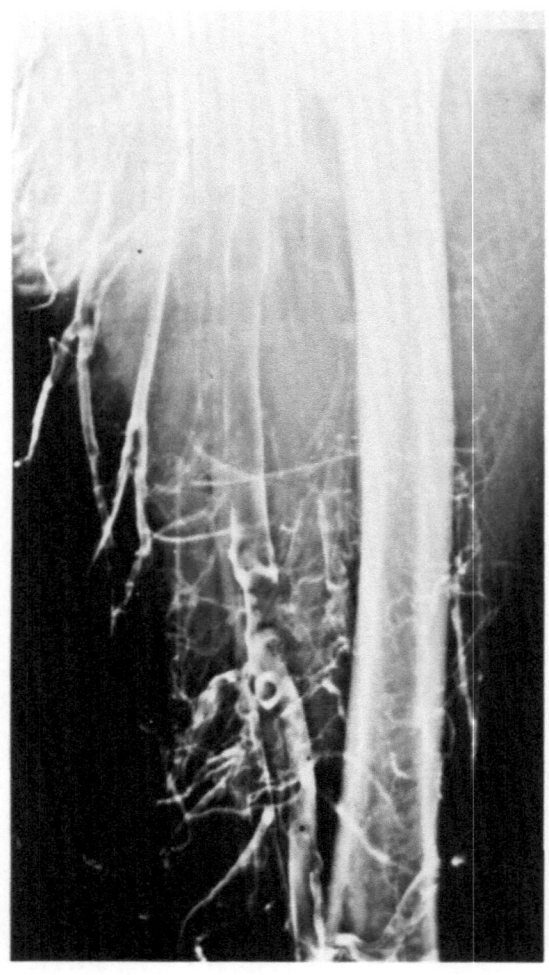

Fig. 113: Left ilio-femoro-popliteal phlebitis. Patient presenting with a retroperitoneal hematoma treated with anticoagulants. Images of the type phlebothrombosis are recorded from the entire left femoro-popliteal axis. Note also the filling defects in the superficial branches of the internal saphenous vein at the medial aspect of the thigh.

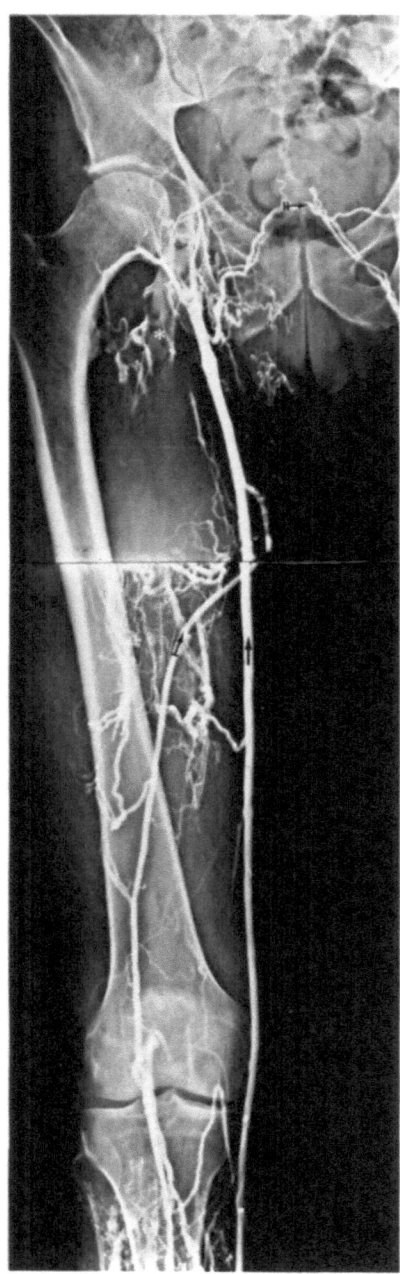

Fig. 114

Figs. 114 and 115:

114: Venogram of the right lower limb. Diffuse phlebitis of all deep veins of the right lower limb. Collateral circulation is mainly through the internal saphenous vein ↑ and an anastomosis at the posterior aspect of the thigh, between the external and the internal saphenous vein ↕. The profunda femoris vein seems to be occluded. Note the reopacification of a large clot in the right common femoral vein ∗. Moderate right to left suprapubic collateral circulation ↕.

115 (see p. 72): Unifemoral left percutaneous ilio-cavography. Note that the head of the thrombus "dribbles" into the inferior vena cava at its origin ❋.

Conclusion: Diffuse ilio-femoro-popliteal phlebitis associated with phlebitis of the calf. The head of the thrombus is situated in the inferior vena cava at its origin. The patient had been "labelled" as follows: isolated sural phlebitis.

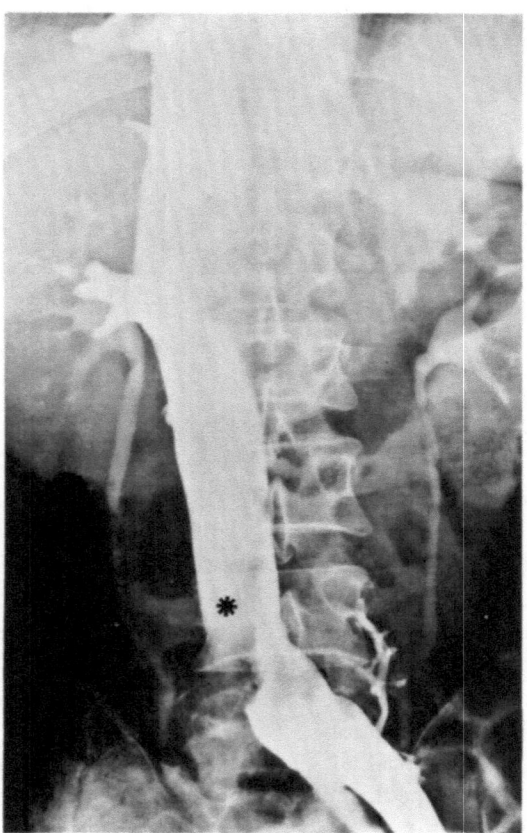

Fig. 115

115: Unifemoral left percutaneous ilio-cavography.
Note that the head of the thrombus "dribbles" into
the inferior vena cava at its origin ✳. (See also
p. 71.)

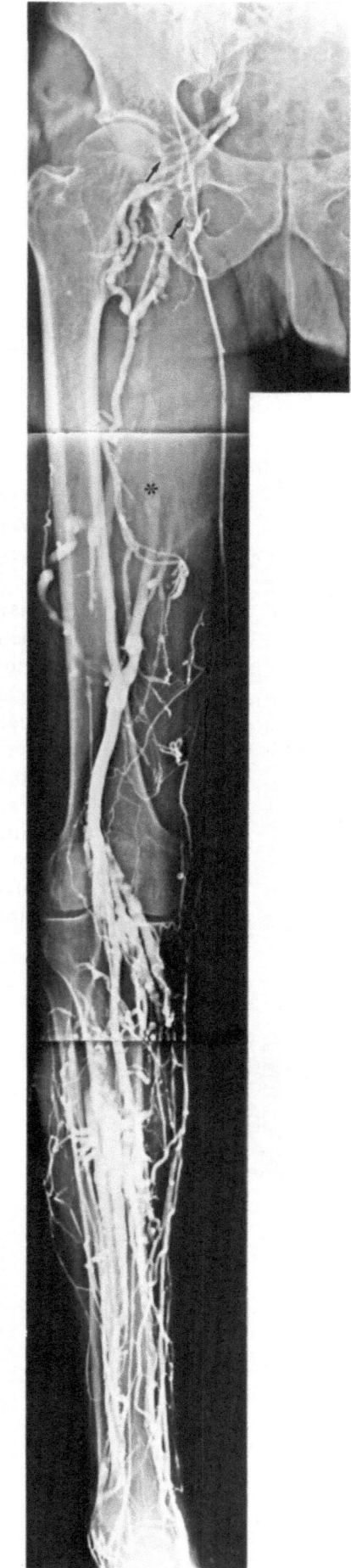

Fig. 116: Venogram of the right lower limb. The
deep veins of the leg are patent. Their upper part is
obscured because the tourniquet had been too
tightly applied. The popliteal vein is free. The
superficial femoral vein is occluded in its upper
part ✳. There is moreover clear obstruction of the
iliac vein, since obturator ↕ and inferior gluteal ↑ collateral circulation reopacified the right hypogastric
system. Right ilio-femoral phlebitis which had been
mistaken clinically for a sural phlebitis.

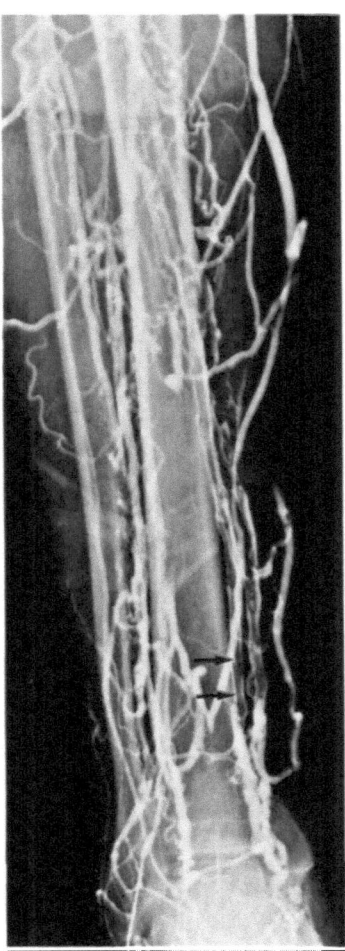

Fig. 117: Sural phlebitis. Venogram of the right lower limb. Note the filling defects ↑↑ in the posterior tibial veins at the lower part of the leg.

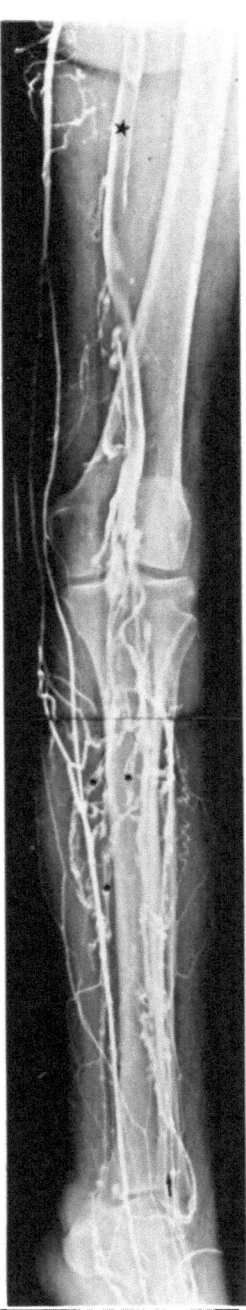

Fig. 118: Acute phlebitis of the left lower limb. Partial occlusion of the deep veins of the leg. The anterior tibial veins ↑ seem to be still permeable and valvulated. Loose thrombi in the muscular branches ✱. Permeability of the lower part of the popliteal vein. Numerous loose thrombus with filling defect in the superficial femoral vein ★.

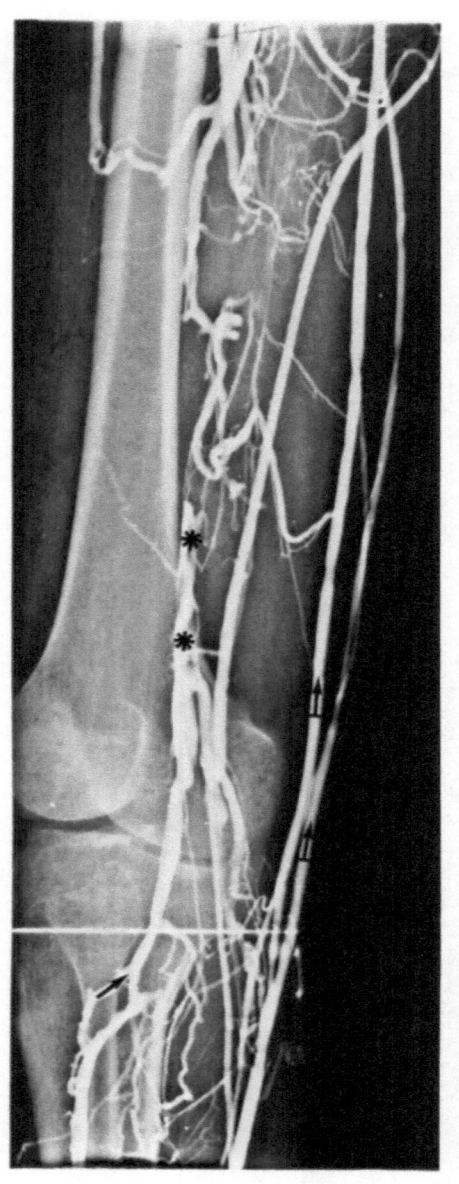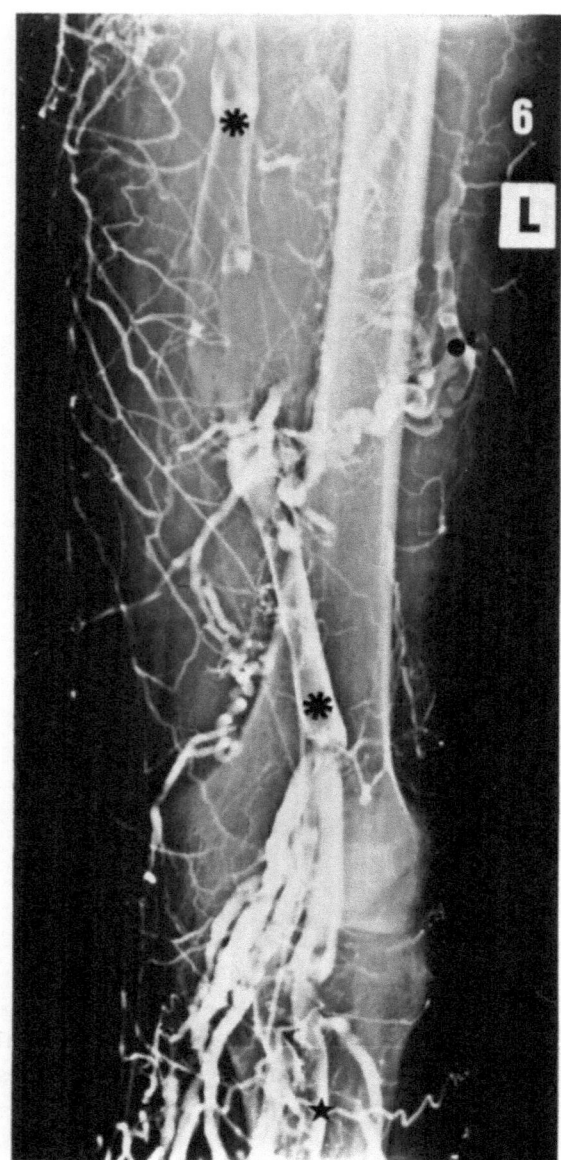

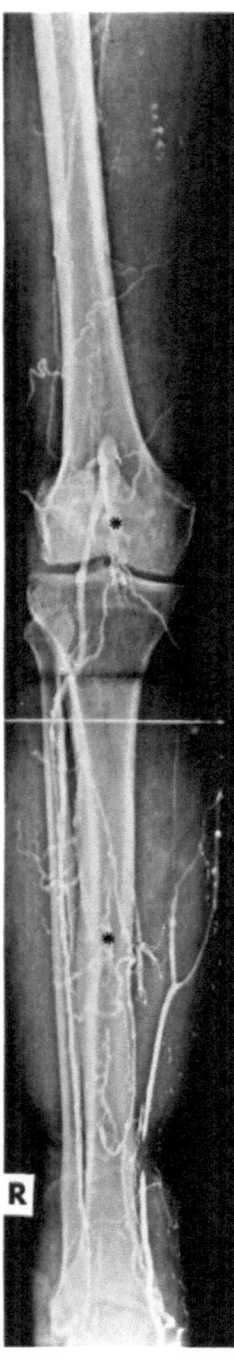

Fig. 121: Acute phlebitis of the right lower limb. A large amount of contrast medium is injected. Nevertheless, there is only very faint opacification of a part of the leg veins which show filling defects * and of the middle part of the popliteal vein which is also occluded with a thrombus *. Above this level there is no opacification of the femoropopliteal axis or of any collateral route. The inferior veno cavography (not shown here) confirms the existence of an associated iliocaval occlusion. The day after, this patient showed signs of ischemic phlebitis and, later, venous gangrene.

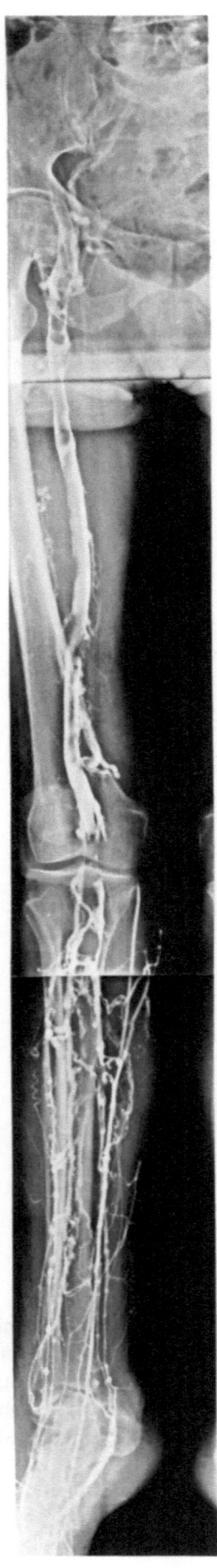

Fig. 122: Acute phlebitis of the right lower limb. Appearance of phlebothrombosis involving at once the deep veins of the leg and the entire femoro-popliteal axis as well as the common femoral vein.

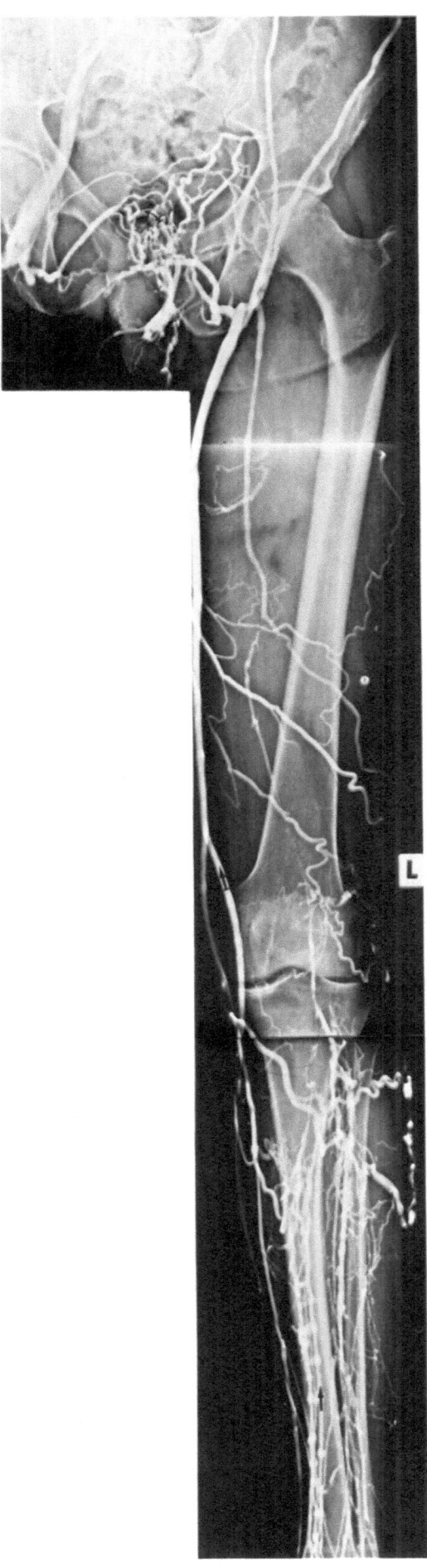

Fig. 123: Acute phlebitis of the left lower limb. Free flow venography with a large amount of contrast medium. The posterior tibial veins ↑ are permeable. The anterior tibial and peroneal veins are occluded. No femoropopliteal opacification. Collateral circulation solely through the internal saphenous vein ↥. Suprapubic and subcutaneous abdominal collateral circulation ↧ toward the right iliac system is proof of associated left iliac occlusion. Clinically this patient had been suspected of isolated sural phlebitis.

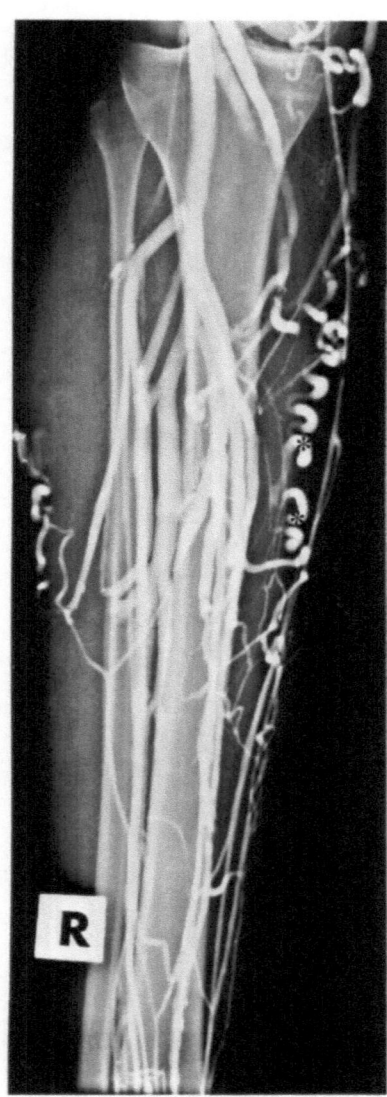

Fig. 124: Sural phlebitis. This patient was treated with heparin as soon as clinical signs were noted. Venogram of the right lower limb. Follow-up investigation after 15 days' treatment with heparin. Complete recanalization of all deep veins of the leg which have however lost their valves. Some varices at the medial aspect of the right calf ●✳✳ .

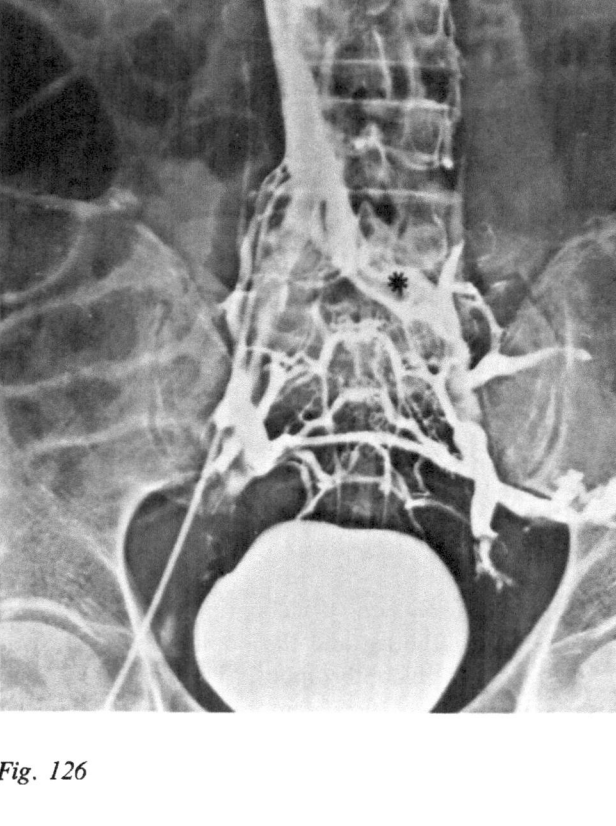

Fig. 126

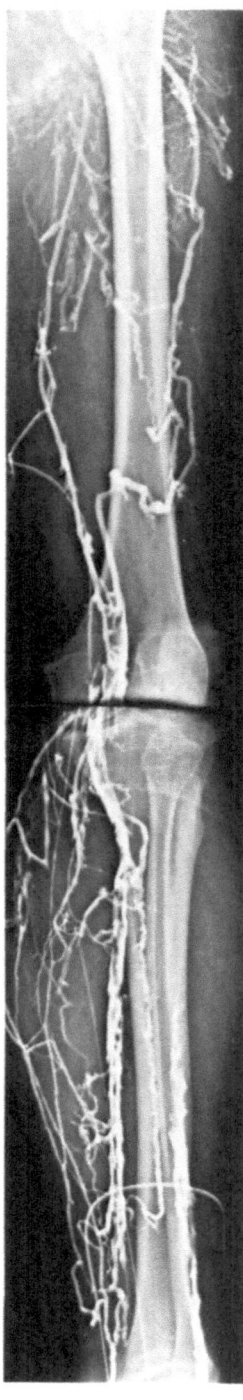

Fig. 125

Figs. 125 and 126: Diffuse acute phlebitis of the ilio-femoro-popliteal axis and of the leg veins.

125: Free flow injection phlebogram of the left lower limb. Huge filling defects in the deep veins of the leg and in the popliteal vein. No opacification of the superficial femoral vein. Collateral derivation via branches of the muscle veins at the medial and lateral aspects of the thigh. No opacification of the common femoral vein. Very important venous stasis.

126: Retrograde left iliac phlebography. Right femoral venous Seldinger. Reflux into the left common iliac vein which shows multiple filling defects and thrombosis ✻. No opacification below this level. This patient's condition has evolved to ischemic phlebitis with acute venous stasis.

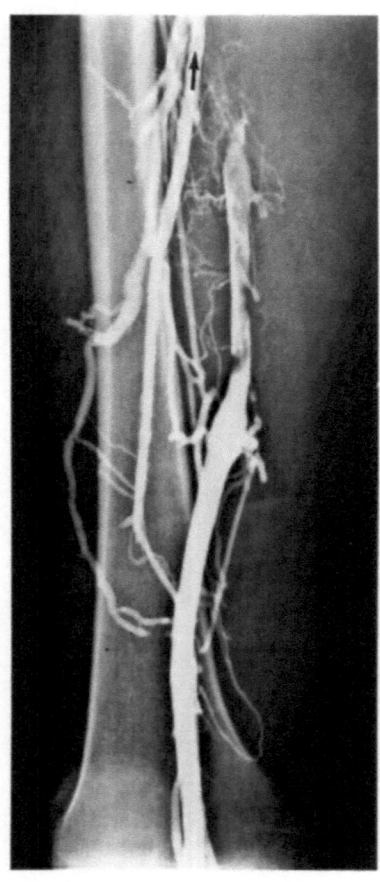

Fig. 127: Phlebography of the right lower limb. The deep veins of the leg and the popliteal vein are permeable. There are signs of phlebothrombosis with free thrombus in the middle part of the superficial femoral vein. Collateral circulation via the profunda femoris vein ↑ which reopacifies perfectly permeable ilio-femoral axis above. (The film is not shown here.)

Chapter 4

ILIOFEMORAL AND ILIOCAVAL PHLEBITES. THROMBOSIS OF THE INFERIOR VENA CAVA

Figures 128–167

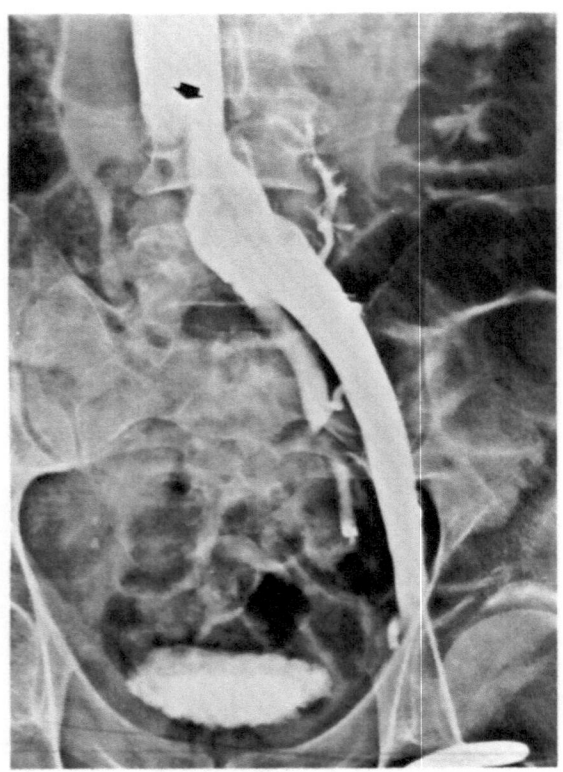

Fig. 128: Right iliocaval phlebitis. Unilateral left investigation. High rate injection which nevertheless succeeds in moulding the upper head of a right iliac thrombus which is located in the inferior vena cava ◄. These findings lead to modifying the surgical procedure in this patient.

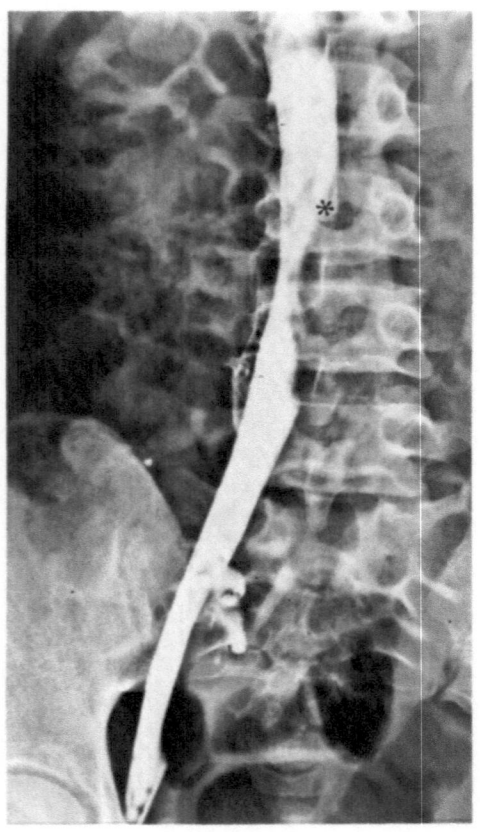

Fig. 129: Left iliac phlebitis with a thrombus extending into the inferior vena cava up to the level of the third lumbar vertebra ✳ . Investigation by unilateral right iliocavography.

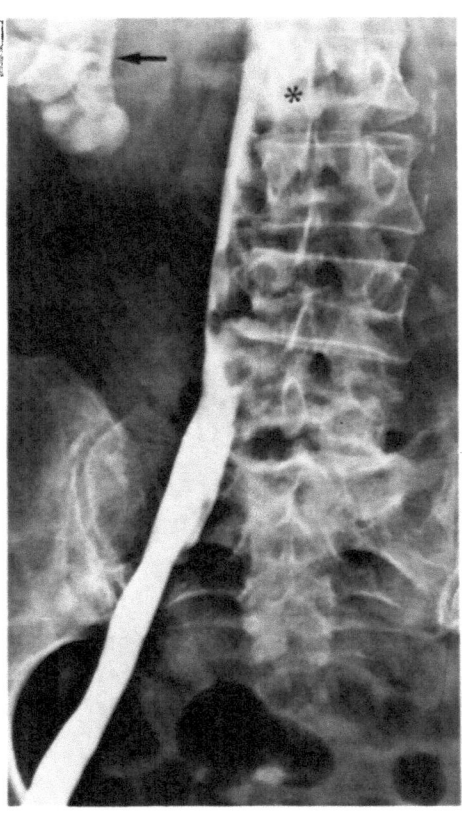

Fig. 130: Left iliocaval phlebitis. Investigation by injection into the right iliac vein; this latter is perfectly permeable. The thrombus occupies the inferior vena cava as far as the renal veins ✳. Note the coralliform nephrolith in the right kidney ↑.

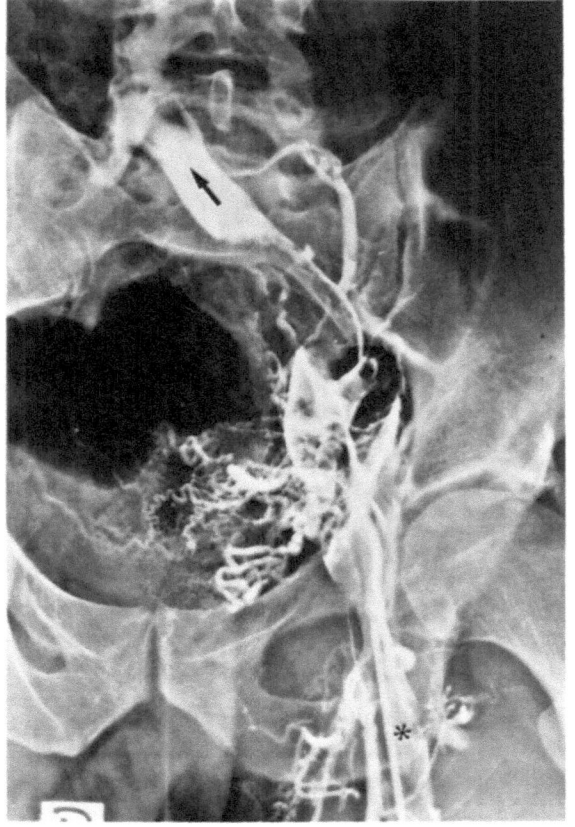

Fig. 131: Left iliofemoral phlebitis. Injection into the thrombus of the left femoral vein with reflux into the common femoral vein, demonstrating the thrombus to be of the phlebothrombotic type ✳. The opacification of the external iliac axis is very fragmentary, the phlebitis is very adhesive; nevertheless there is filling of the left common iliac vein which seems to be permeable ↑. Failure of the right femoral catheterization: this technique does not show whether there is a thrombus in the inferior cava.

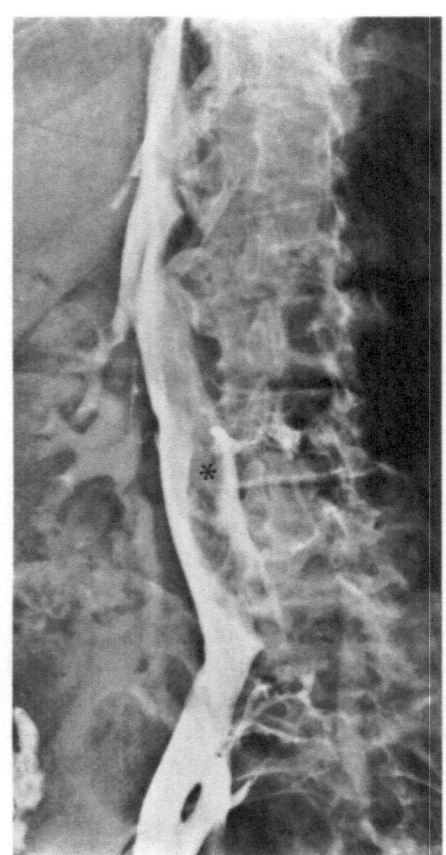

Fig. 132: Left iliocaval phlebitis. Note that the left anterior oblique projection demonstrates clearly an enormous loose thrombus * in the infrarenal inferior vena cava. Right femoral catheterization.

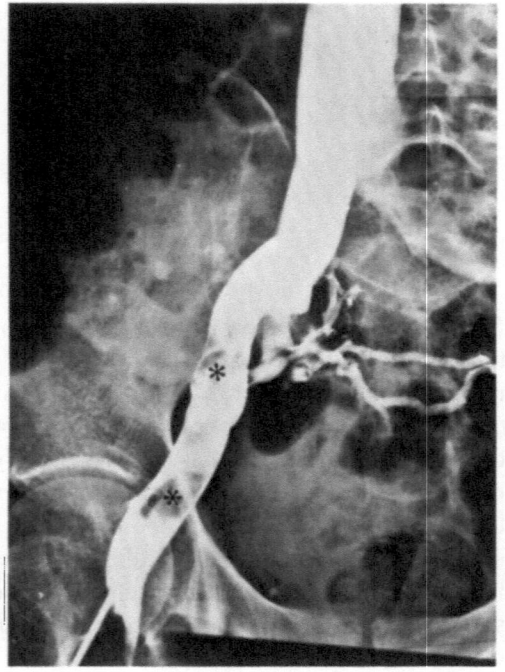

Fig. 133: Right unifemoral percutaneous iliocavography. Multiple filling defects* of the phlebothrombotic type on the whole right iliac axis, without any associated thrombosis of the inferior vena cava.

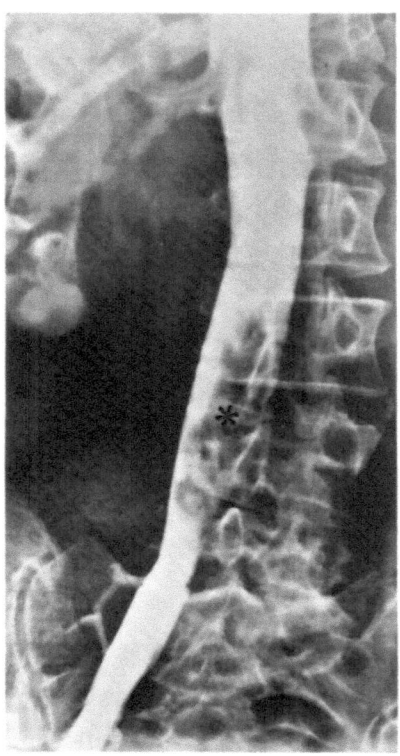

Fig. 134: Left iliocaval phlebitis with enormous thrombus in the infrarenal inferior vena cava ∗. Right femoral injection. Right anterior oblique projection (same patient as Fig. 132). Thrombus "seems" lower.

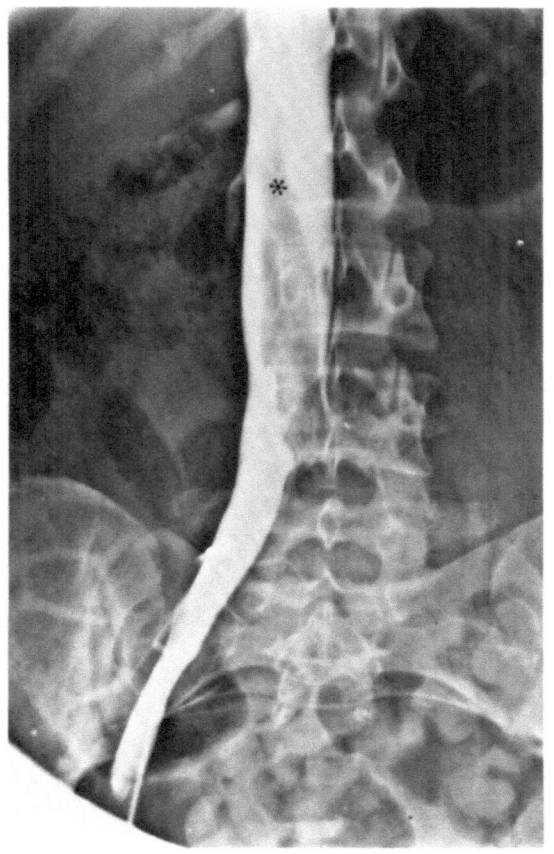

Fig. 135: Left iliocaval phlebitis with a thrombus in the inferior vena cava extending as far as the right renal vein ∗. Right femoral catheterization.

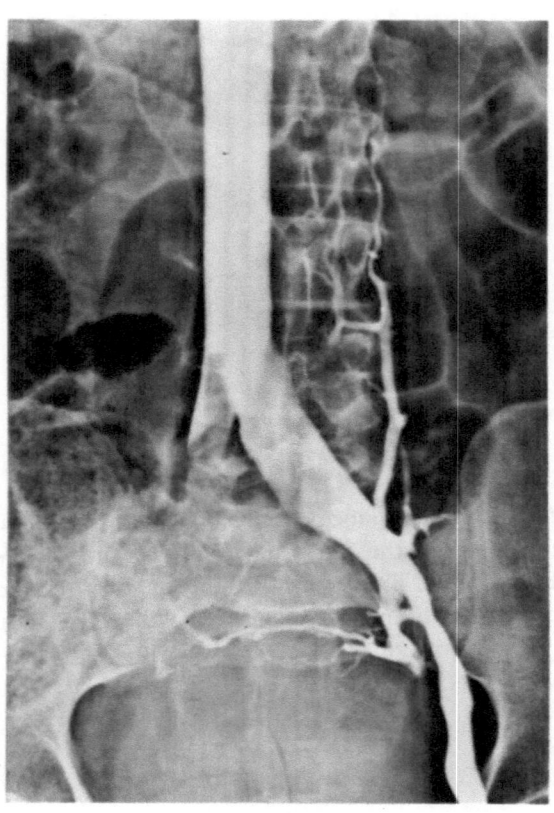

Fig. 136: Right ilio-caval phlebitis. Left femora catheterization. Slight reflux into the common iliac vein allows outlining of the head of the iliac thrombus which is situated just at the origin of the inferior vena cava.

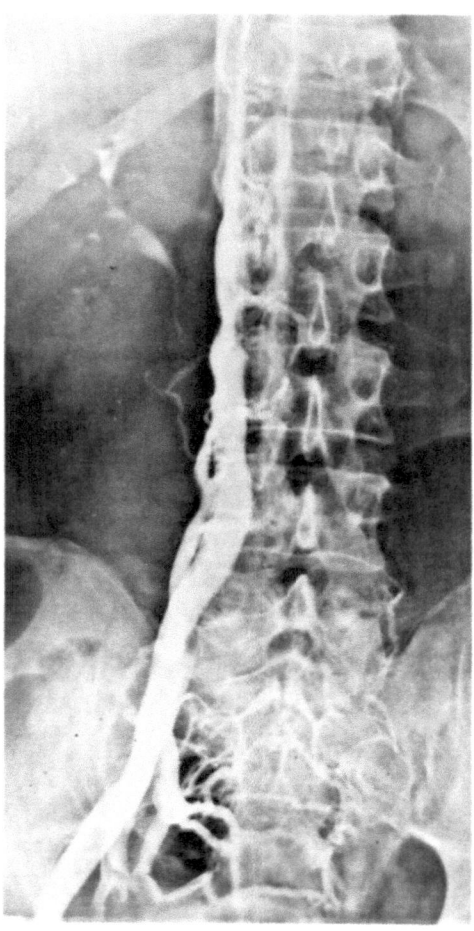 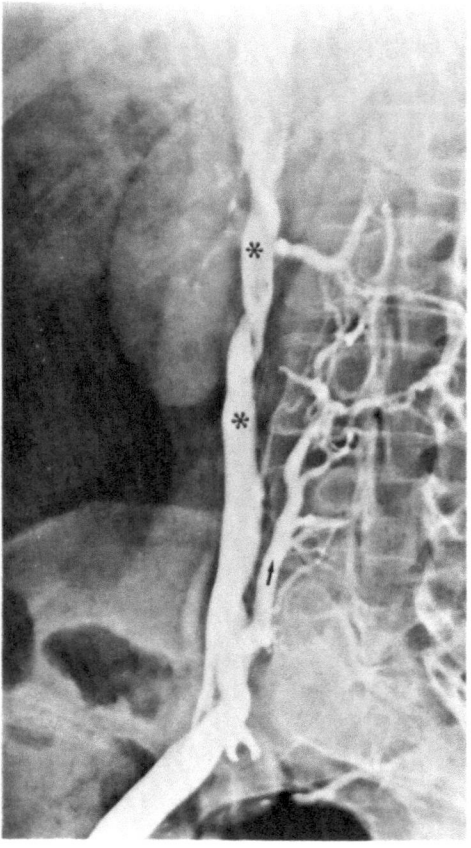

Fig. 137   *Fig. 138*

Figs. 137 and 138: Value of the left anterior oblique projection for the demonstration of inferior venal caval loose thrombi. Left iliocaval phlebitis. Right femoral injection.

137: Frontal projection. Patency of the right iliac axis. The inferior vena cava seems to be opacified partly along the right aspect of the spine. Opacification of intra and extraspinal plexus.

138: Left anterior oblique projection. Opacification of the right ascending lumbar vein and the spinal plexuses ↑. This projection clears the inferior vena cava from the spine, rules out extrinsic compression, and demonstrates the lamellar appearance of the entire infrarenal part of the inferior vena cava ∗∗. The diagnosis was: chronic iliocaval phlebitis with recanalization. At surgery: *Recent* loose lamellar thrombus of the phlebothrombotic type on the posterior aspect of the inferior vena cava, which has thus been ill-demonstrated on the frontal projection (137) taken with the patient in the supine position. This points out the importance of the left anterior oblique projection for demonstrating, on one hand, thrombi located on the posterior aspect of the inferior vena cava, and on the other hand determining, for example, whether it is a matter of intracaval thrombosis or of extrinsic compression by retroperitoneal adenopathies.

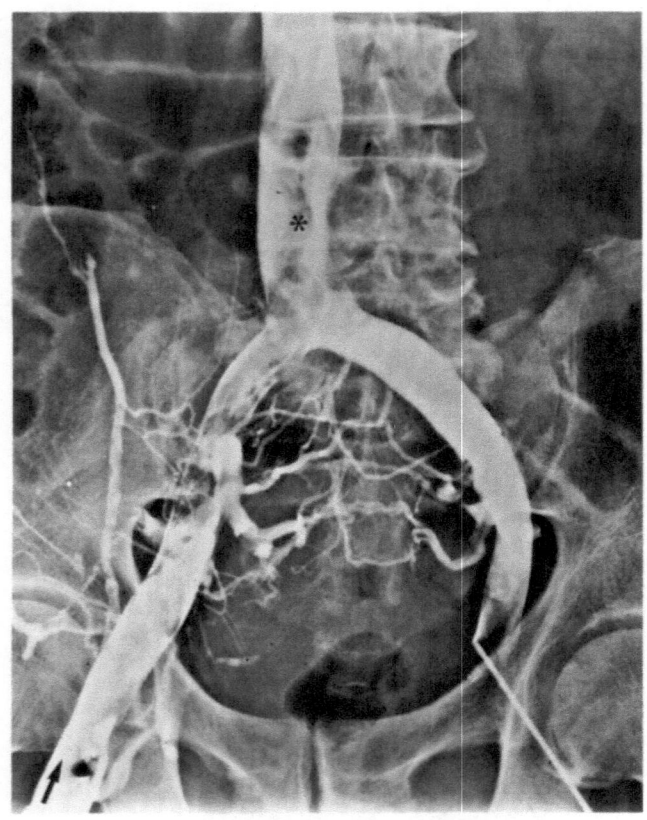

Fig. 139: Bifemoral percutaneous cavography. Puncture into a right iliofemoral thrombus ↟. The iliac phlebitis is of the phlebothrombotic type and involves the inferior vena cava. There is a voluminous "snake-head"∗ like image in the infrarenal segment of the inferior vena cava. Typical appearance of a very emboligenic phlebothrombosis.

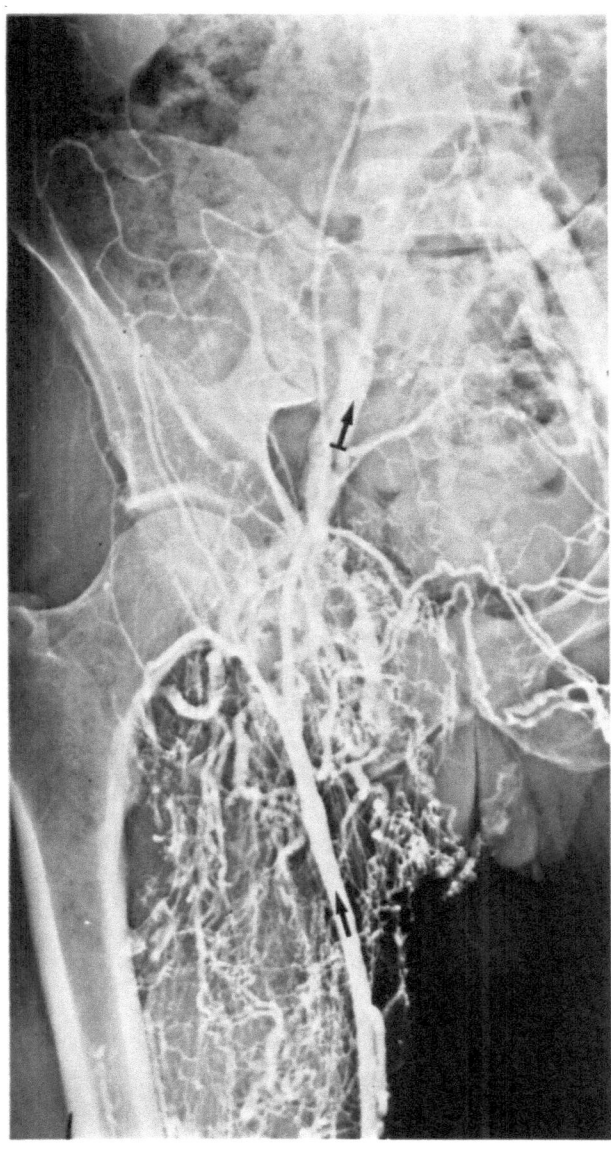

Fig. 140: Right iliofemoral phlebitis. Free circulation venogram of the right lower limb performed with a large amount of contrast medium. The deep venous circulation of the right lower limb is totally occluded (including the profunda femoris vein). Collateral circulation occurs only through the internal saphenous system ↑ and produces only very faint opacification of the right hypogastric venous system ↕. Contralateral derivation toward the left through veins of the Retzius space.

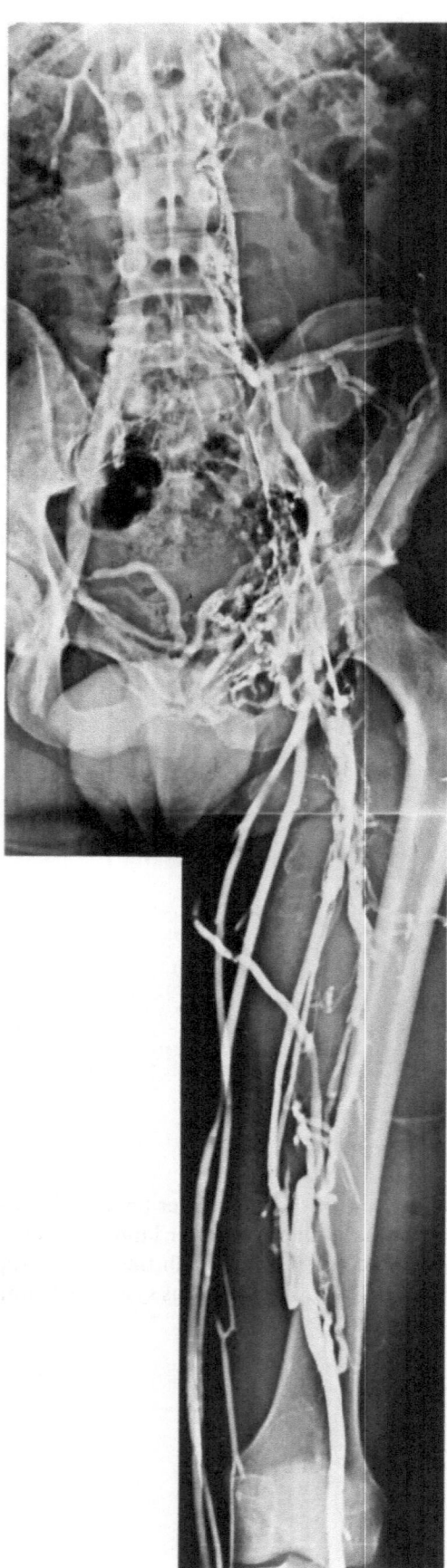

Fig. 141: Left iliofemoral phlebitis extended to the left common iliac vein. The suprapubic collateral circulation reopacifies the right iliac system. Note duplication of the internal saphenous vein, a rather common occurrence. There are also homolateral collateral derivations in the left iliac muscle.

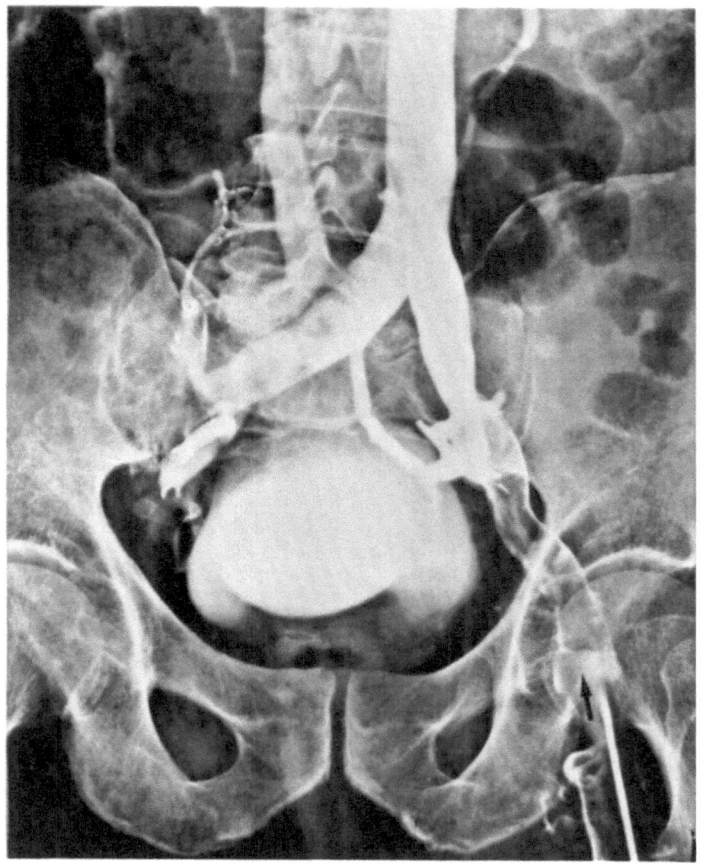

Fig. 142: Left iliofemoral phlebitis. Puncture into a thrombus in the left femoral vein ↑. Duplication of inferior vena cava. Iliofemoral phlebitis associated with a congenital anomaly of the inferior vena cava.

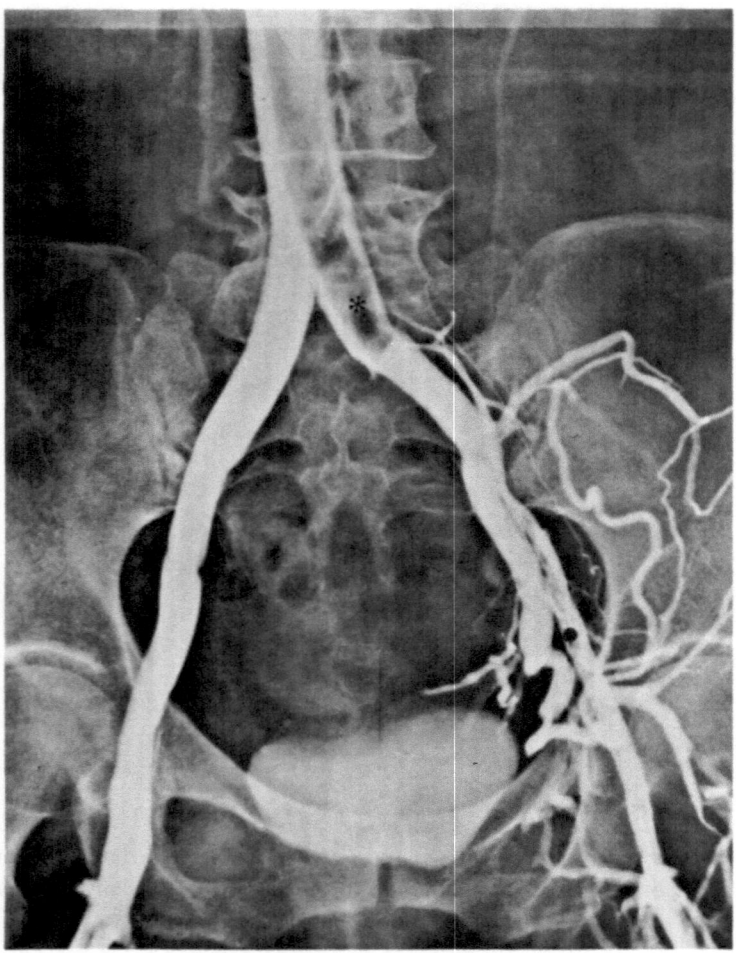

Fig. 143

Figs. 143 and 144: This patient has a history of numerous phlebitis of the left lower limb. Pulmonary embolism in spite of anticoagulant treatment.

143: Bifemoral percutaneous cavography. Centering on the pelvis. Left iliofemoral chronic phlebitis with a grid-like appearance of the left external iliac vein ●. There is already a filling defect ✳ in the left common iliac vein and on the lower part of the inferior vena cava.

144: Same patient. Centering on the abdomen. The thrombus ✳ extends as far as the interrenal portion of the inferior vena cava. Very interesting case, showing the development of phlebothrombosis in a case of iliofemoral chronic phlebitis. It is easy to imagine the mechanism of the pulmonary embolism in this patient under anticoagulant therapy. Interest of cavography for the diagnosis of pulmonary embolism: It is not sufficient to perform only venography of the lower limb; in this case it would not have revealed the origin and the topography of the thrombus.

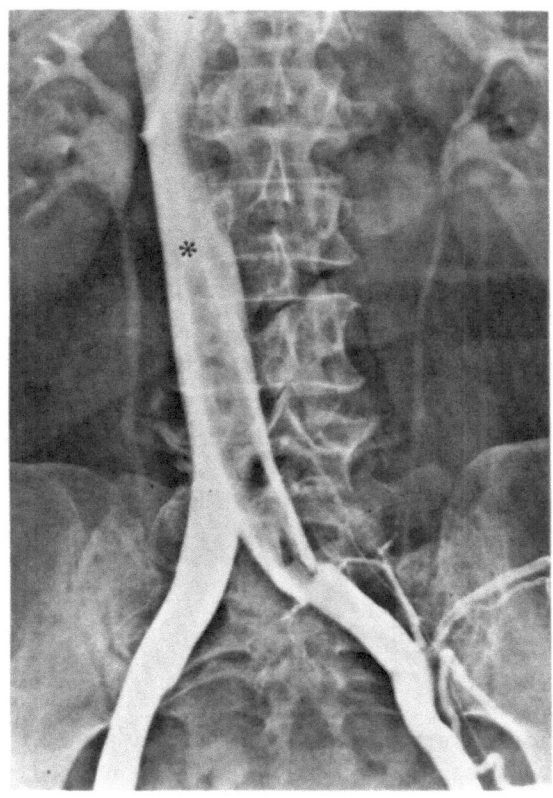

Fig. 144

Fig. 145

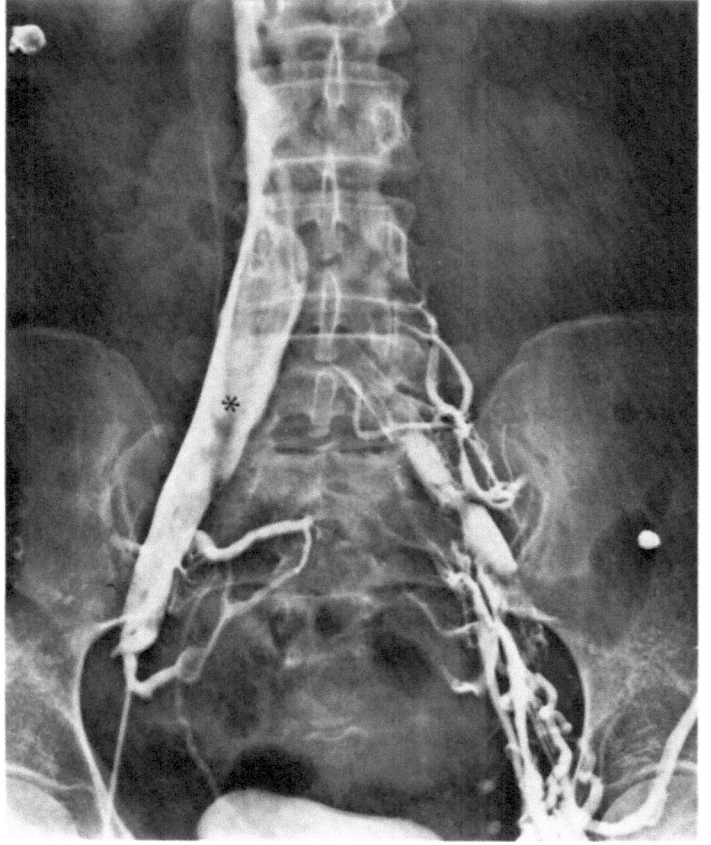

Figs. 145 and 146: Bifemoral percutaneous cavography. Left iliac adhesive phlebitis. Right iliocaval phlebothrombosis. Voluminous thrombus which has its origin in the right iliac vein ∗ and extends as far as the interrenal segment of the inferior vena cava ∗, well demonstrated in Fig. 146 (see p. 94) corresponding to centering onto the abdomen.

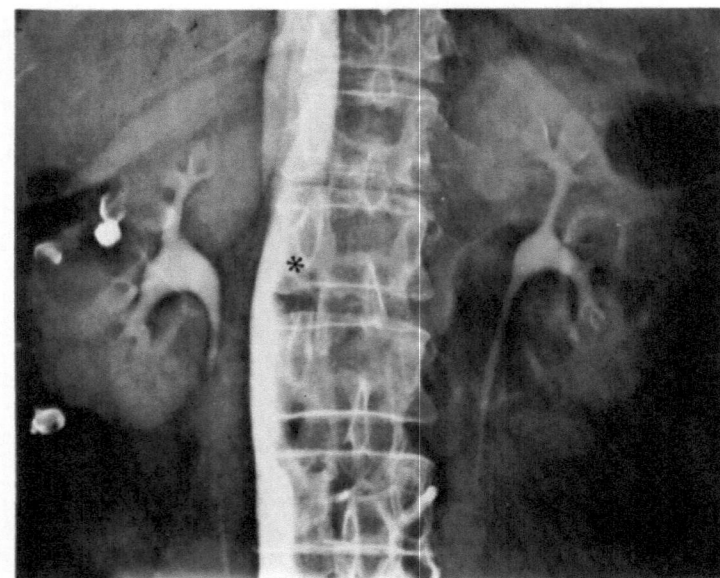

Fig. 146

Figs. 145 (see p. 93) *and 146:* Bifemoral percutaneous cavography. Left iliac adhesive phlebitis. Right iliocaval phlebothrombosis. Voluminous thrombus which has its origin in the right iliac vein ∗ and extends as far as the interrenal segment of the inferior vena cava ∗ , well demonstrated in Fig. 146 corresponding to centering onto the abdomen.

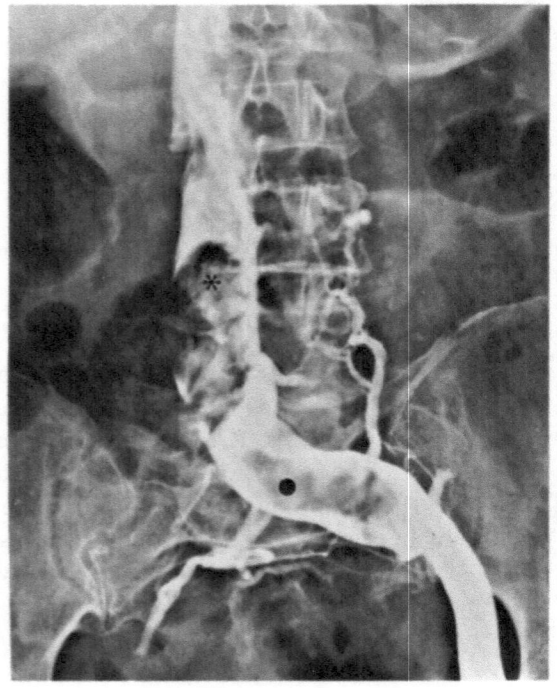

Fig. 147: Clinical signs of right iliofemoral phlebitis. Left unifemoral cavography. This investigation demonstrates on the one hand an iliac thrombus extending as far as the infrarenal inferior vena cava ∗ , and on the other hand, a voluminous thrombus in the left common iliac vein ●.

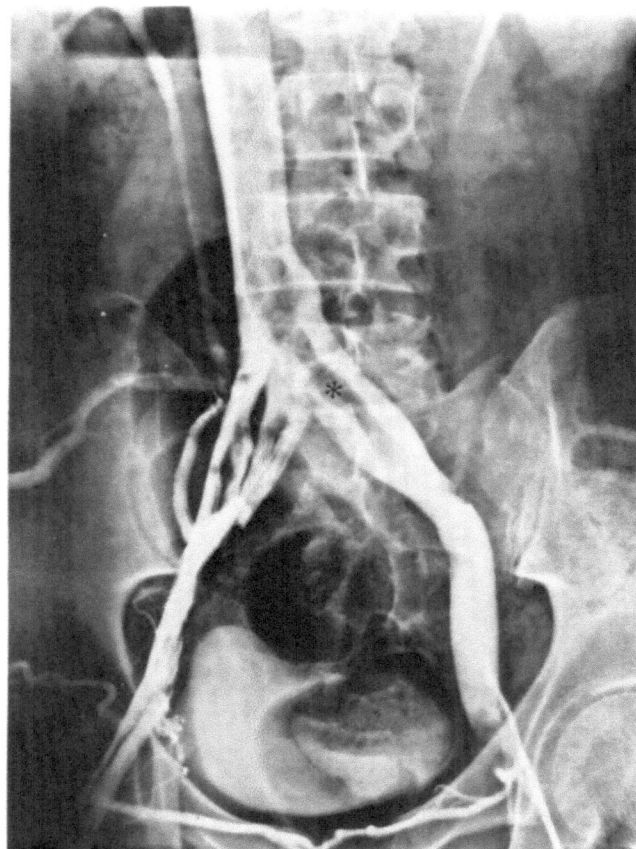

Fig. 148

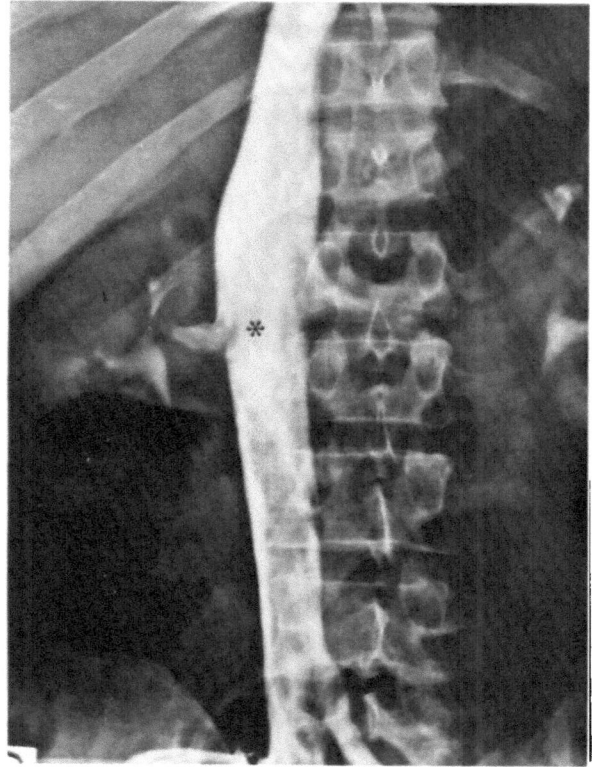

Fig. 149

Figs. 148 and 149: Bifemoral percutaneous cavography. Right iliac chronic phlebitis with duplication of the right common iliac vein. This patient has a history of pulmonary embolisms. Reason for the *bi*femoral percutaneous cavography: this technique demonstrates that the pulmonary embolism does not originate from the right phlebitis but from the left common iliac vein which contains a voluminous thrombus * extending as far as the interrenal segment of the inferior vena cava *; this is clearly demonstrated on the film centered onto the abdomen (149).

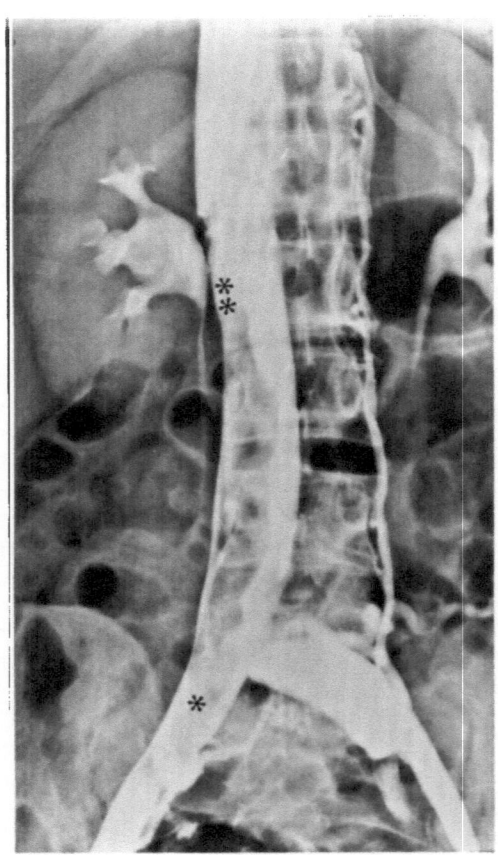

Fig. 150: Bifemoral percutaneous cavography. Ilio-inferior caval phlebitis, originating from the right common iliac vein ∗ . The thrombus extends as far as the right renal vein ∗∗ .

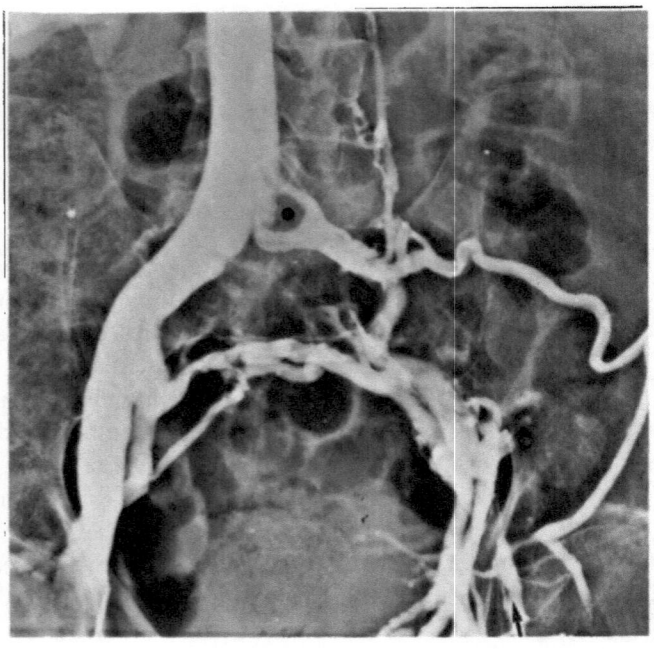

Fig. 151: Left iliac phlebitis. Puncture into the thrombus on the left ↑. The presacral and iliac collateral circulation reopacifies the terminal portion of the left common iliac vein which is the site of a huge synechia ●. Cockett's syndrome associated with underlying iliac phlebitis.

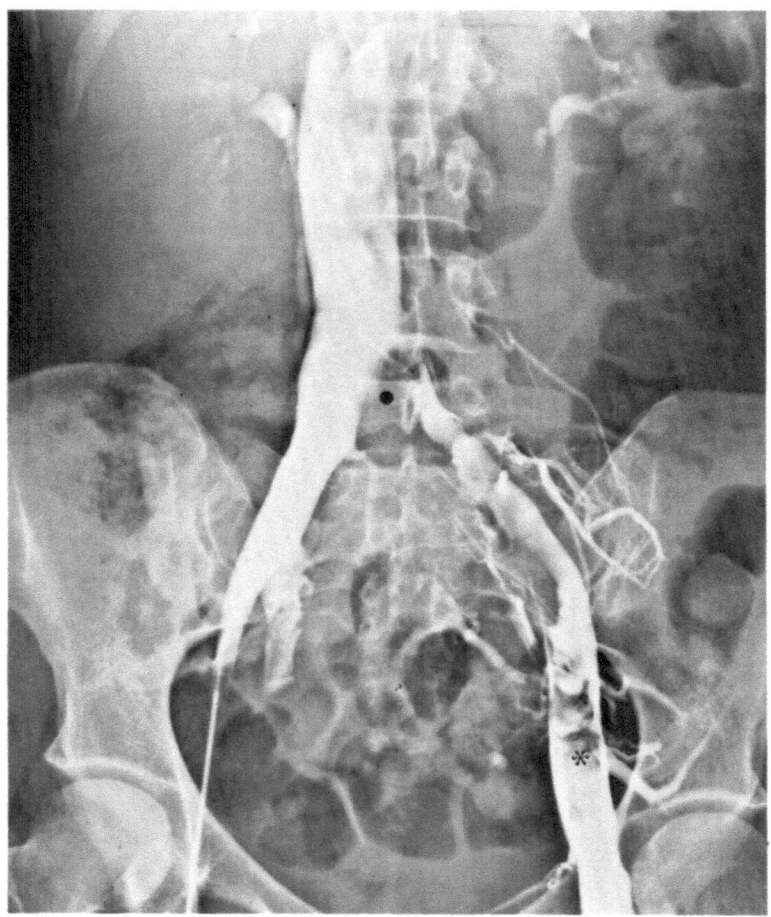

Fig. 152: Left iliac phlebitis. Loose thrombus in the left external iliac vein∗. Fenestration of the terminal ● portion of the left common iliac vein. Diagnosis made during operation: voluminous loose thrombus below the synechia in a Cockett's syndrome of the left common iliac vein.

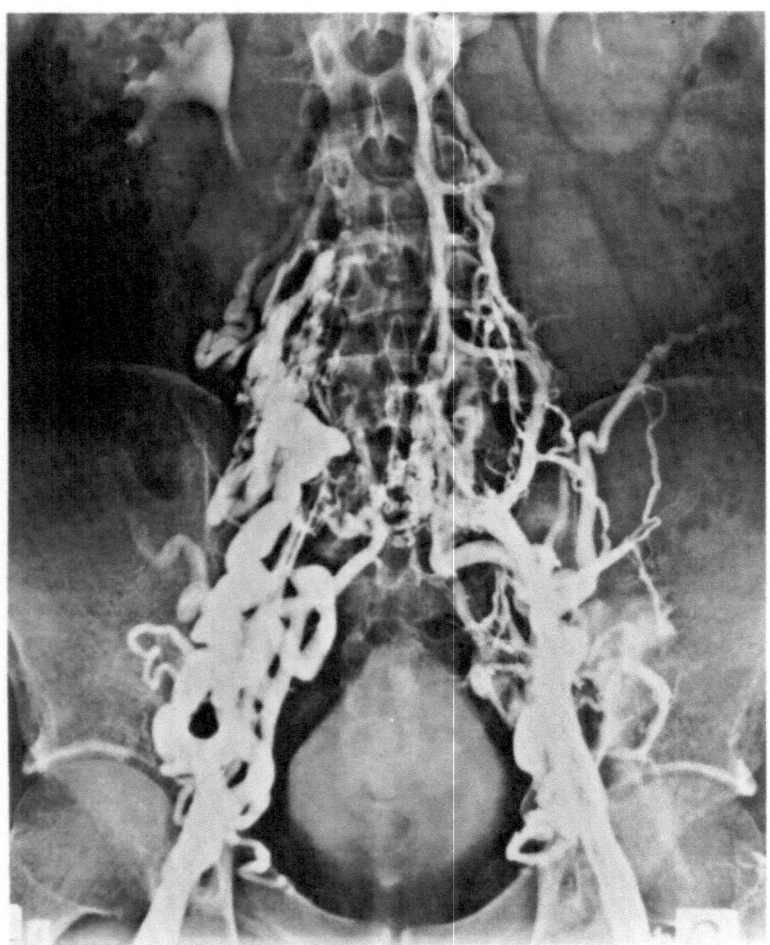

Fig. 153

Figs. 153 and 154: Bilateral ilio-caval phlebitis. Figure 153 corresponds to a bifemoral percutaneous cavography with puncture into a bilateral thrombus. Rather poorly developed collateral circulation does not allow demonstration of the level of the head of the thrombus in the thrombus in the inferior vena cava. *154:* Descending cavography through percutaneous brachial approach. The thrombosis does not reach the segment of the renal veins but terminates in the infrarenal portion of the inferior vena cava.

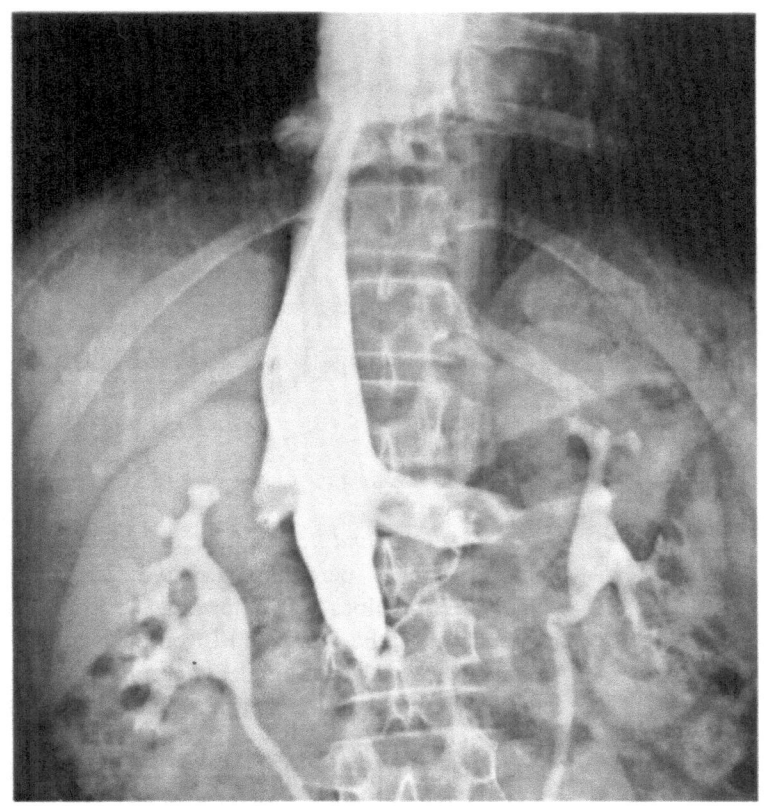

Fig. 154

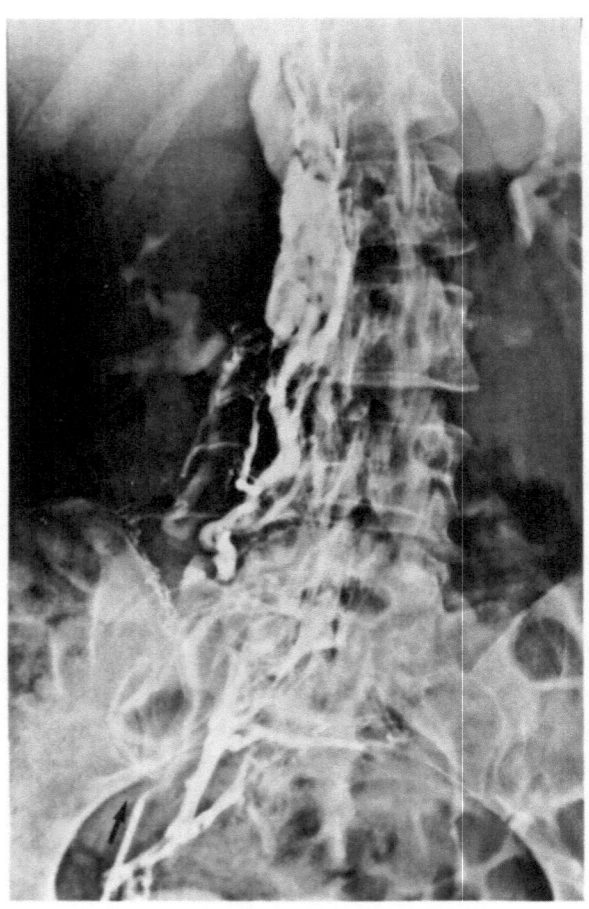

Fig. 155

Figs. 155, 156 and 157: Iliocaval phlebitis. Uni-femoral right ↑ percutaneous cavography (155). This injection does not determine accurately the upper level of the intracaval thrombus.

156 and 157: Descending cavography ↓ by per-cutaneous brachial approach; frontal (156) and lateral (157) views. The site of occlusion is the infrarenal portion of the inferior vena cava. The interrenal and the retrohepatic segments are free, as demonstrated in Fig. 157, which shows moreover a reflux into the left renal vein ↑.

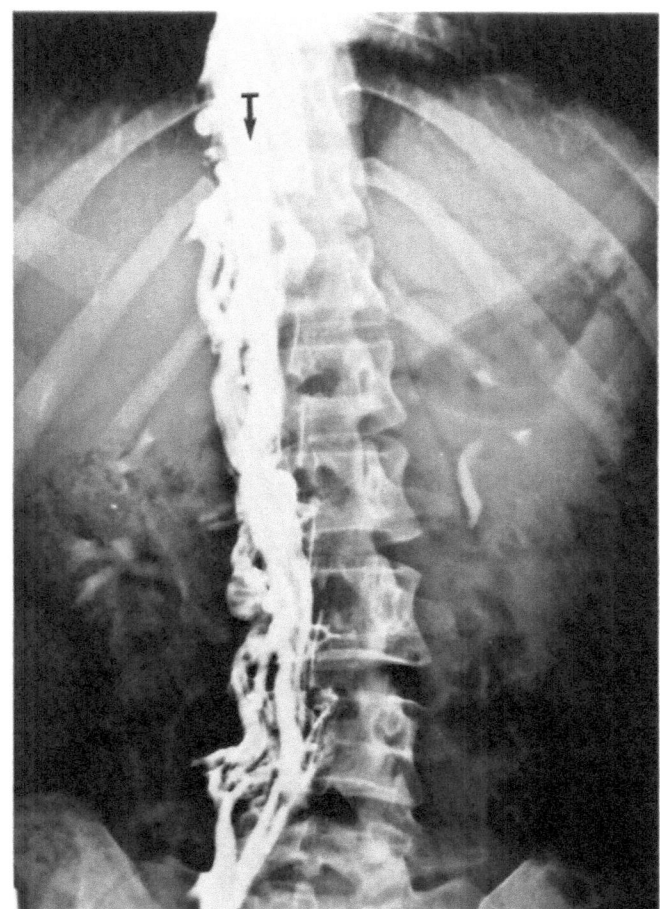

Fig. 156

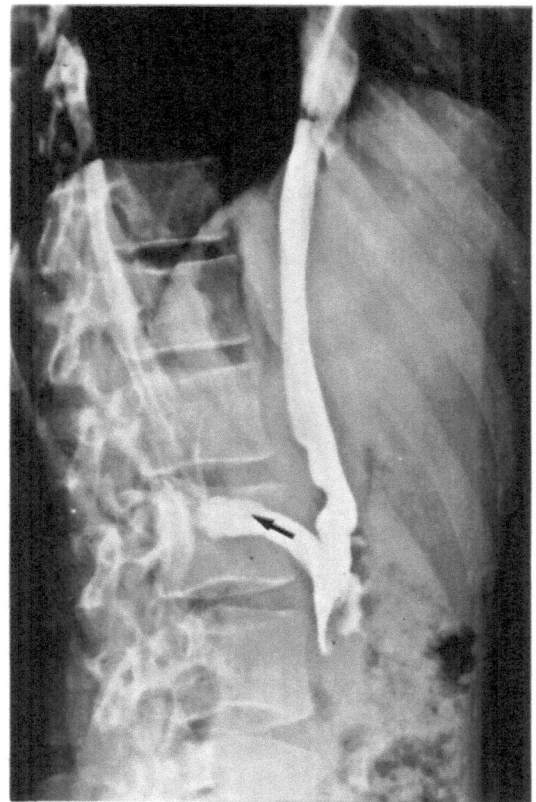

Fig. 157

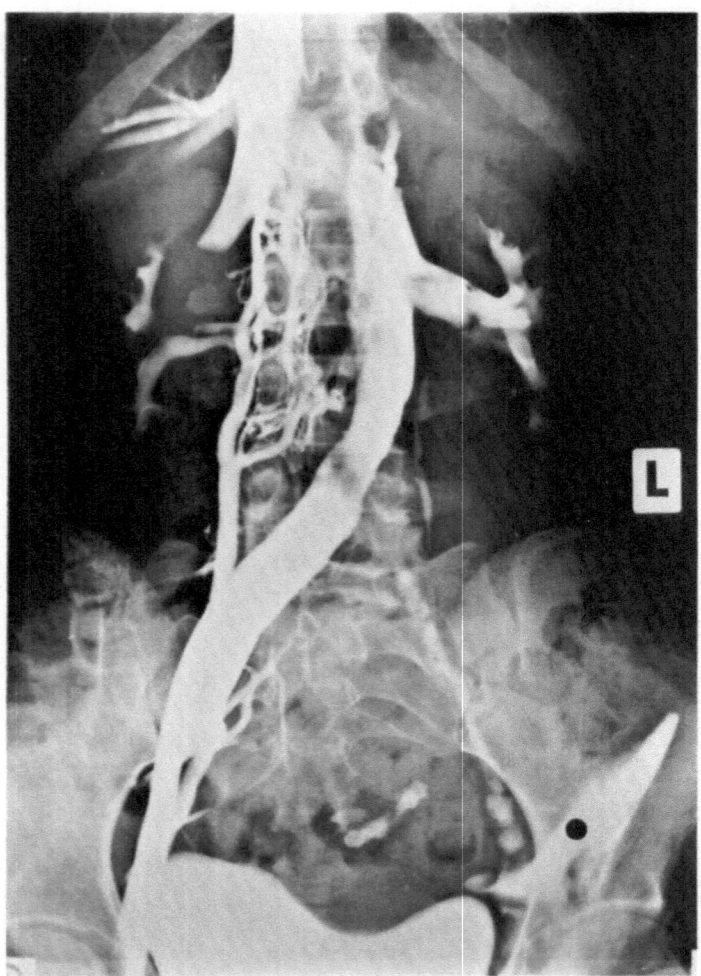

Fig. 158: Left iliac phlebitis. Failure of an attempted percutaneous catheterization (note extravasation of contrast medium ● on the left iliac vein). The right unifemoral percutaneous cavography shows a leftsided inferior vena cava (L). Conclusion: left iliac phlebitis associated with a congenital anomaly of the inferior vena cava.

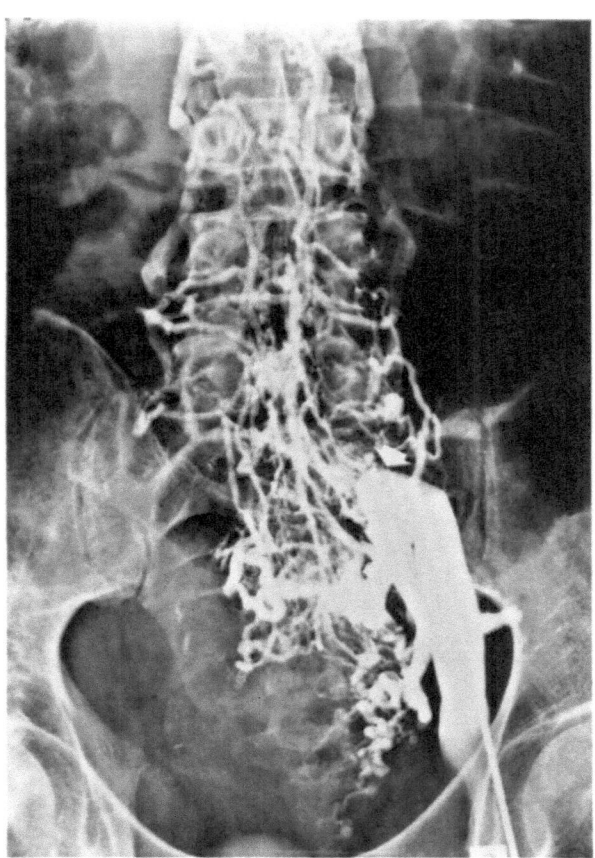

Fig. 159: Patient admitted to hospital for bilateral edema of the lower limbs. No pathologic history. Left unifemoral cavography. Failure of the catheterization on the right side. Complete obstruction ⬥ of the left common iliac axis and of the infrarenal segment of the inferior vena cava. Operation report: carcinoma of the right kidney with inferior vena caval thrombosis. In this case inferior vena caval thrombosis was the syndrome of a carcinoma of the kidney.

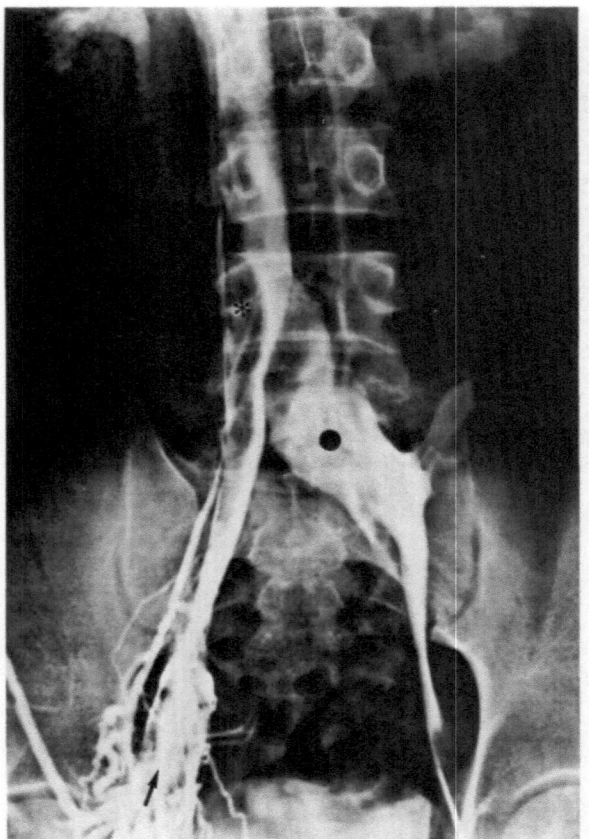 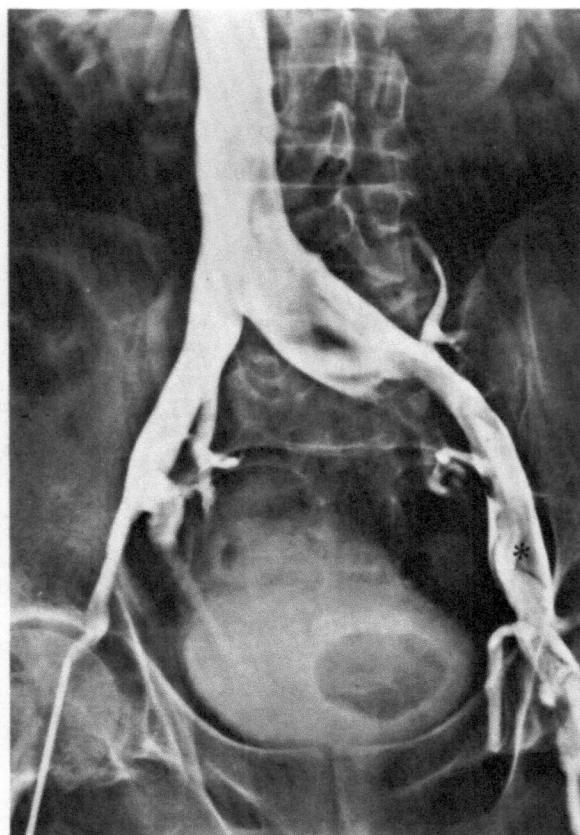

Fig. 160: Bifemoral percutaneous cavography. Puncture into a right femoral thrombus. Voluminous loose thrombus * above a grid-like appearance of the right external iliac vein. The thrombus extends as far as the infrarenal portion of the inferior vena cava. Note the associated Cockett's syndrome with flattening and pseudo-widening of the left common iliac vein ●.

Fig. 161: Cockett s syndrome associated with below iliac phlebitis * of the phlebothrombotic type.

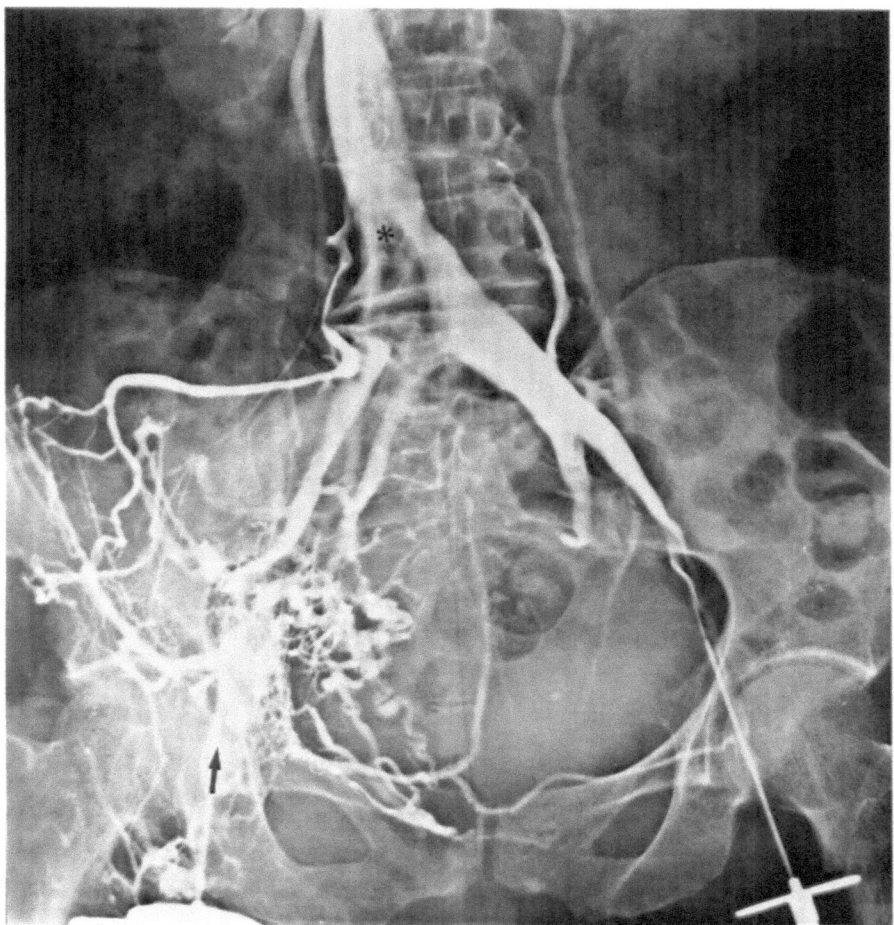

Fig. 162

Figs. 162 and 163: Bifemoral percutaneous cavography. Frontal projection (162). Left anterior oblique projection (163 — see p. 106). Left anterior oblique projection (163). Puncture into a femoral thrombus on the right ⇡. The collateral circulation and the left injection outline the head of the thrombus * which is situated in the infrarenal portion of the inferior vena cava at its origin.

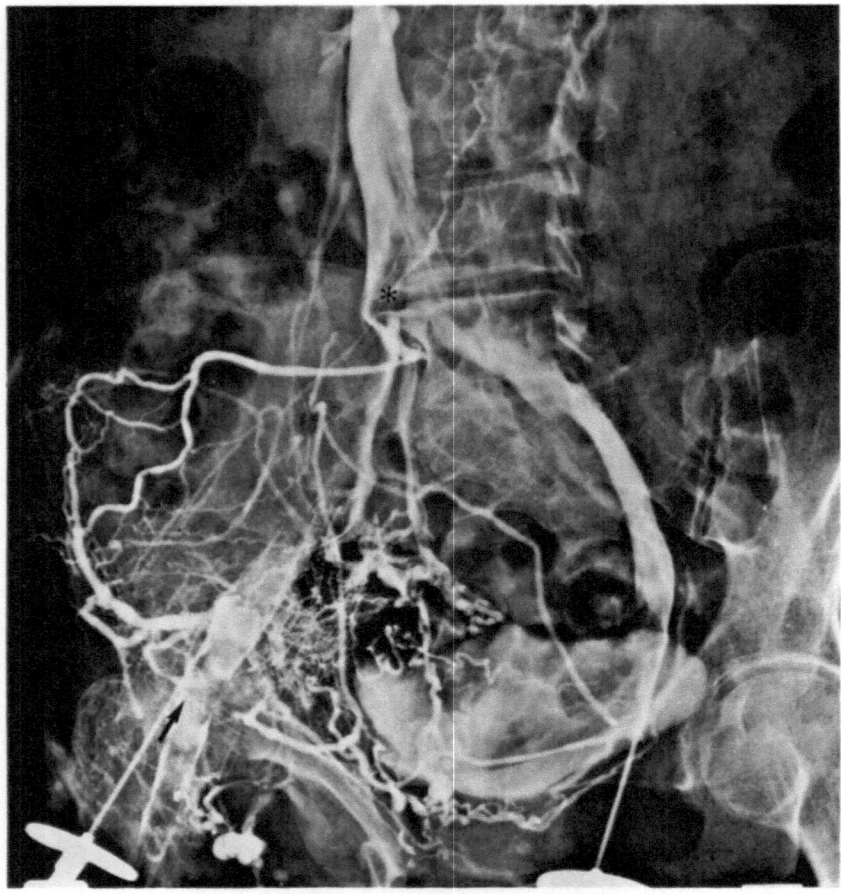

Fig. 163

Figs. 162 and 163: Bifemoral percutaneous cavography. Frontal projection (162 — see p. 105). Left anterior oblique projection (163). Left anterior oblique projection (163). Puncture into a femoral thrombus on the right ↑. The collateral circulation and the left injection outline the head of the thrombus * which is situated in the infrarenal portion of the inferior vena cava at its origin.

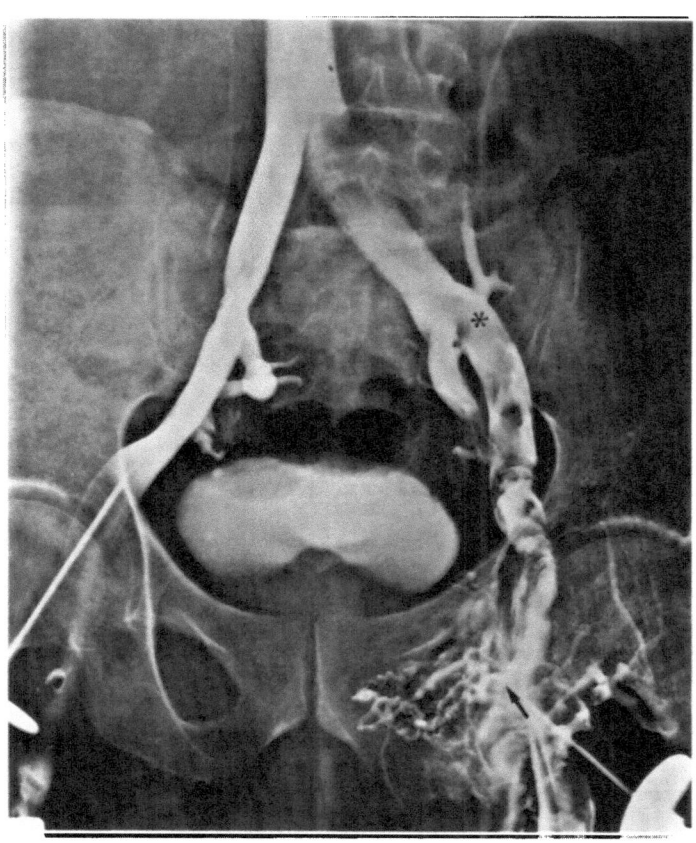

Fig. 164: Left iliofemoral phlebitis. Bifemoral percutaneous cavography. Puncture in the femoral thrombus on the left ↑. The injection delineates the head of the thrombus * which does not extend beyond the left external iliac vein.

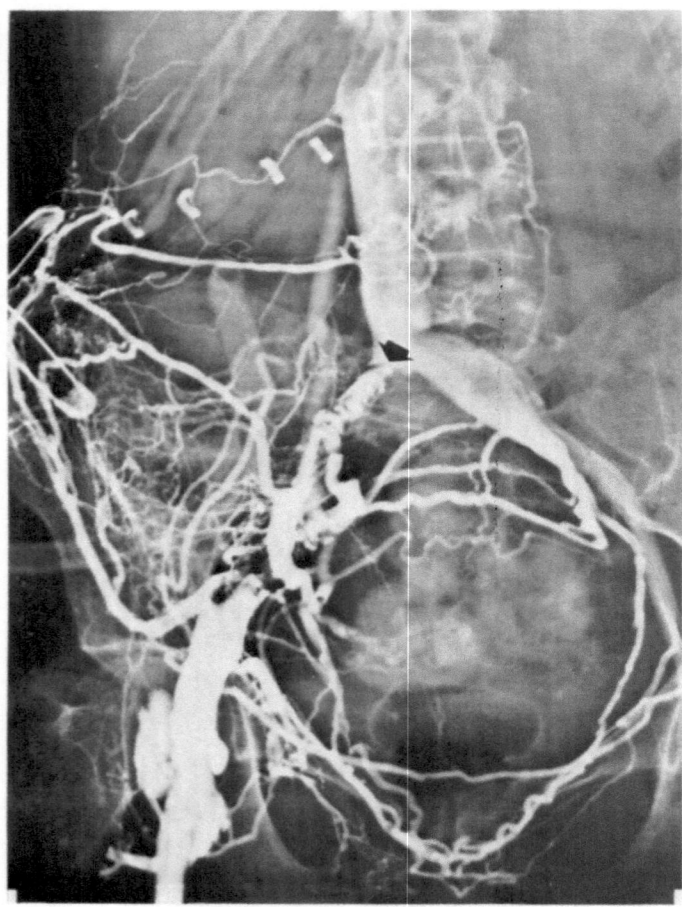

Fig. 165: Right iliac phlebitis. Right femoral catheterization with small extravasation of contrast medium. Opacification of numerous suprapubic and iliac collateral channels. The collateral circulation delineates the upper level of the obstruction, which does not extend beyond the termination of the right common iliac vein. The thrombus is thus not intracaval ◂. Post-operative iliac phlebitis.

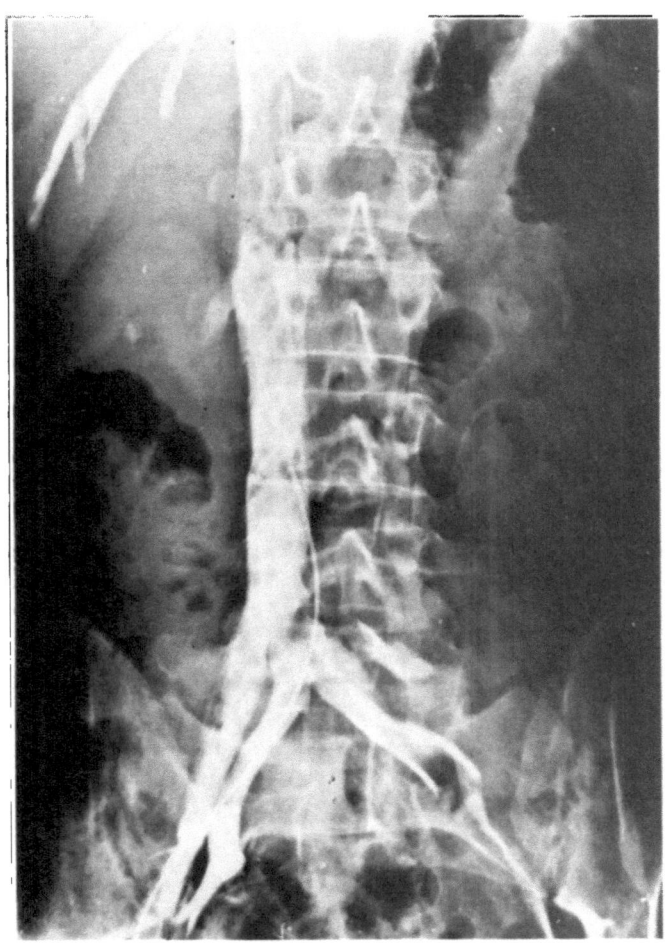

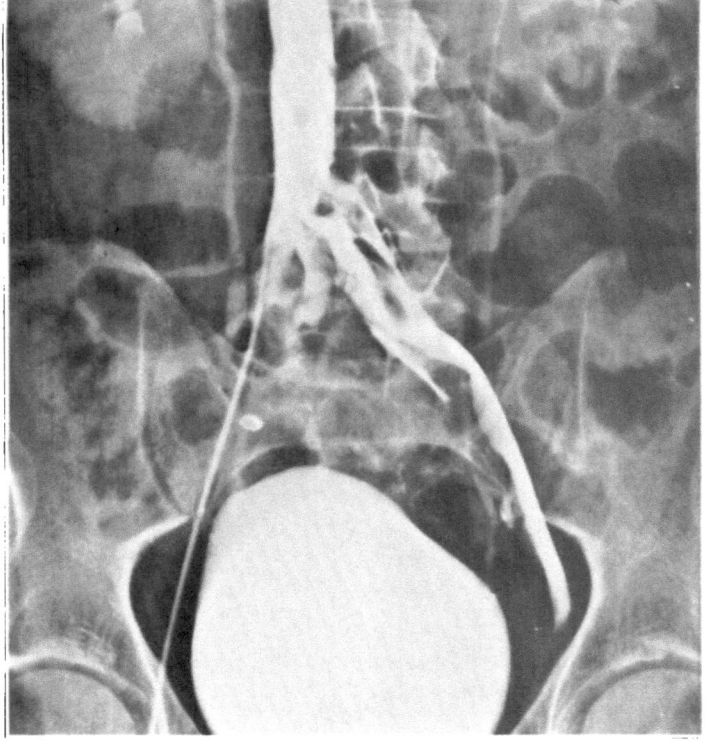

Figs. 166 and 167: Left iliac phlebitis. Cavography through right iliofemoral percutaneous catheterization.

166: Filling of the inferior vena cava showing duplication of the right iliac vein. Reflux into the left iliac vein, showing the absence of flow in this venous axis.

167: Retrograde left iliac venography. A preshaped catheter is positioned at the termination of the left common iliac vein. This projection shows the left iliac thrombosis to be very extensive.

Chapter 5

COLLATERAL CIRCULATION IN CASE OF OBLITERATION OF THE VEINS OF THE LOWER LIMBS AND THE ILIAC VEINS

Figures 168–203

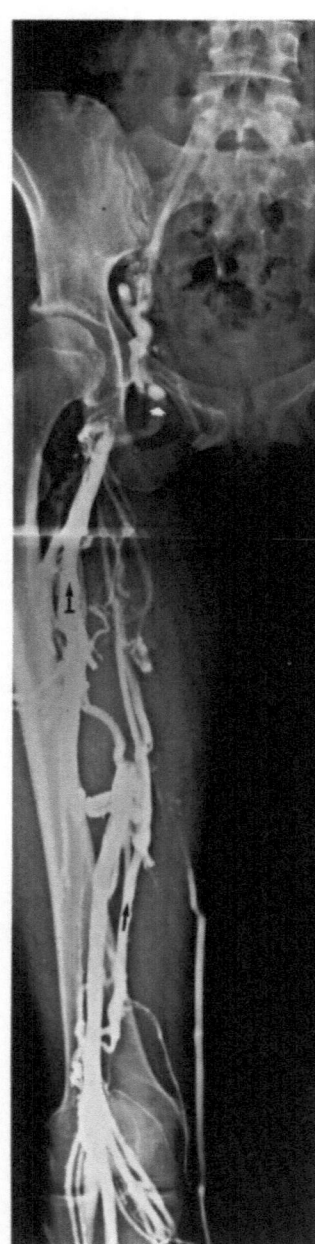

Fig. 168: Collateral circulation in a case of obstruction of the superficial and of the common femoral veins. The internal saphenous vein functions as collateral as far as the lower third of the thigh. It is then occluded. The collateral circulation is mainly via a retro-adductor ↑ vein which drains into the profunda femoris vein ↥, then via branches of the right hypogastric venous system, namely the obturator vein ◂, which reopacifies the right common iliac vein. Obstruction thus involves the external iliac vein, the common femoral vein and the upper part of the right superficial femoral vein.

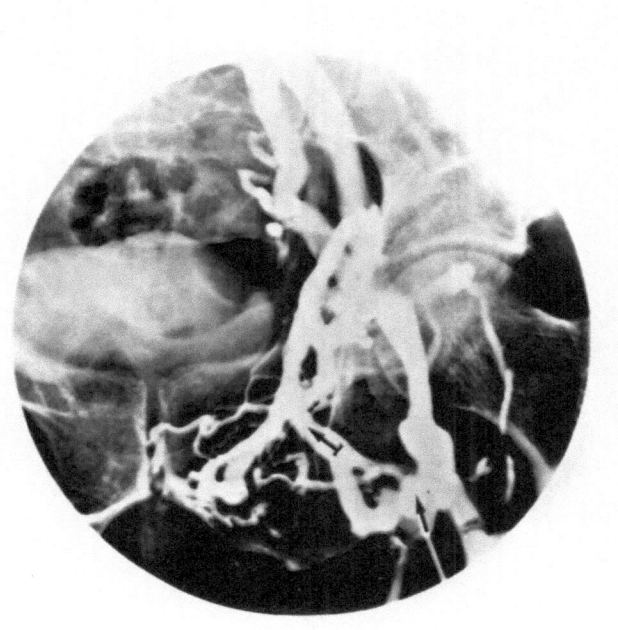

Fig. 169: Percutaneous catheterization of the termination of the internal saphenous vein ↑. Reflux into the profunda femoris vein, with opacification of obturator ↓ branches with reopacification of the left internal iliac vein. The left common femoral vein is partly opacified; it is very stenosed. Post-traumatic phlebitis (following surgery).

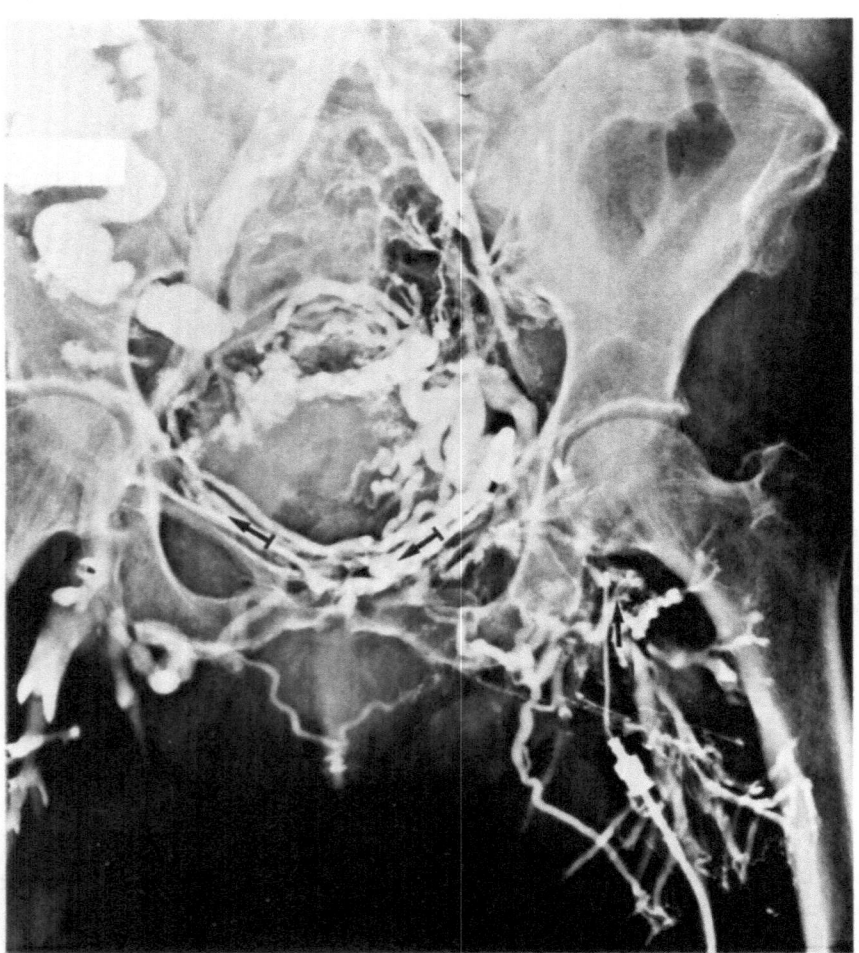

Fig. 170: Left iliac phlebitis. Puncture into the thrombus on the left ↡. Reflux in the branches of the left profunda femoris vein. Supra and retropubic collateral circulation ↡ opacifying the right iliac axis. Dilatation of presacral plexuses which also function as left to right collateral circulation.

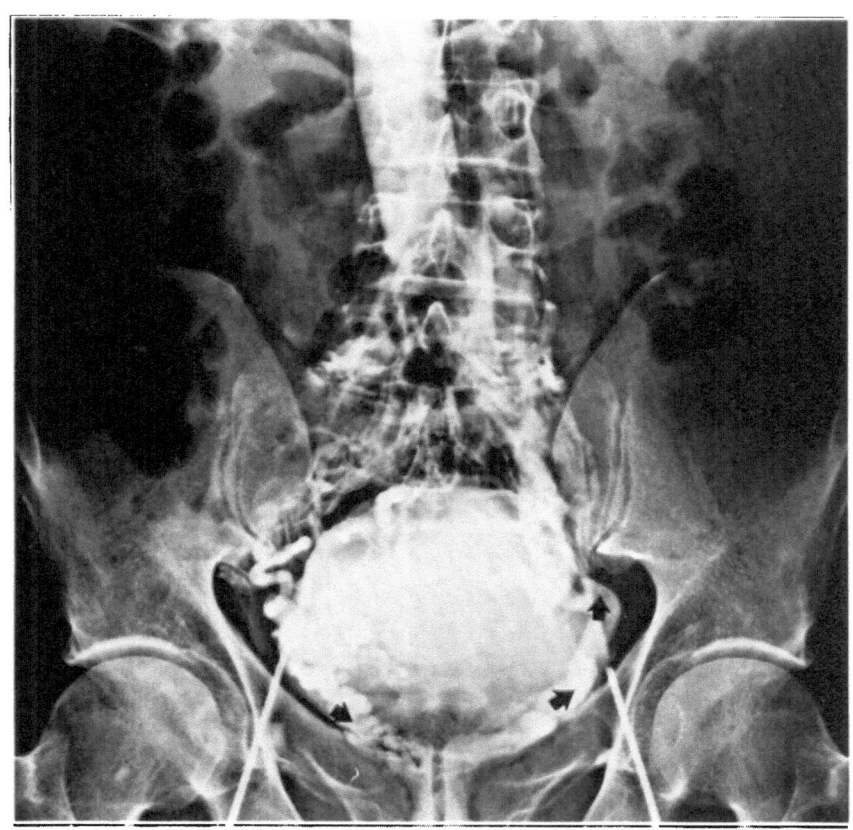

Fig. 171: Right iliac chronis phlebitis. Very marked right to left ♠ suprapubic collateral circulation.

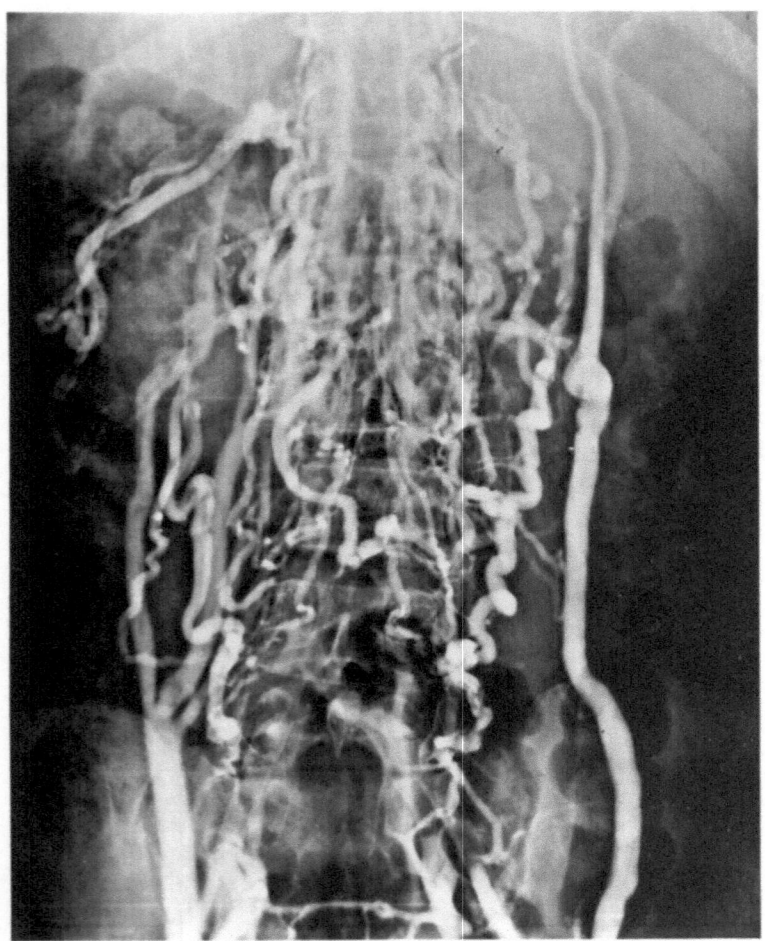

Fig. 172: Very old ilio-inferior caval obstruction with large abdomino-thoracic superficial collateral channels. The anterolateral veins of the abdomen drain toward the axillary veins.

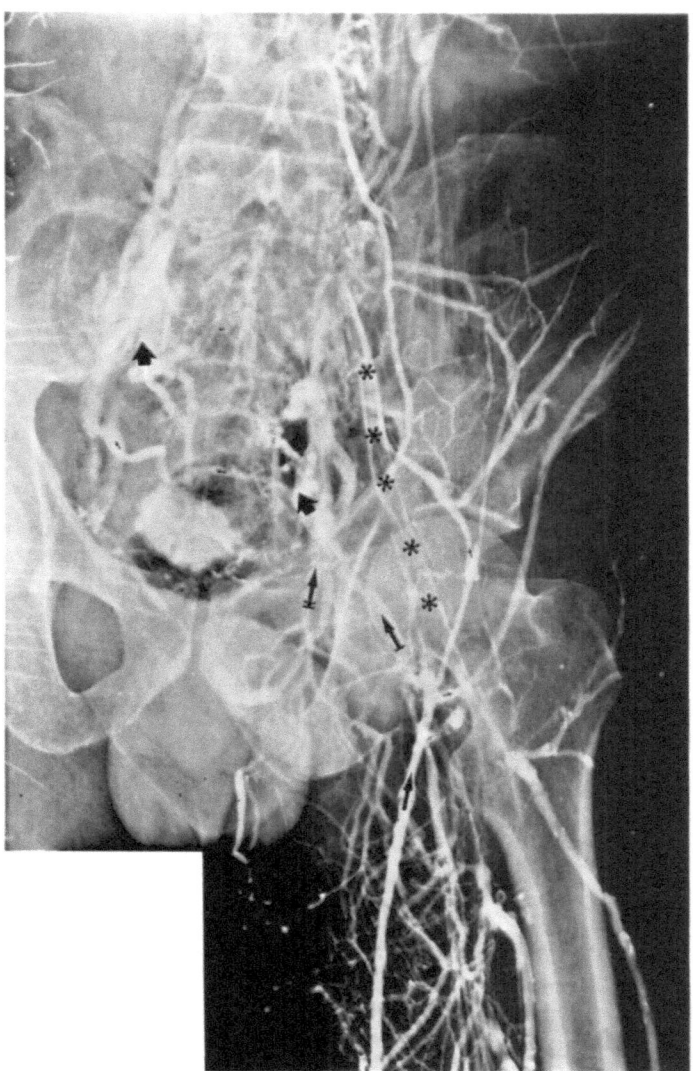

Fig. 173: Diffuse phlebitis of all deep veins of the right lower limb associated with iliac phlebitis. The left iliofemoral system is outlined by the contrast medium **. The collateral circulation is via the internal saphenous vein on the one hand, and on the other hand, the inferior gluteal ↑ and obturator veins ↑ first into the left ♦ and second into the right hypogastric ♦ system. The left common iliac vein is occluded and there is left–right derivation via the presacral plexuses. The importance of the superficial abdominal collateral circulation suggests that there is an associated inferior vena caval thrombosis.

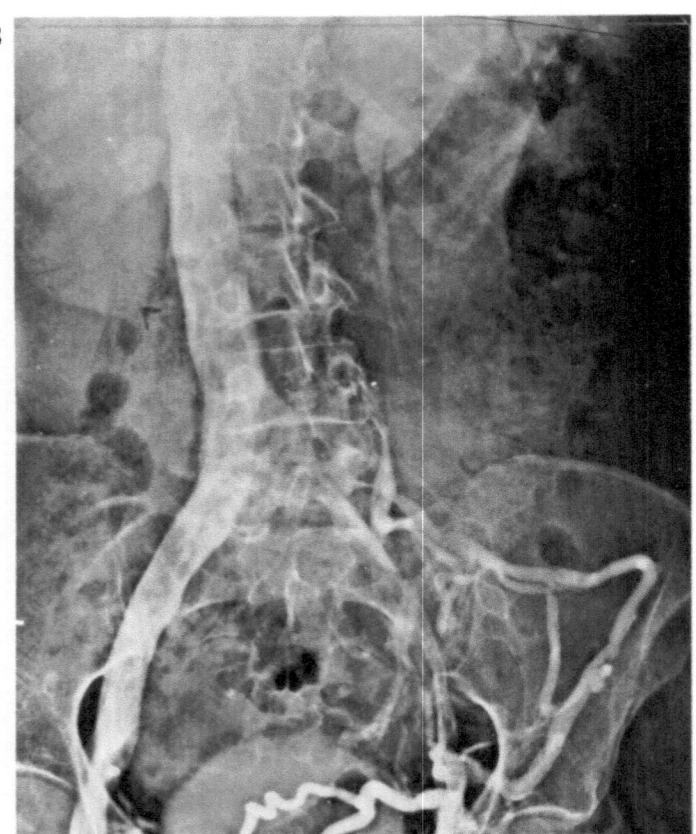

Fig. 174

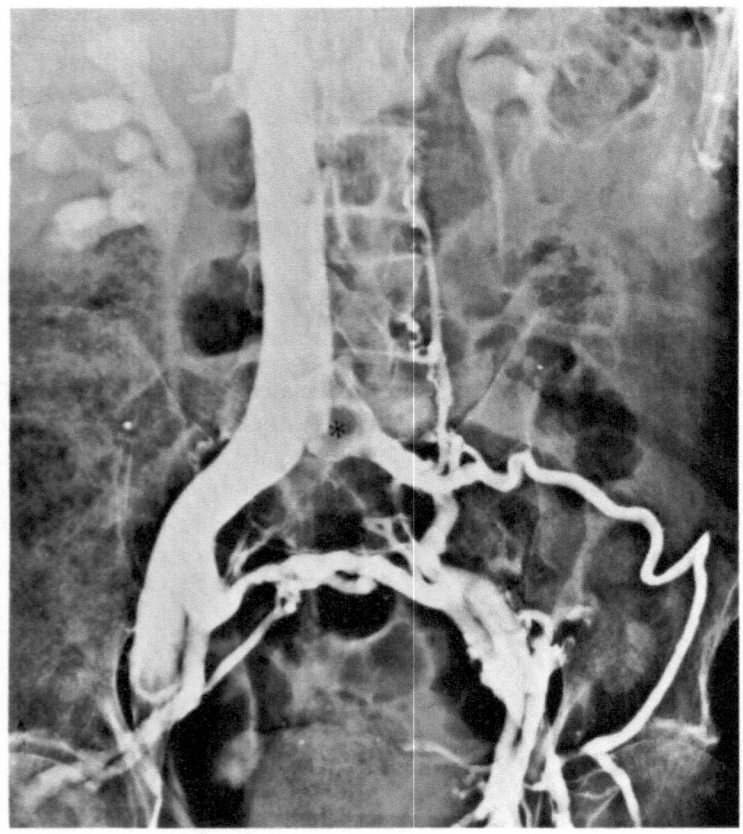

Fig. 175

Figs. 174 and 175: Same patient, presenting with left iliac phlebitis. Figure 174 corresponds to the centering onto the pelvis of a phlebogram of the left lower limb, carried out with free circulation. Figure 175 shows a bifemoral percutaneous cavography with punture into the saphenous on the left side. Note the quality of the contrast in Fig. 175, which affirms the patency of the inferior vena cava. Cockett's syndrome * with underlying thrombosis.

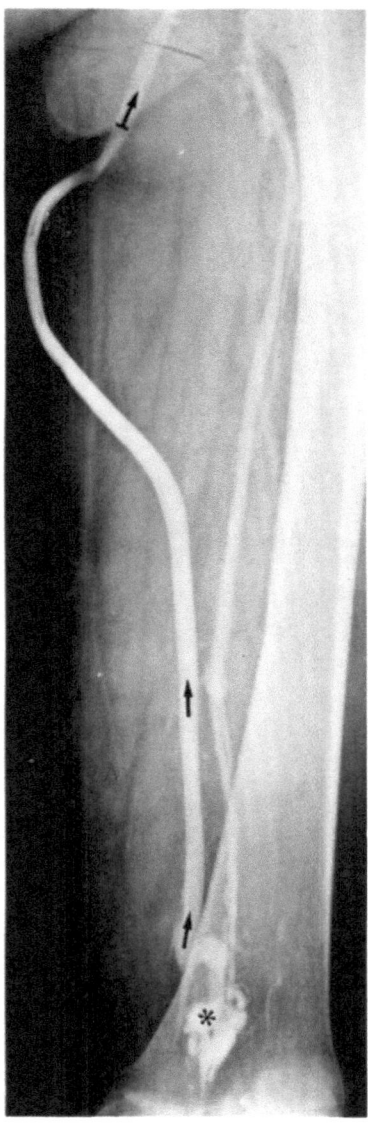

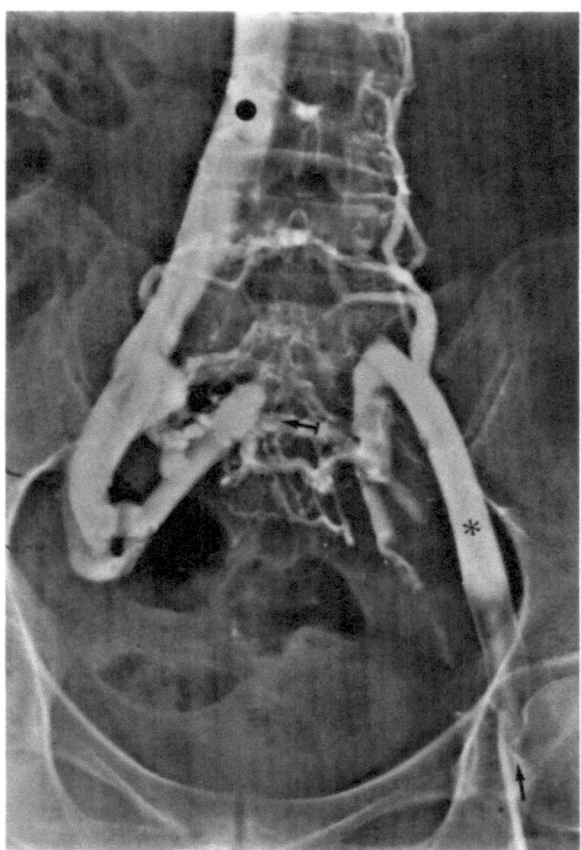

Fig. 177: Short obliteration of the left common iliac vein with a patent left external iliac vein *. Left unifemoral cavography ↿. Very strong presacral ↕ collateral circulation which reopacifies the free inferior vena cava ●.

Fig. 176: Superficial collateral circulation ↕ between the two saphenous veins. This is a case of a superficial anastomosis branching from the termination of the external saphenous vein* at the level of the popliteal space, winding along the posterior and medial aspect of the thigh and joining the internal saphenous vein ↕ above. In France, it is called the vein of Giacomini.

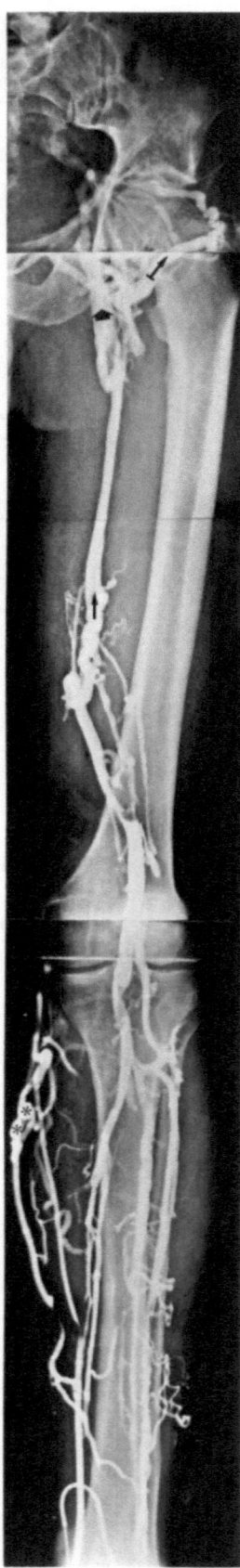

Fig. 178: Collateral circulation in a case of occlusion of the superficial femoral vein and of the left iliofemoral axis. The popliteal vein is patent at the level of Hunter's canal; collateral circulation is through the retro-adductor vein ⬆ and then through the profunda femoris vein ◄. The common femoral vein and the left external iliac veins are obstructed as witnessed by the collateral circulation around the neck of femur ⬆ and through the left obturator and inferior gluteal veins. Note also the varices on the leg, proof of ancient phlebitic occlusion of the deep leg veins, which are also valveless * *.

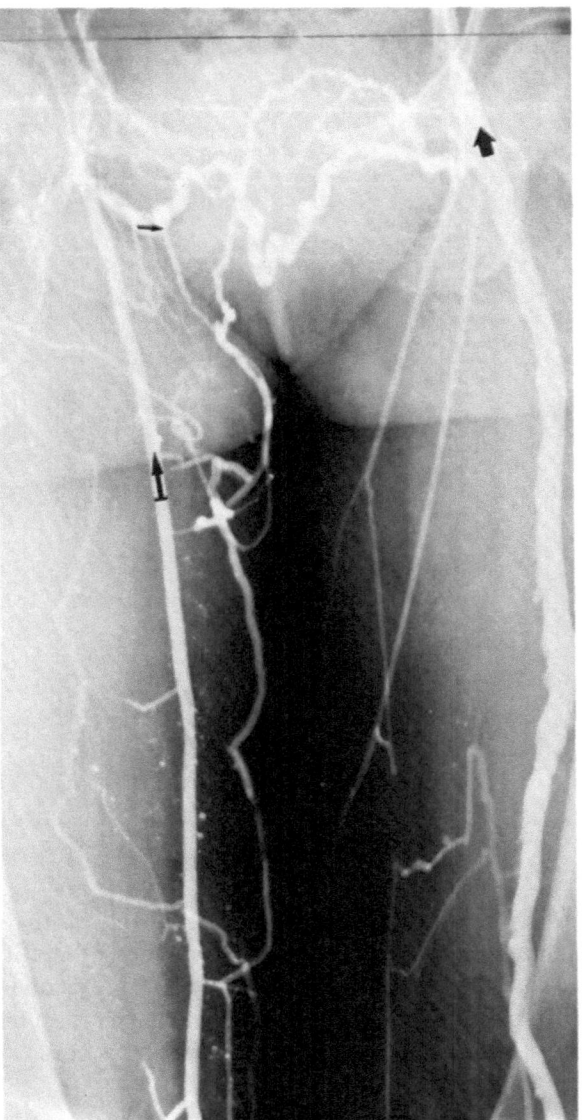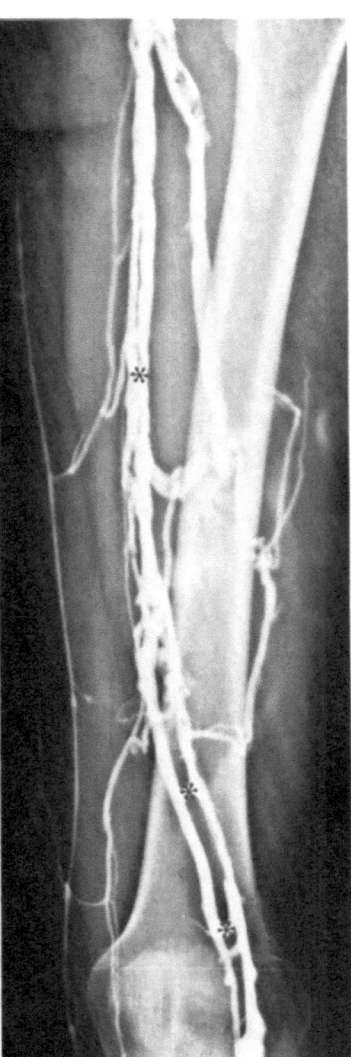

Fig. 179: Venography of both lower limbs. Normal appearance of the left ♠ superficial femoral vein. On the right side complete occlusion of the deep venous pathway. Only the internal saphenous vein ↑ ensures the collateral circulation. Right-to-left ↑ suprapubic derivation, proof of right iliac phlebitis. It is a case of a physiological equivalent of a Palma intervention.

Fig. 180: Collateral circulation of the femoro-popliteal system, corresponding to venae comitantes, anastomosed in a ladder-like manner * all along the superficial femoral arteriovenous pedicle. These veins may reach quite a large caliber; they are one of the collateral routes of the venous flow in the lower limb.

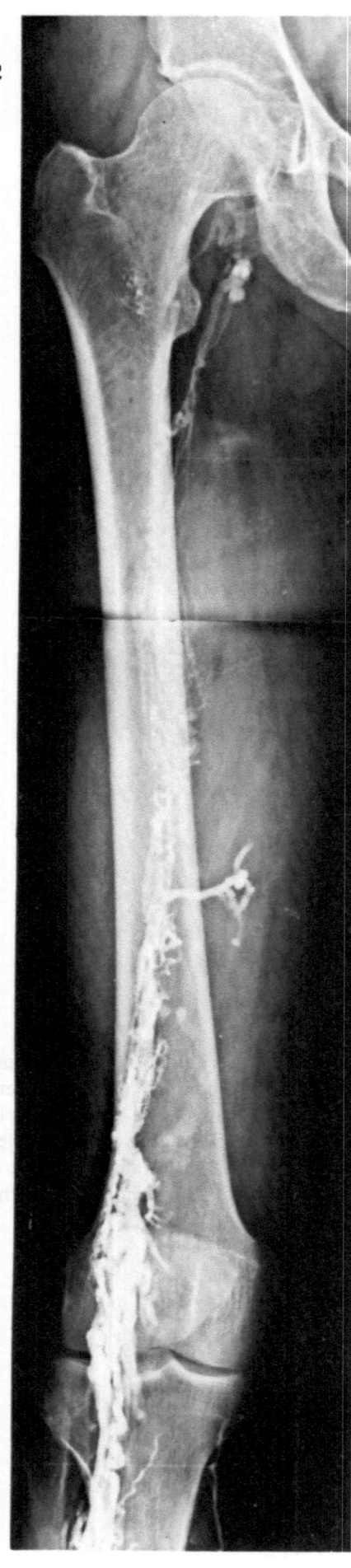

Fig. 181: Very uncommon collateral pathway, with very low circulation rate, at the evel of the right lower limb; it corresponds to small veins arround the sciatic nerve and on the posterior aspect of the thigh. The usual collateral routes are all occluded in this patient who has acute venous stasis.

123

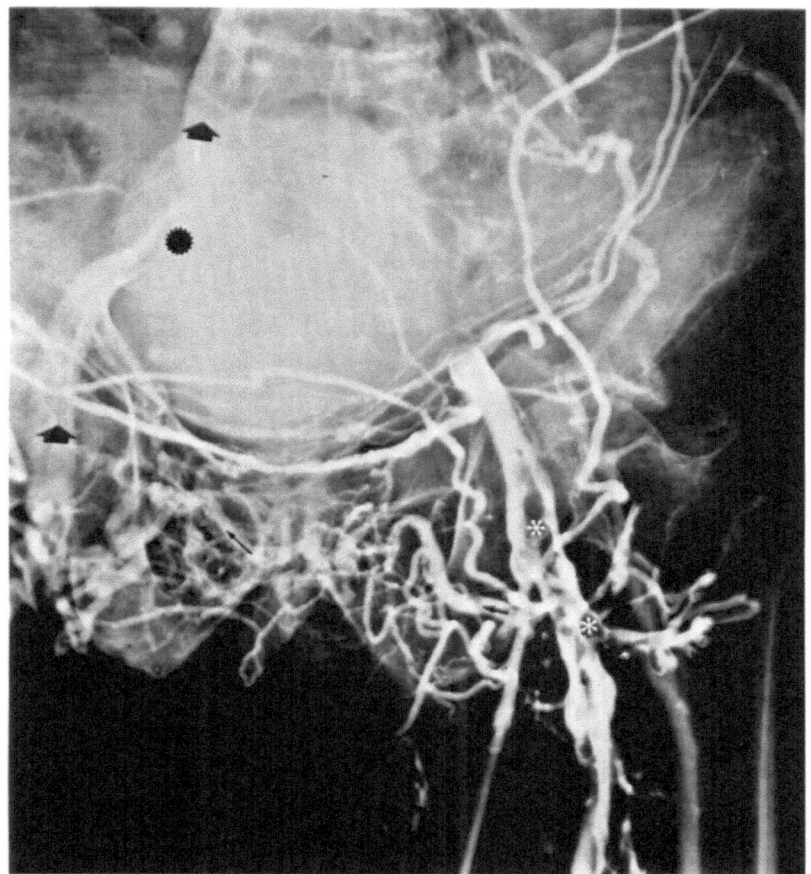

Fig. 182: Free low injection phlebography of the left lower limb. Large amount of contrast medium. Centering on the pelvis. Huge thrombus in the common femoral vein *. Collateral circulation through retropubic veins reopacifying the right iliac axis ▲ which is, however, stenosed in the lesser pelvis ●. Phlebitis by extrinsic compression due to pelvic adenopathies.

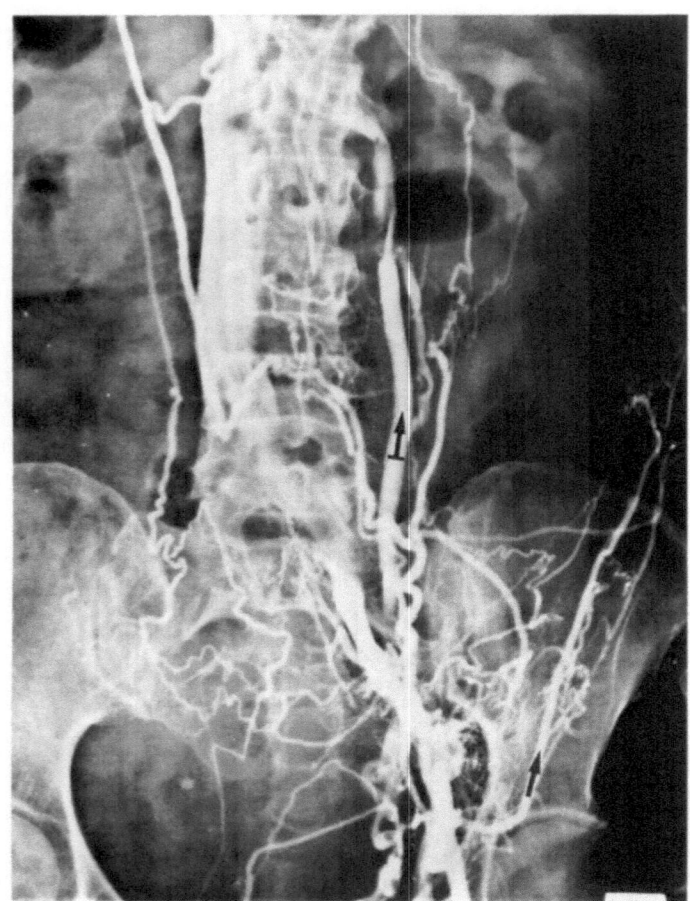

Fig. 183: Left iliac phlebitis. Left femoral injection into the thrombus. Opacification of superficial abdominal collateral circulation ↑. Opacification of some veins of the left hypogastric system, which opacifies a left ovarian vein ↑ emptying into the left renal vein.

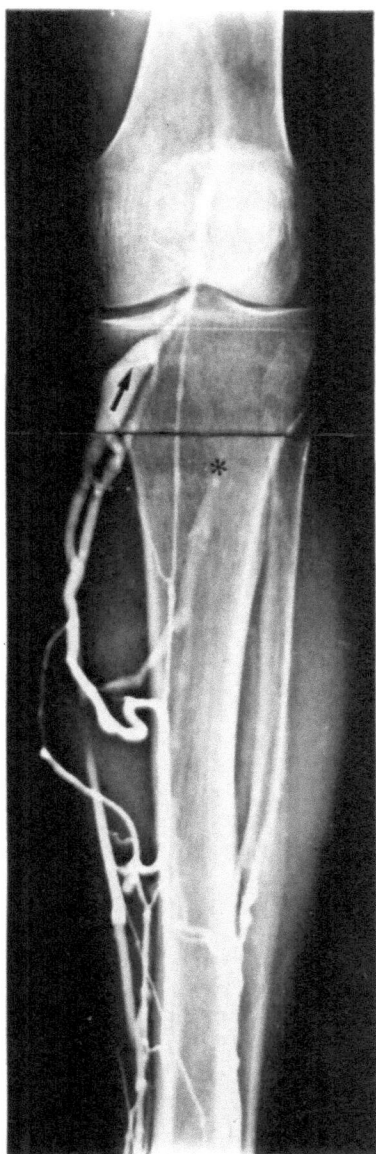

Fig. 184

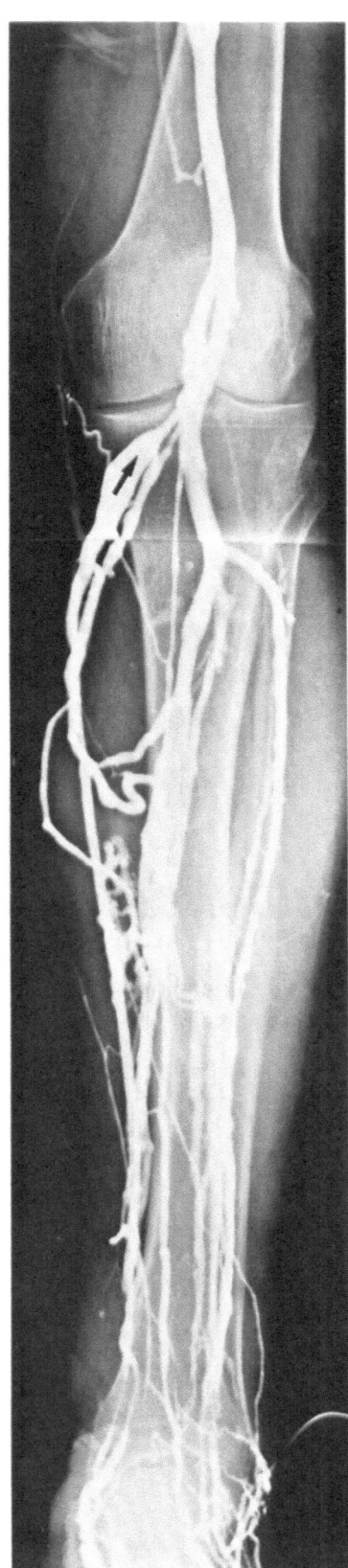

Figs. 184 and 185: A rather common collateral route at the level of the leg: the internal gastrocnemial vein ↑. This opacifies first (Fig. 184) showing a certain degree of compression of the tibio-peroneal trunk ∗ . These veins have competent valves; there is no reflux. When there are no valves, one can observe varices of the leg branched onto these internal gastrocnemial veins.

Fig. 185

126

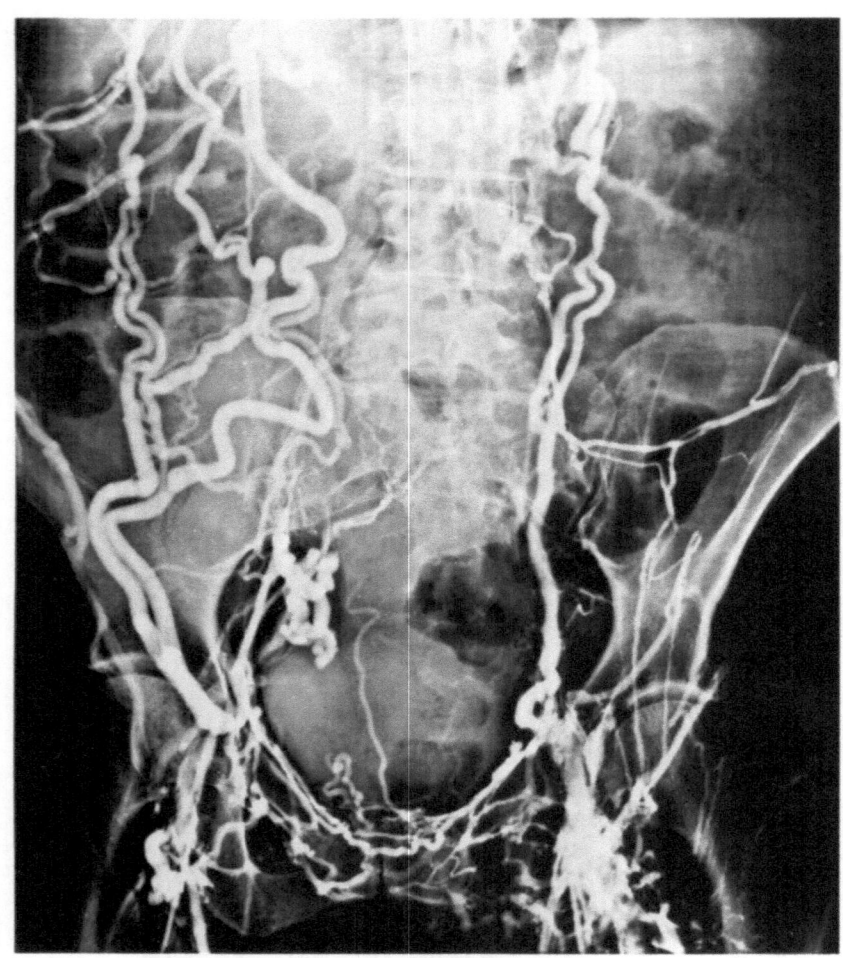

Fig. 186: Very old ilio-inferior caval obstruction, with very marked superficial, mainly thoraco-abdominal collateral circulation.

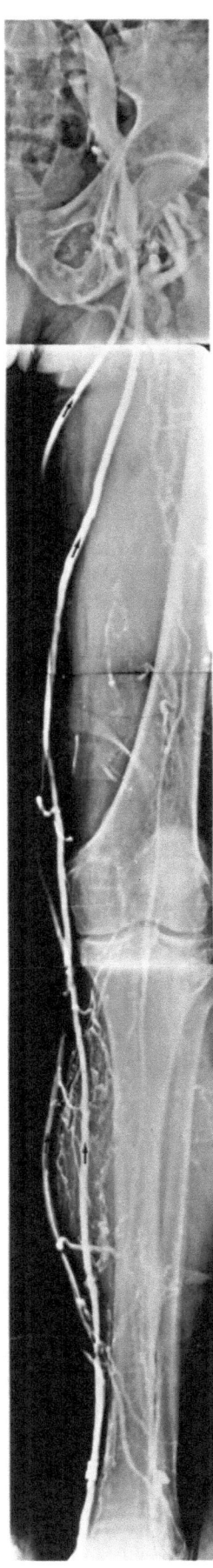

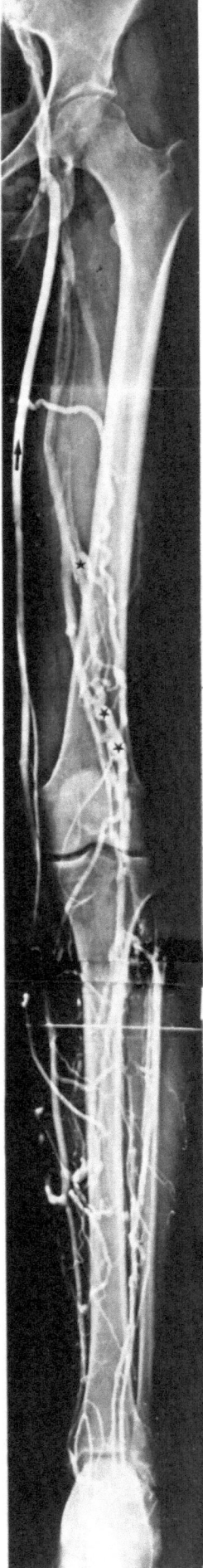

Fig. 187: Extended phlebitis of all veins of the left lower limb. The only collateral route is represented by the internal saphenous system which corresponds to several veins ↑, as is most often the case. Complete obliteration of all deep veins, including the profunda femoris vein.

Fig. 188: Extended obstruction of all deep veins of the left lower limb ⋆. Collateral circulation is mainly through the internal saphenous and some venae comitantes, anastomosed like a ladder on the course of the superficial femoral pedicle.

128

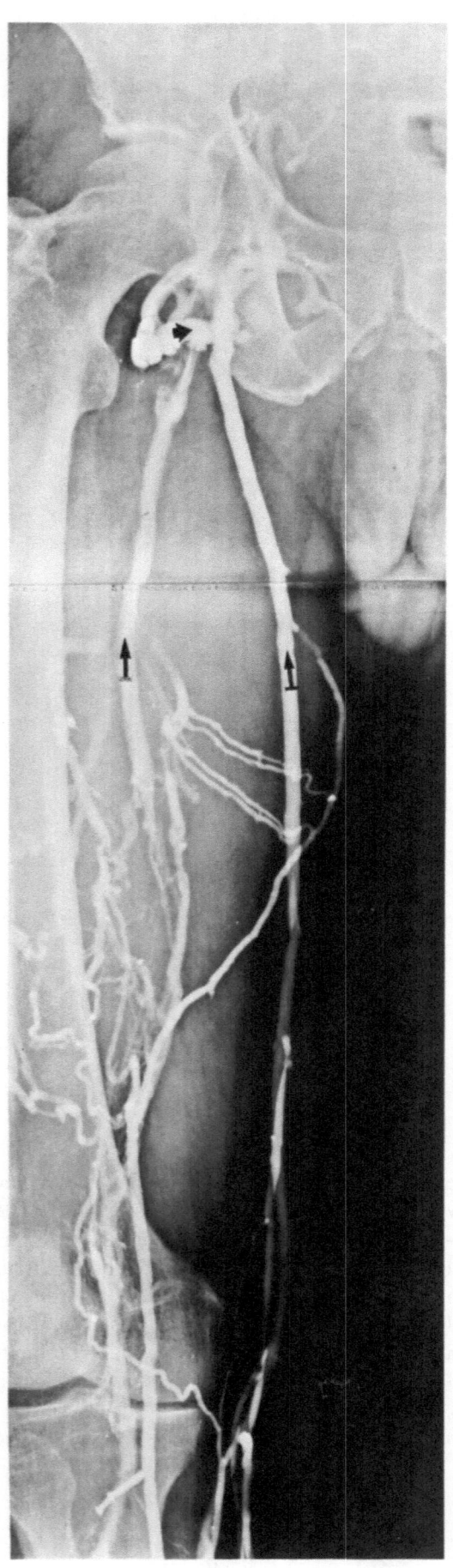

Fig. 189: Femoropopliteal obstruction. Collateral circulation via the profunda femoris vein ↑ and the internal saphenous vein ↥. Associated right external iliac obstruction, as demonstrated by the collateral circulation branched onto the anastomoses ♠ of the profunda femoris vein and of the right hypogastric system through the inferior gluteal and the right obturator vein.

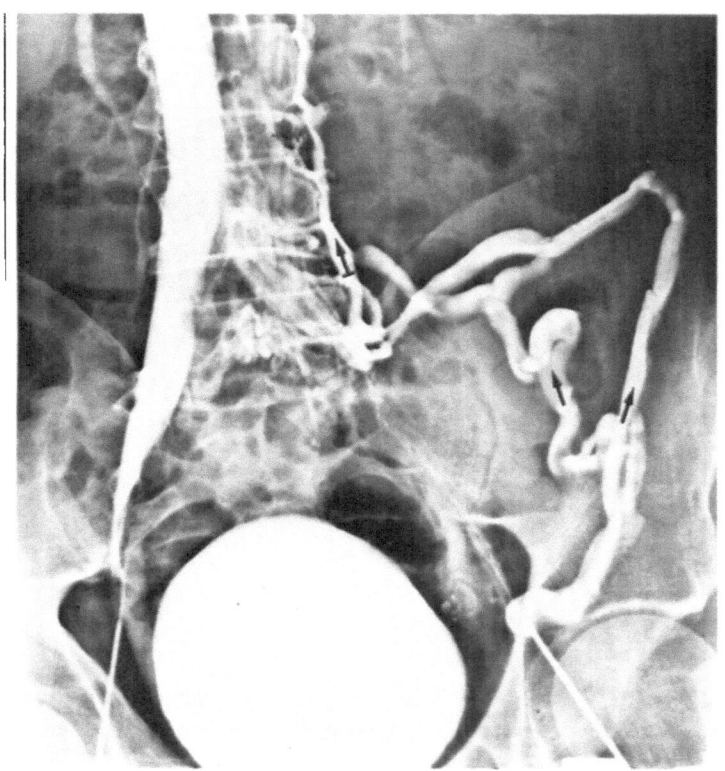

Fig. 190: Left iliac phlebitis. collateral circulation through the deep iliac ↑ circumflex veins, reanastomosing the lumbar ascending vein ↑ and allowing opacification of the left common iliac vein which shows multiple synechias. Cockett's syndrome with underlying iliac phlebitis.

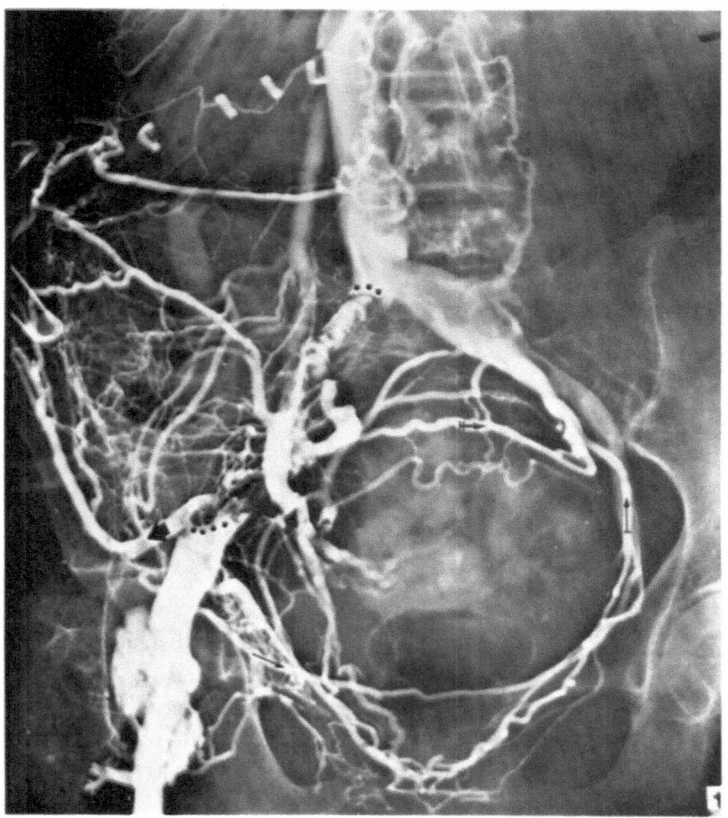

Fig. 191: Right iliac phlebitis. Collateral circulation via the deep iliac circumflex vein ♠ and the retrosymphysial veins ↑. Partial opacification of the left hypogastric system ↓. Right–left drainage through the presacral plexuses ↓. Note the head of the thrombus which does not touch the inferior vena cava ● ● ●.

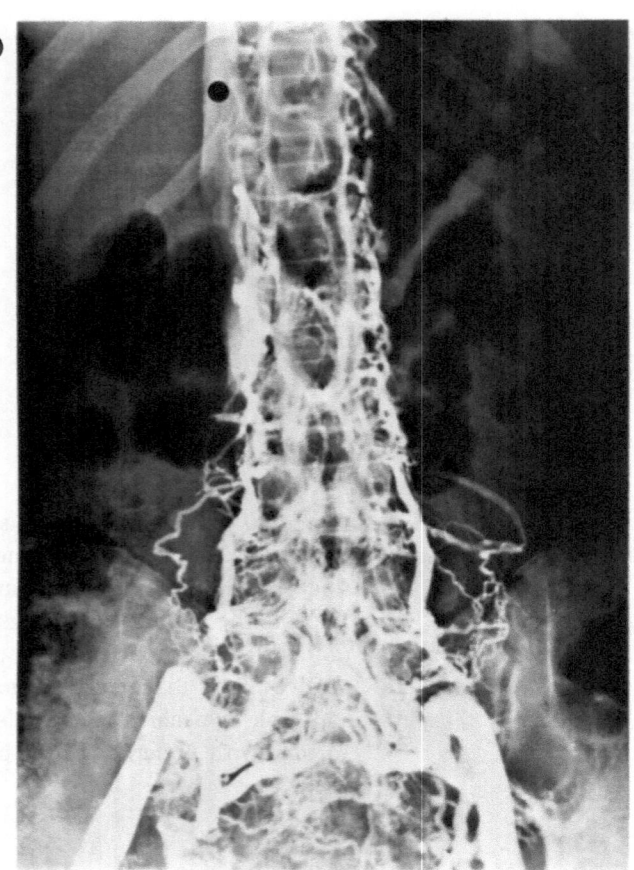

Fig. 192: Inferior vena caval obstruction. Collateral circulation is mainly via the intra and extraspinal plexuses which reopacify the retrohepatic portion of the inferior vena cava which is free ●. Plication of the inferior vena cava.

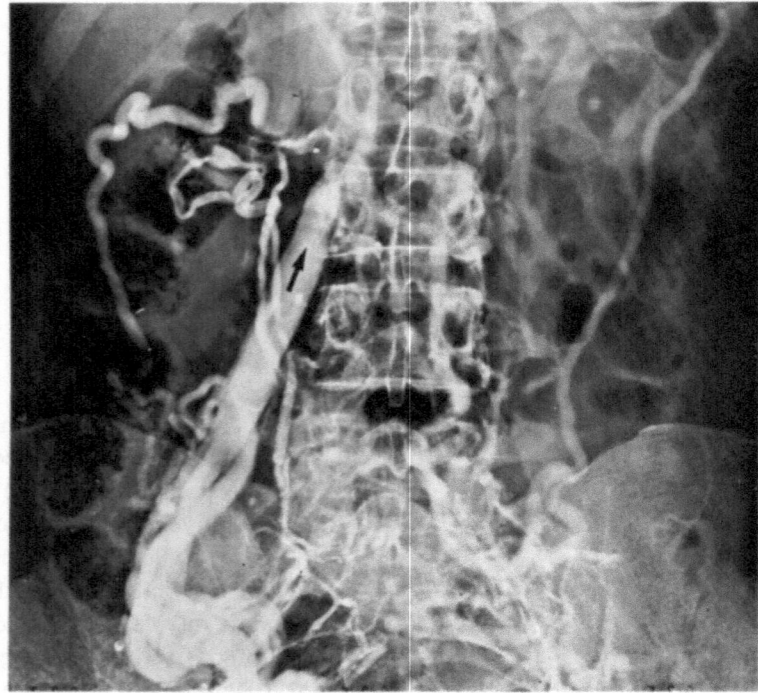

Fig. 193: Obstruction of the infrarenal segment of the inferior vena cava. Collateral circulation through a large right ovarian vein ↑ which joins the cava just below the right renal vein.

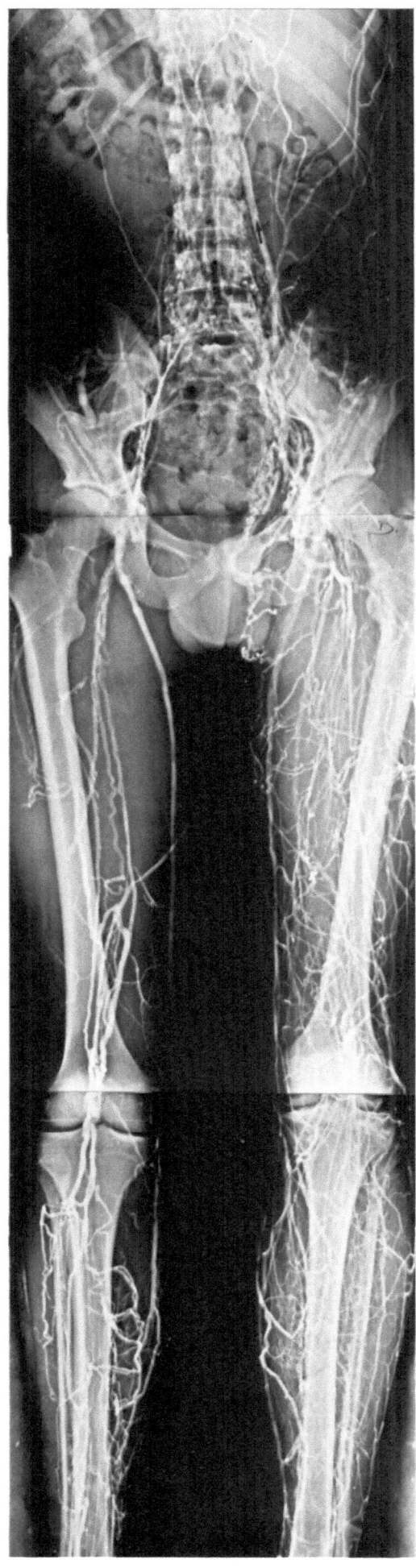

Fig. 194: Venography of both lower limbs. Complete obstruction of the entire deep venous system of both lower limbs, of both iliac axes, and of the infrarenal segment of the inferior vena cava. Note the filling of a left spermatic vein ↑ in this 20-year-old male who had Behçet's disease.

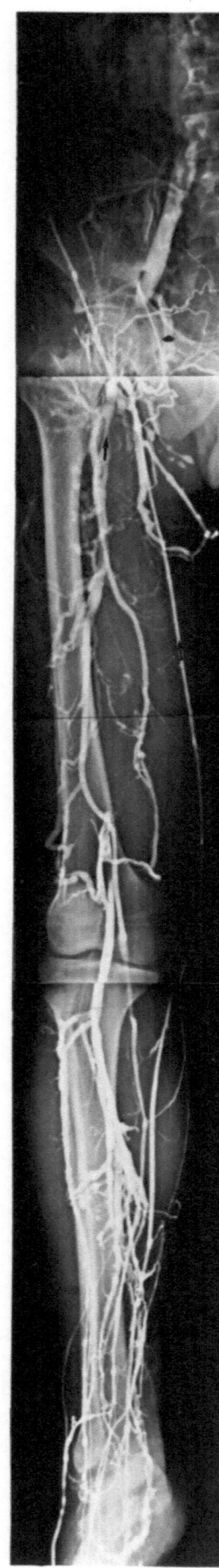

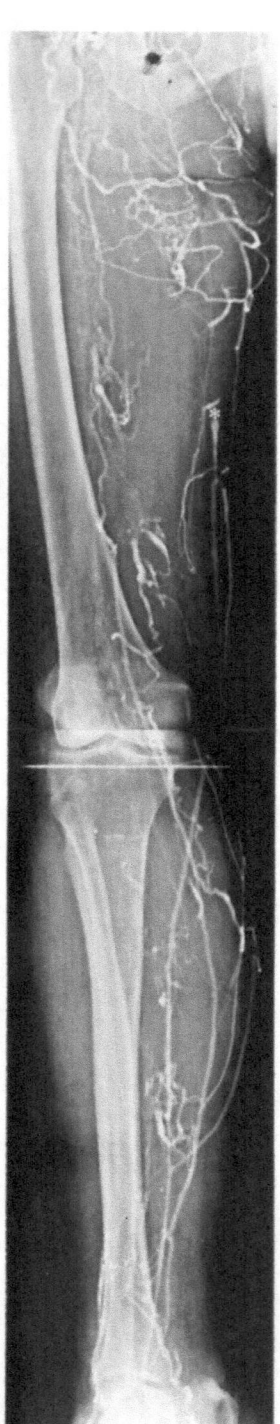

Fig. 195: Femoropopliteal obstruction involving the common femoral vein. The collateral circulation is via the profunda femoris vein ↑, the internal saphenous ↕, which is slender, and the anastomoses between the branches of the profunda and the left hypogastric system, namely the obturator vein ↩.

Fig. 196: Complete obstruction of the entire deep venous system of the right lower limb. The collateral circulation is partly superficial, partly internal saphenous, in so far as the internal saphenous is obstructed in its upper part. Patient with acute venous stasis.

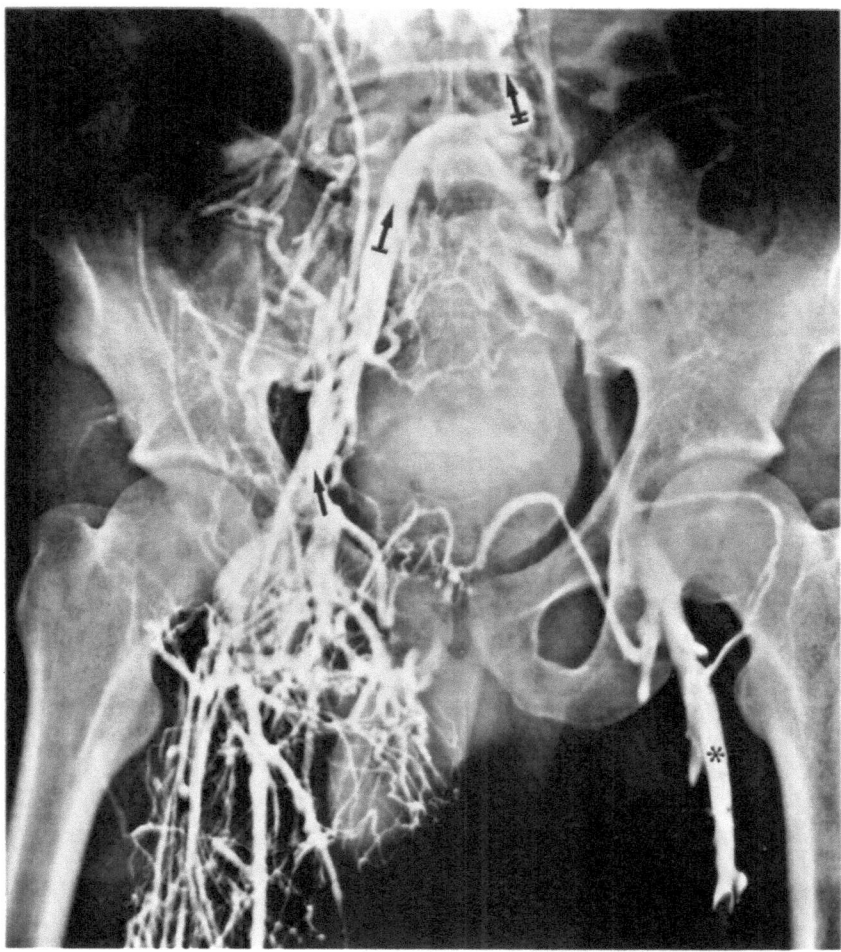

Fig. 197: Right iliac phlebitis. Venogram of the right lower limb with free flow injection; centering onto the lesser pelvis. Complete obstruction of the deep venous system of the right leg. The profunda femoris vein is obstructed; only the superficial veins and the internal saphenous vein function as collateral circulation. Reopacification of the right hypogastric system ↑, and then of the right common iliac vein ↕. Reflux into the left superficial femoral vein ∗, due to right–left suprapubic anastomoses. Note also the occlusion of the inferior vena cava. The opacified structure which continues the right common iliac vein is not the inferior vena cava but a vein of the azygos system ↨ which fills via the extraspinal plexuses.

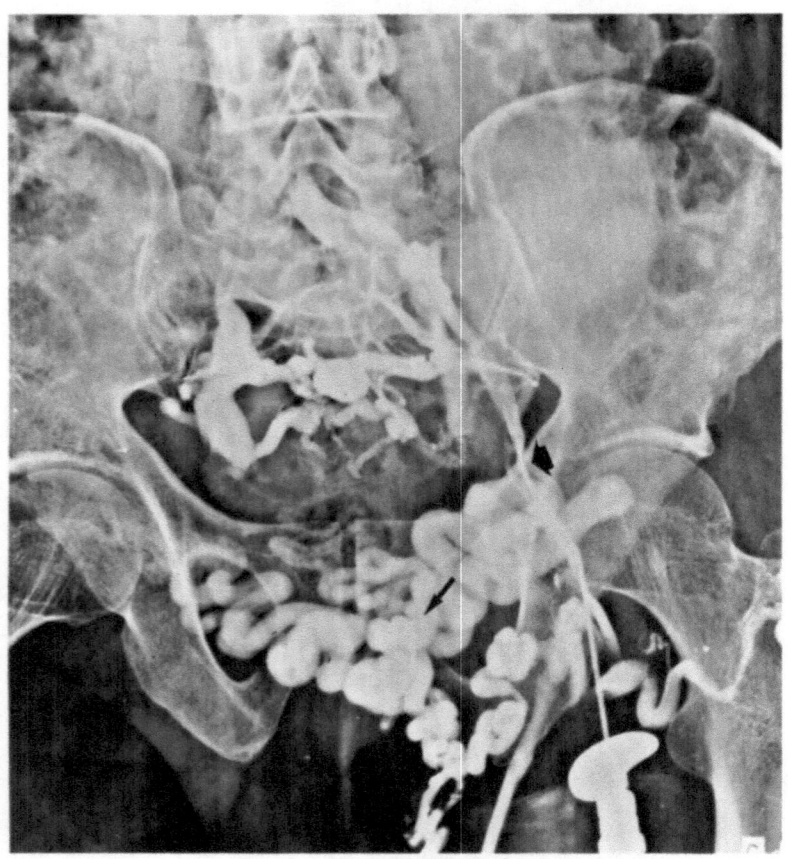

Fig. 198: Stenosis of the left external iliac vein ◄. Voluminous vulvar ↑ and suprapubic varices.

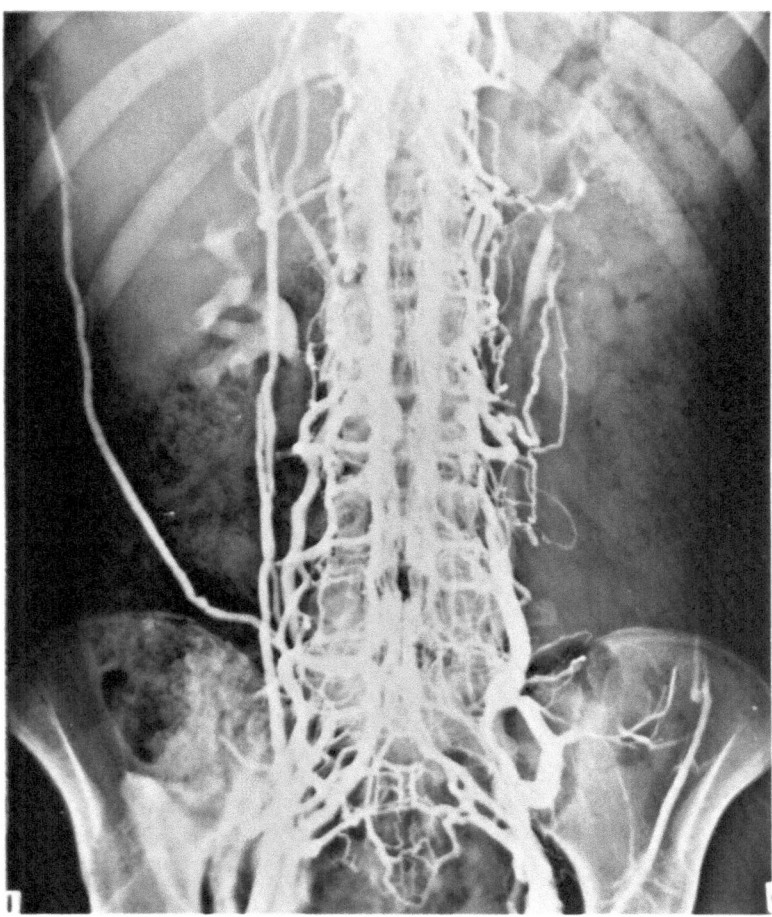

Fig. 199: Very old ilio-inferior caval obstruction with superficial collateral circulation but mainly via the intra and extraspinal plexuses. The retrohepatic segment of the inferior vena cava is obstructed and there is an associated Budd-Chiari syndrome.

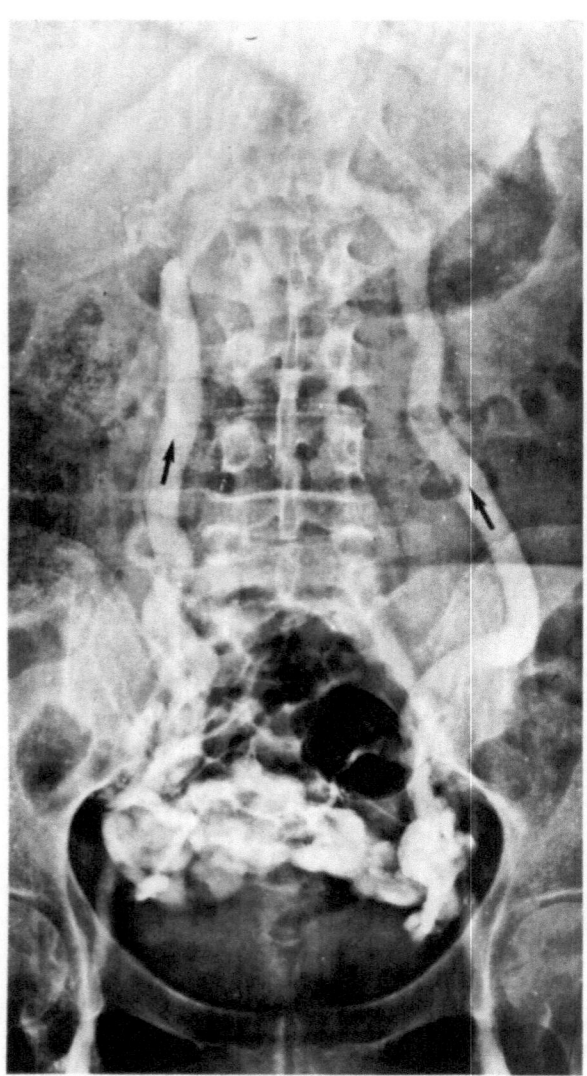

Fig. 200

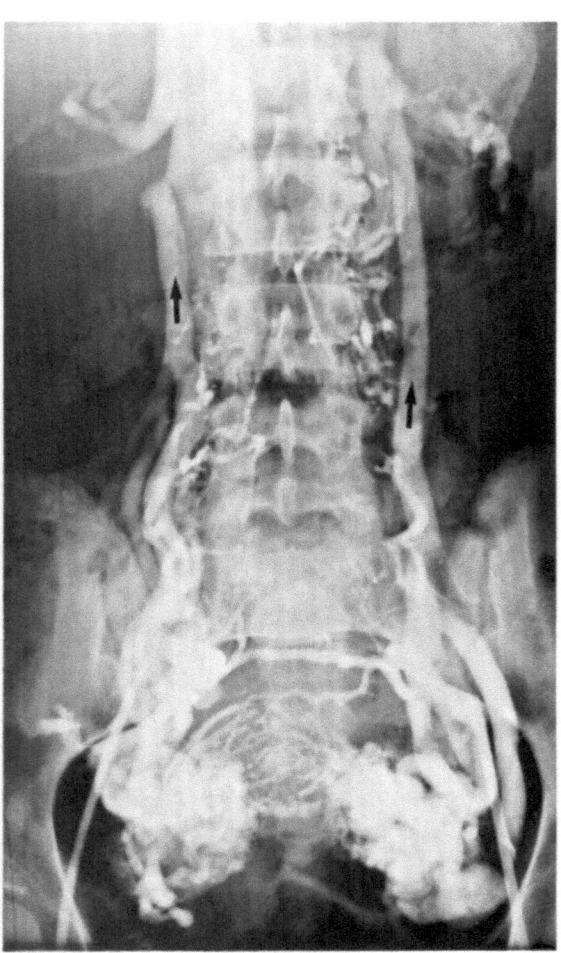

Fig. 201

Figs. 200 and 201: Two ovarian veins ↑ of very large caliber which function as collaterals in a case of occlusion of the infrarenal inferior vena cava. Figure 200 depicts a venogram of the inferior limb and Fig. 201 a bifemoral percutaneous cavogram.

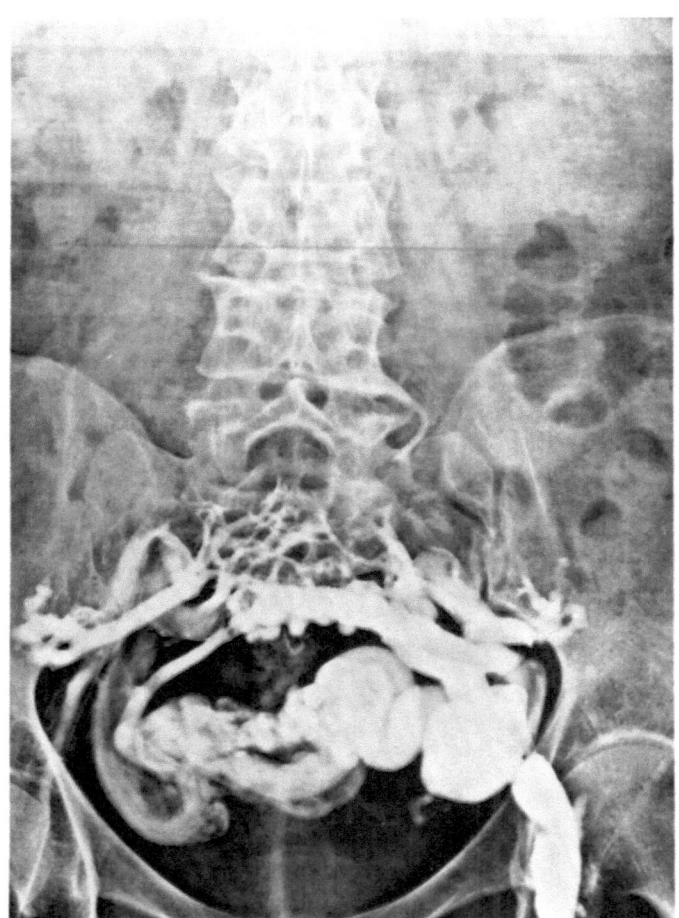 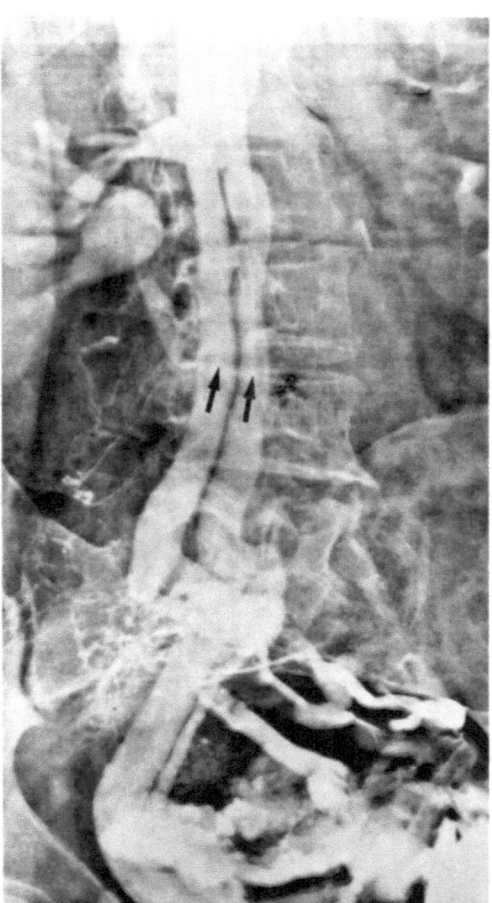

Fig. 202   *Fig. 203*

Figs. 202 and 203: The infrarenal segment of the inferior vena cava is occluded. Left unilateral catheterization with small extravasation of the contrast medium. Frontal projection (Fig. 202: opacification of voluminous pelvic varices in a female patient.) Figure 203 depicts an oblique projection demonstrating the collateral drainage through a duplicated ↑↑ right ovarian vein. No filling of the left ovarian vein, since there is a thrombosis of the left renal vein (verified at autopsy).

Chapter 6

SURGERY IN ILIOFEMORAL PHLEBITES

Figures 204–224

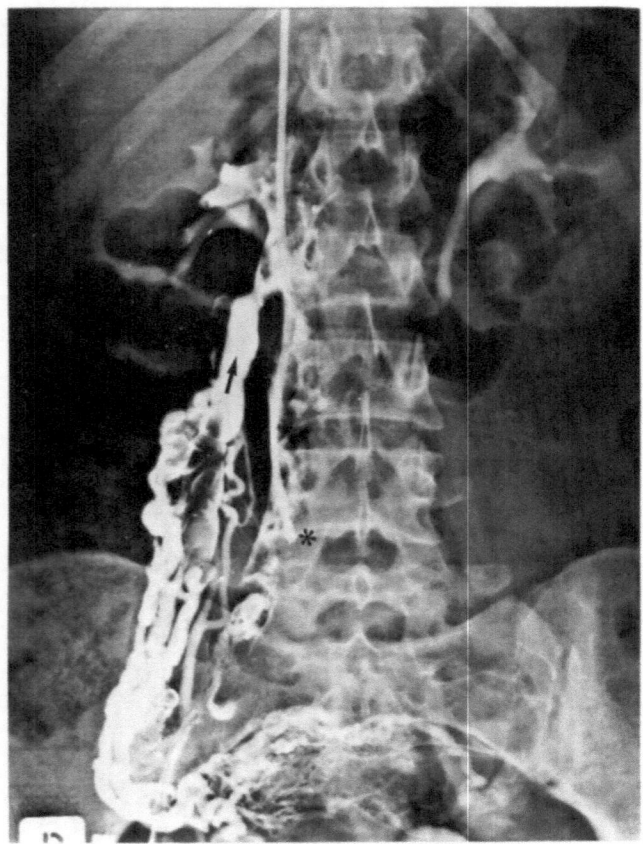

Fig. 204: Descending cavography with percutaneous brachial catheterization. This patient had numerous pulmonary embolisms. Placement of a clip on the infrarenal segment of the inferior vena cava. The catheter passes through the teeth of the Teflon clip and is situated in the infrarenal portion of the inferior vena cava ∗ . Diffuse thrombosis below the clip. The injection demonstrates the thrombosis of the infrarenal segment of the inferior vena cava extending also into the only still patent collateral pathway, a large right ⇟ ovarian vein (site of a very large thrombus).

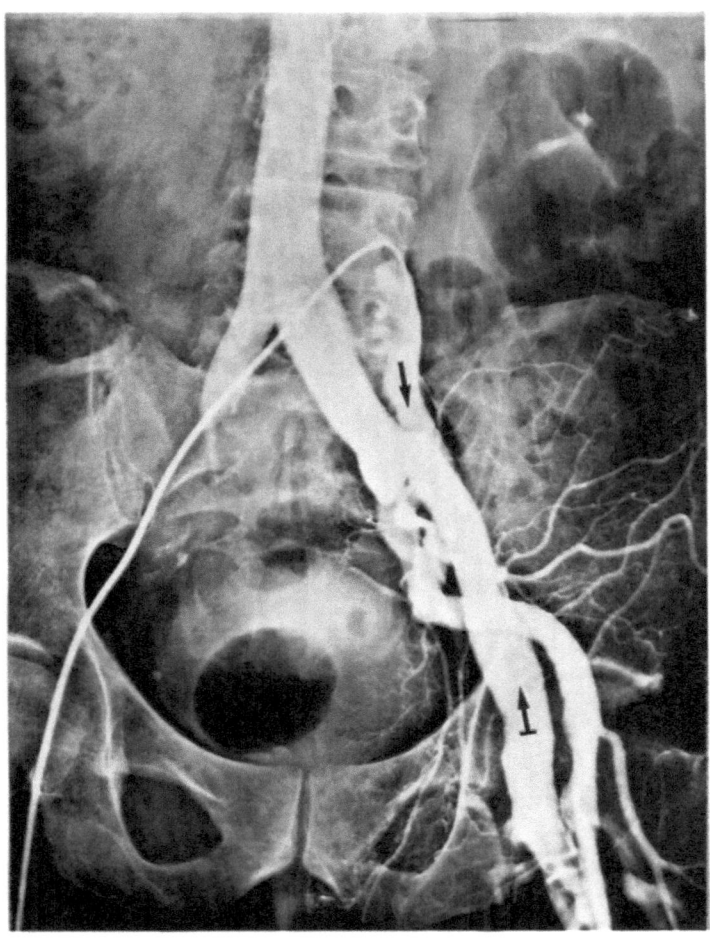

Fig. 205

Figs. 205, 206, 207 and 208: Operative treatment in left iliac phlebitis: thrombectomy associated with arterialization at the Scarpa's triangle.

205 and 206: Left iliac arteriography through right femoral Seldinger. Control of the arterialization. Successive opacification (205) of the left iliac artery ↿, then of the left iliac ⇃ venous system which is perfectly permeable.

206 (see p. 142): Another control 10 days later because of the occurrence of edema of the left lower limb. Same technique. Late phase of the seriography. The left iliac vein is patent ⇃ but there is complete thrombosis of the inferior vena cava * below the Teflon clip positioned on the infrarenal segment.

207 and 208 (see p. 142): Right unifemoral cavography in the same patient demonstrates obstruction of the infrarenal inferior vena cava extending to the right common iliac vein. Marked parietal collateral circulation. It is thus a matter of failure of the operative treatment with diffuse thrombosis below a caval clip; arterialization is incapable of maintaining the patency of the inferior vena cava, although the left common iliac vein remains patent.

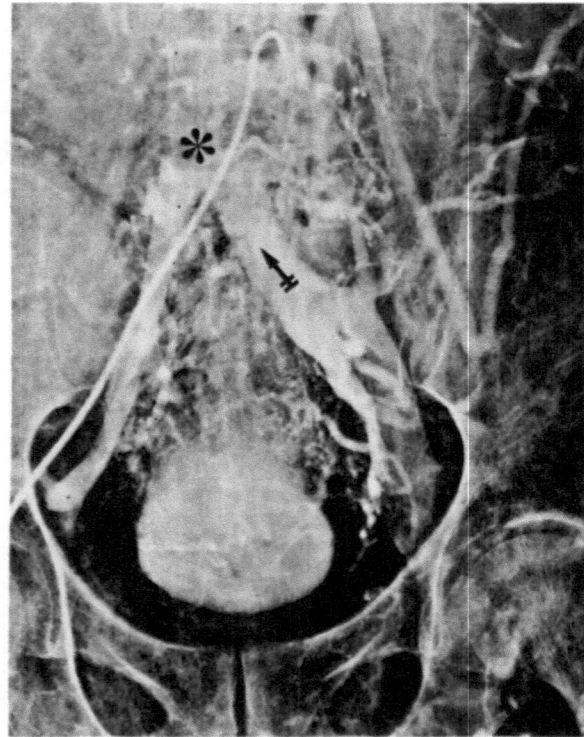

Fig. 206

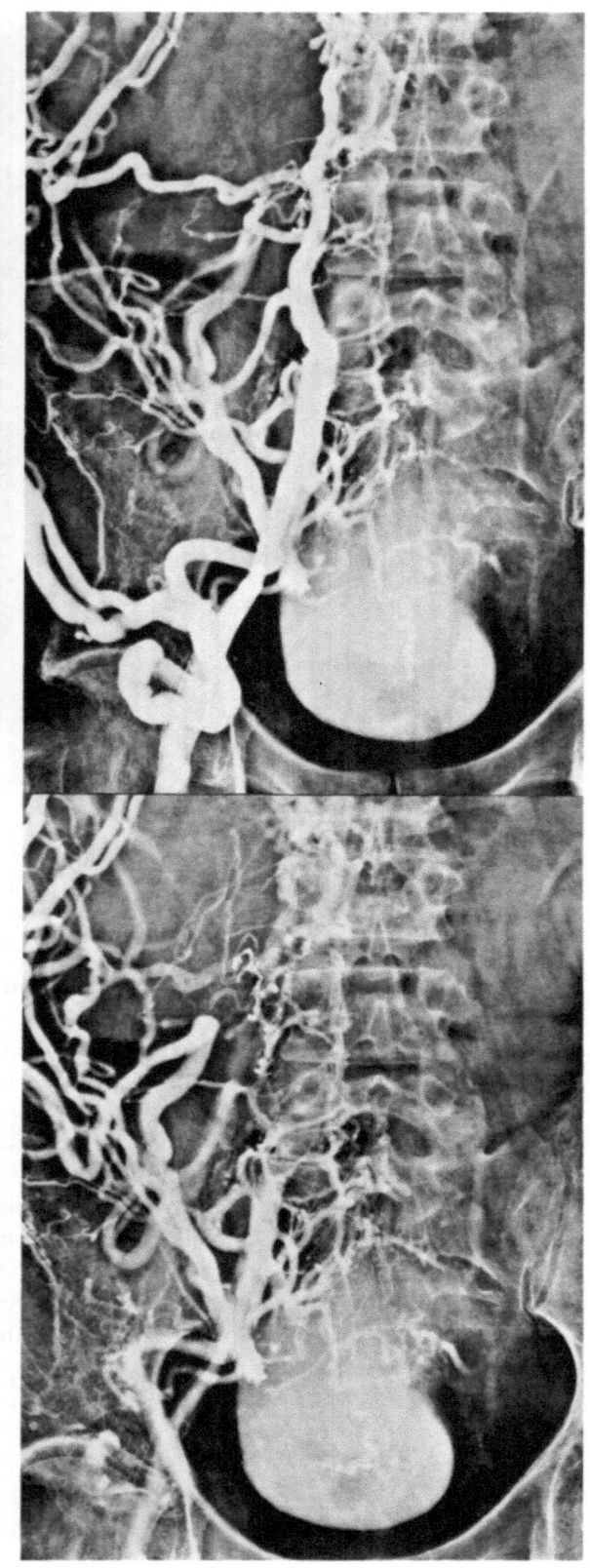

Fig. 207

Fig. 208

205 (see p. 141) *and 206:* Left iliac arteriography through right femoral Seldinger. Control of the arterialization. Successive opacification (205) of the left iliac artery ⬆, then of the left iliac ⬇ venous system which is perfectly permeable.

206: Another control 10 days later because of the occurrence of edema of the left lower limb. Same technique. Late phase of the seriography. The left iliac vein is patent ⬇ but there is complete thrombosis of the inferior vena cava * below the Teflon clip positioned on the infrarenal segment.

207 and 208: Right unifemoral cavography in the same patient demonstrates obstruction of the infrarenal inferior vena cava extending to the right common iliac vein. Marked parietal collateral circulation. It is thus a matter of failure of the operative treatment with diffuse thrombosis below a caval clip; arterialization is incapable of maintaining the patency of the inferior vena cava, although the left common iliac vein remains patent.

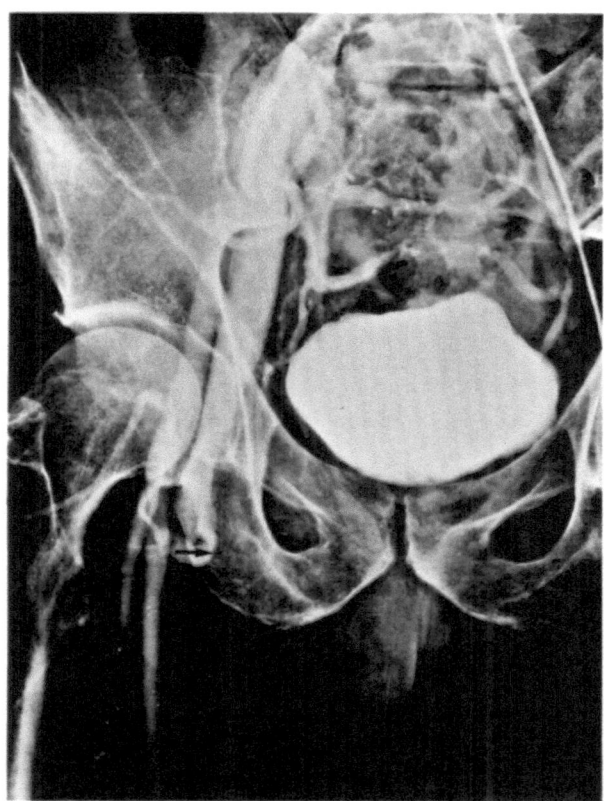

Fig. 209: Right iliac phlebitis. Thrombectomy; arterialization at the right Scarpa's triangle. Control of the arteriovenous fistula and of the right iliac patency. Note that the internal saphenous vein ↑ serves for the arteriovenous fistula at the right Scarpa's triangle.

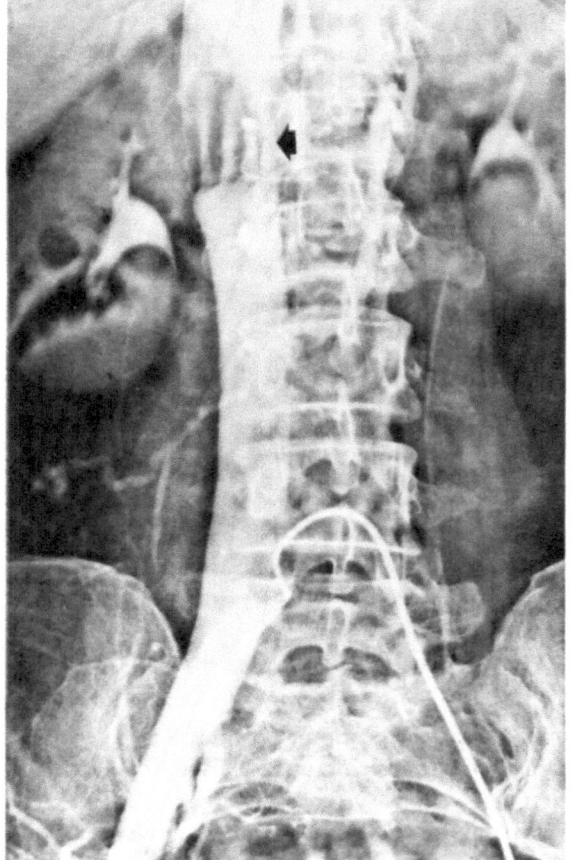

Fig. 210: Right iliac phlebitis in a patient who underwent thrombectomy and arterialization at the level of the right Scarpa's triangle. Teflon clip on the infrarenal inferior vena cava ◄. Control by descending right iliac arteriography (left femoral arterial Seldinger).

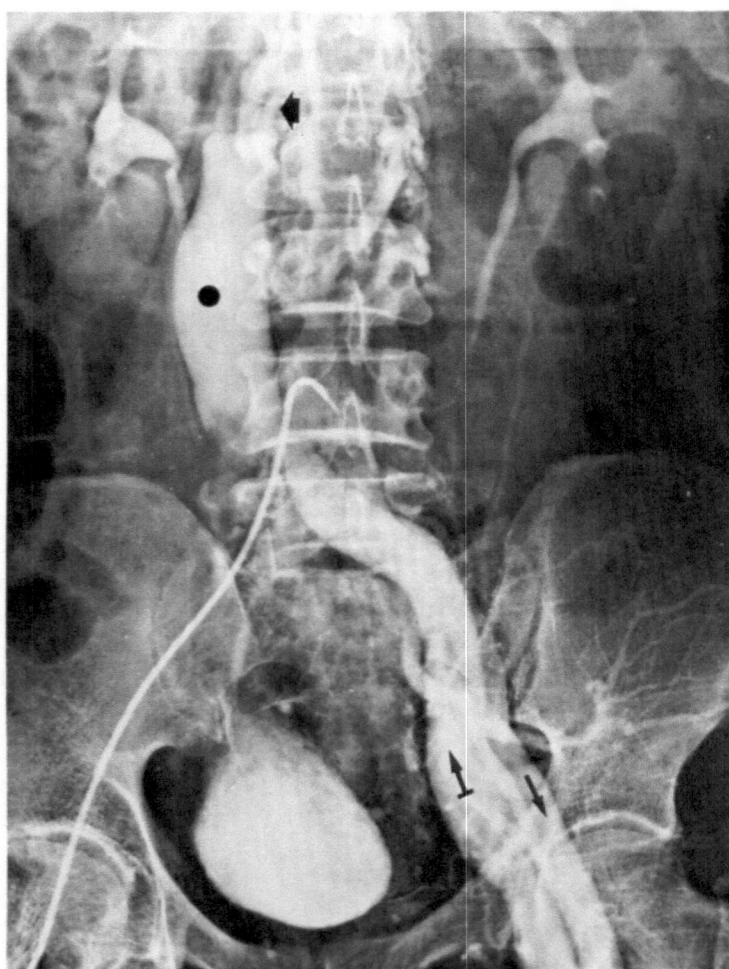

Fig. 211

Figs. 211 and 212: Left iliac phlebitis with thrombectomy and arterialization at the left Scarpa's triangle. Teflon clip on the infrarenal inferior vena cava. Descending left iliac arteriography by right femoral arterial Seldinger. Opacification of the left iliac artery ↿, of the left iliac venous system ↥ through the arteriovenous fistule and, finally, of the inferior vena cava ● with the clip ⬧, providing a "fenestrated" appearance to the infrarenal inferior vena cava.

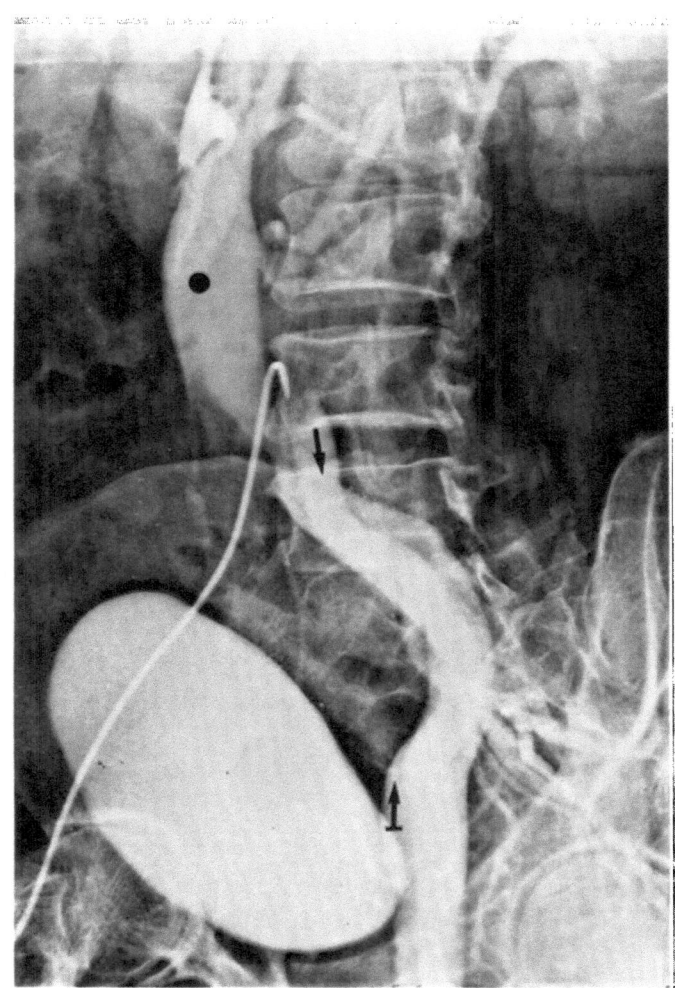

Fig. 212

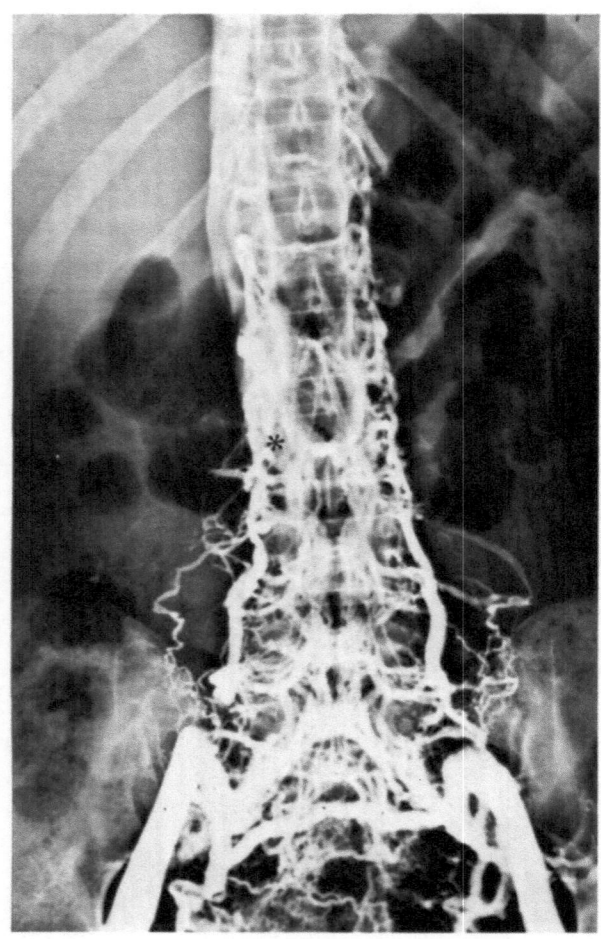

Fig. 213: Plication of the inferior vena cava in a patient with a history of numerous pulmonary embolisms. Note the diffuse obstruction of the infrarenal inferior vena cava∗ in this type of operative treatment. The two iliac veins remain patent in their external iliac portion. Note the marked opacification of the presacral plexuses and of the intra- and extraspinal venous system.

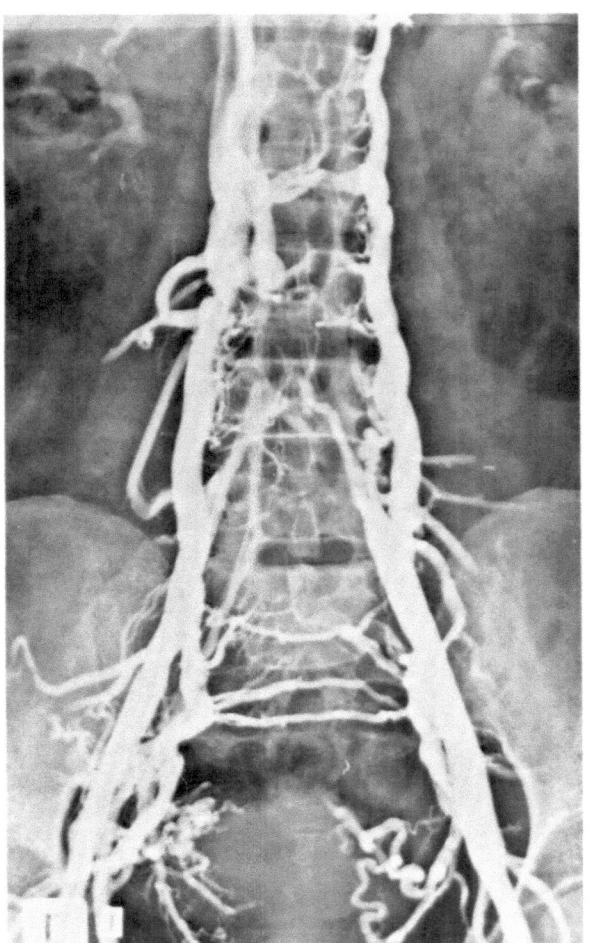 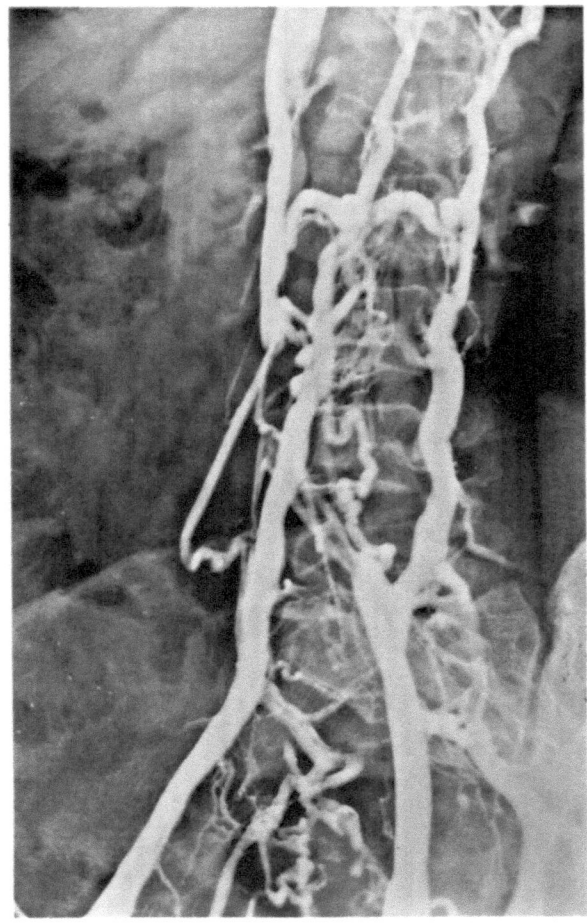

Fig. 214 *Fig. 215*

Figs. 214 and 215: Ligation of the infrarenal inferior vena cava. Collateral circulation develops from the two ascending lumbar veins and from the iliolumbar veins. Left anterior oblique projection (215) demonstrating the collateral circulation. This patient had multiple pulmonary embolisms. Note that the ligation of the infeior vena cava cuts off a great part of the infrarenal inferior caval flow, contrary to the Teflon clips which often keep the infrarenal inferior vena cava perfectly free.

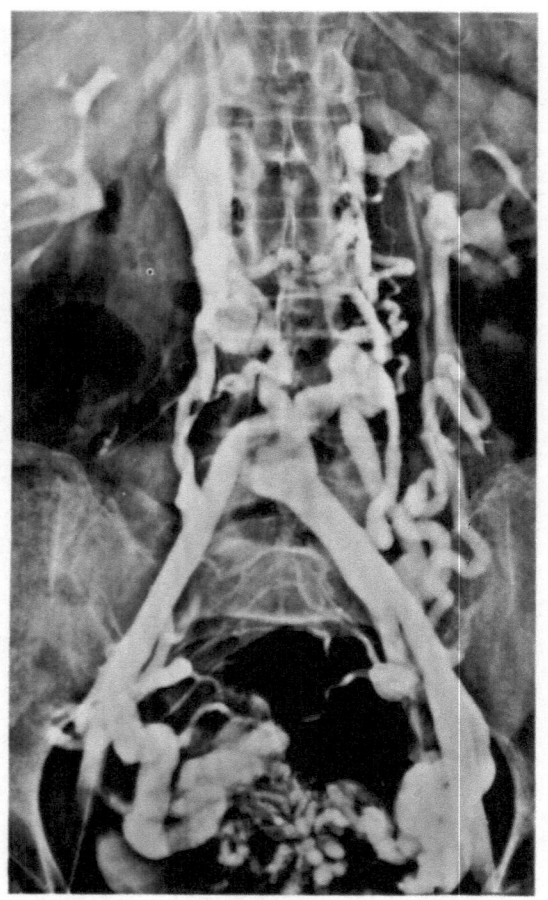

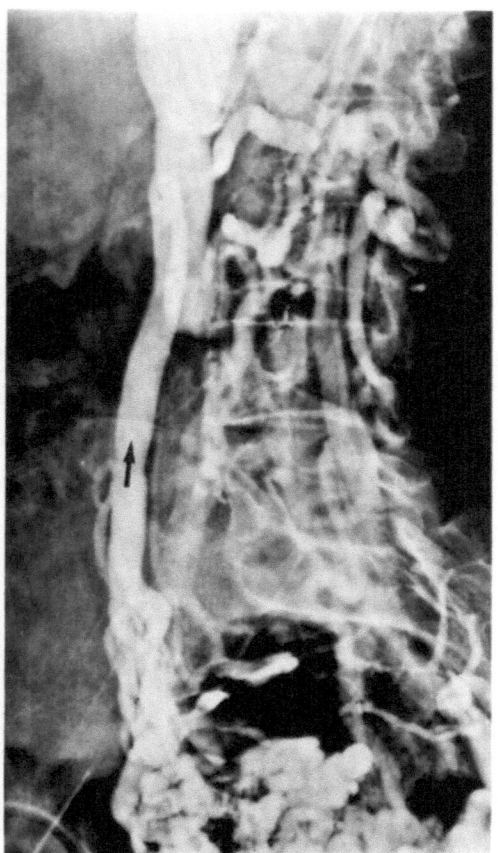

Fig. 216

Fig. 217

Figs. 216 and 217: Ligation of the infrarenal inferior vena cava in a patient who had numerous pulmonary embolisms. With this technique the inferior vena cava is constantly occluded below the plication, as it is with plication. Note on the left anterior oblique projection (217) the opacification of a large gonadic ↑ vein through the uterine plexuses.

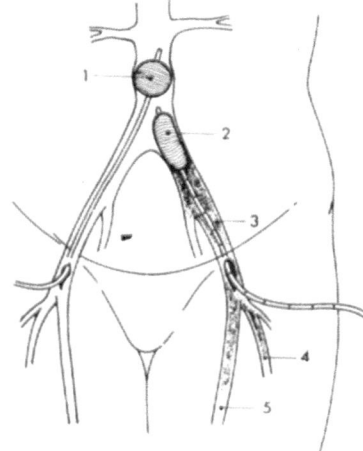

1. Foley catheter.
2. Fogarty catheter.
3. Common femoral vein.
4. Profunda fistula.
5. Superficial femoral vein.

Fig. 218: Diagram showing the operative technique of left iliac venous thrombectomy by means of a balloon catheter. Note the balloon in the infrarenal segment of the inferior vena cava (1) which has been placed via the right iliac vein as a protection against pulmonary migration during surgery. (From H. Haimovici, Vascular Surgery, published by McGraw-Hill, New York.)

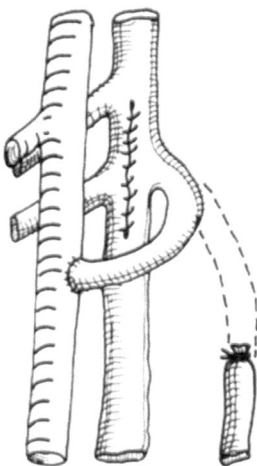

Fig. 219: Diagram showing the operative technique of arterio-venous fistula at the Scarpa's triangle (right) using the internal saphenous.

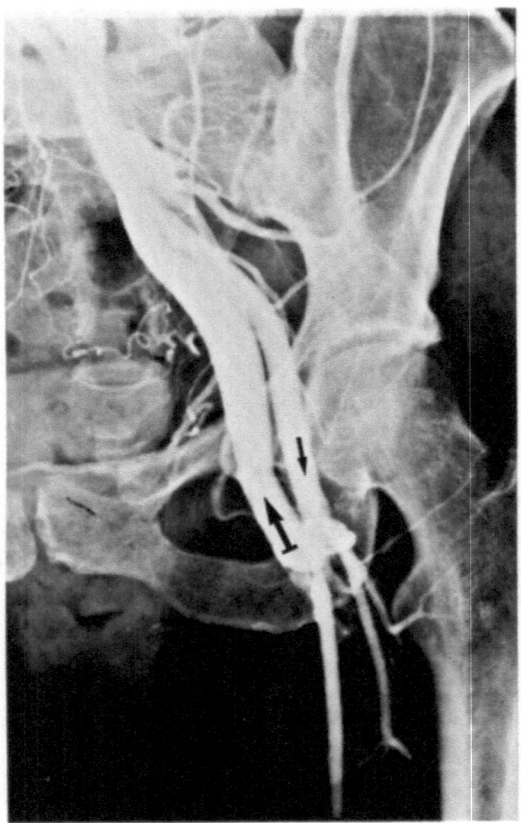

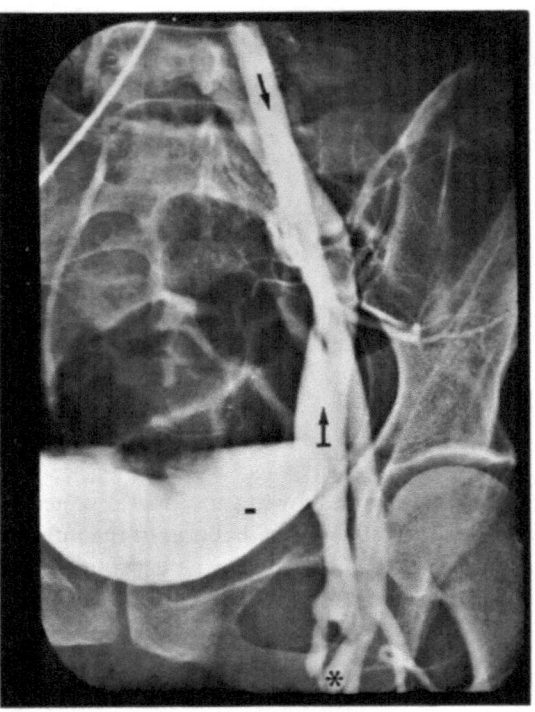

Fig. 221

Fig. 220: Check arteriogram of a temporary arterio-venous fistula at the left Scarpa's triangle in a case of left iliac phlebitis. Note the successive opacification of the left iliofemoral artery ↿, the arteriovenous fistula and finally the left iliac venous system ↕ draining upwardly.

Figs. 221, 222, 223 and 224: Left iliac phlebitis. Thrombectomy associated with arteriovenous fistula at the left Scarpa's triangle. Checking by a descending left iliac arteriography (right arterial femoral Seldinger type injection). Successive opacification of the left iliac artery ↿, of the arteriovenous fistula ∗ and, finally, of the left iliac venous system ↕ which drains upwardly. There is, however, a persistent Cockett's syndrome at the termination of the left common iliac vein, as demonstrated in Fig. 223 and 224, which show a very faint opacification of the inferior vena cava via the left iliac venous system; the inferior vena cava ● is opacified mainly by the presacral plexuses ↟ which drain the iliac venous blood from left to right ⋆. Conclusion: Left iliac venous thrombectomy and arteriovenous fistula at the Scarpa's triangle: good results but persistence of a compression syndrome of the left iliac vein which was not treated operatively at the same time.

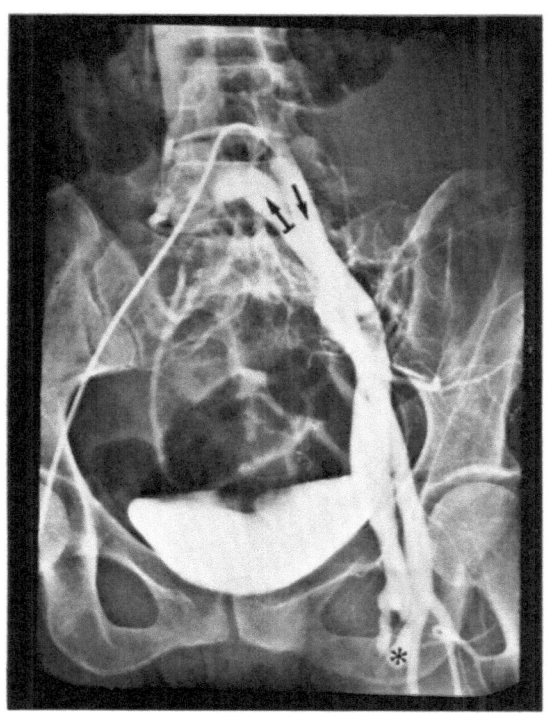

Fig. 222

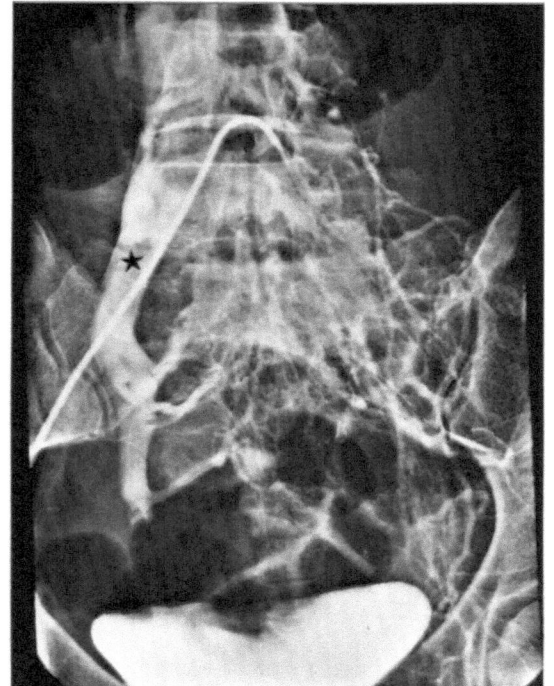

Fig. 224

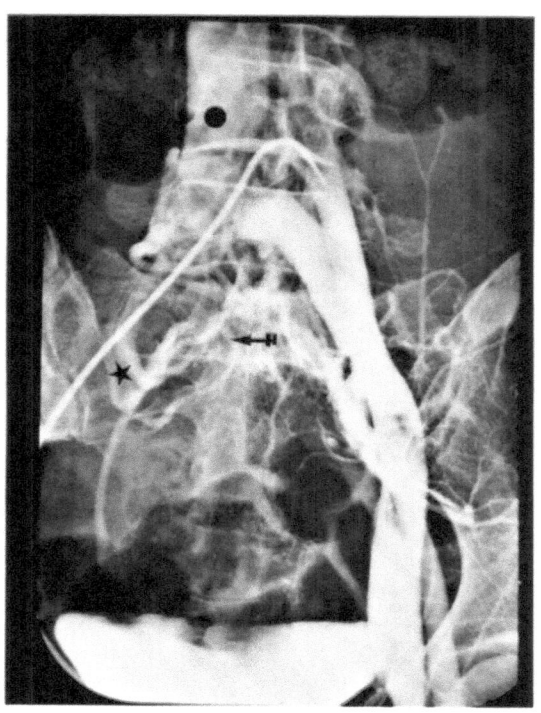

Fig. 223

Chapter 7

CHRONIC PHLEBITIS AND SURGERY
IN CHRONIC PHLEBITIS

Figures 225–285

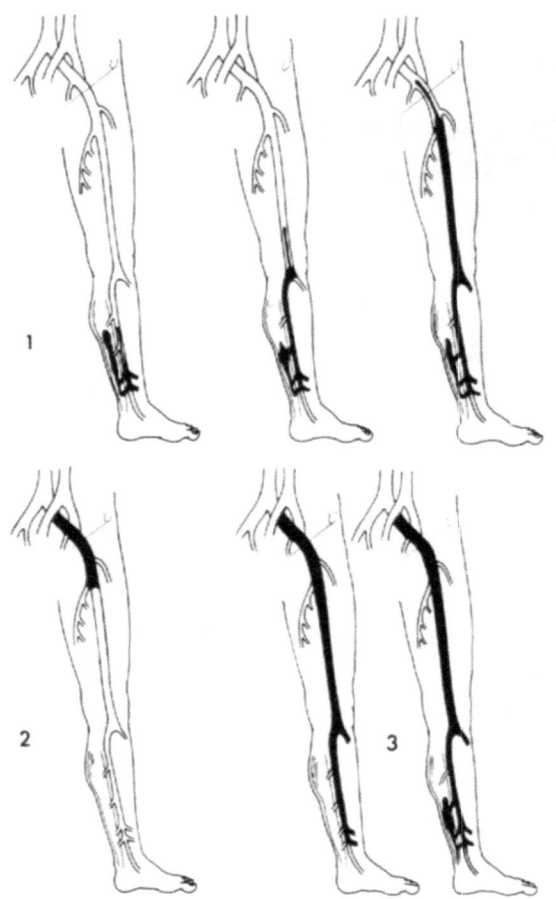

Fig. 225: The three main types of post-thrombotic syndrome: *Type 1:* post-phlebitic syndrome by involvement of the deep veins located below the inguinal ligament. *Type 2:* post-phlebitic syndrome by isolated iliac phlebitis. *Type 3:* post-phlebitic syndrome by diffuse involvement of all veins of the lower limb, including the iliac venous system. (Redrawn from H. Dodd and F.B. Cockett, p. 263, figs. 17 and 19.)

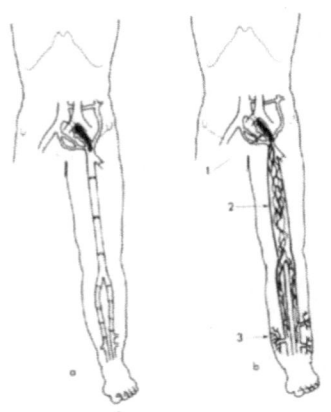

Fig. 226: Final stages in ilio-femoral phlebitis. (a) Thrombosis of iliac segment only, with good collateral circulation and without destruction of peripheral valves. (b) Associated ilio-femoral and sural diffuse thrombosis. Iliac obstruction plus destruction of the distal valves producing all symptoms of the post-phlebitic syndrome, i.e. swelling, pain and ulceration at ankle. (Redrawn from H. Dodd and F.B. Cockett, p. 233, fig. 16.10.)

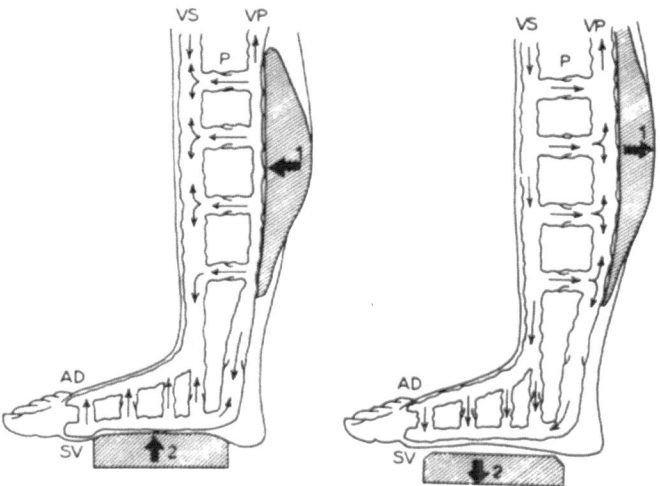

Fig. 227: Diagram showing the influence of upright position and walking on to venous return to the lower limbs in the post-phlebitic syndrome.

On the left: active phase.

♠ 2. · Flattening of the plantar veins.

♠ 1. Muscular contraction compresses the deep veins, ensures deep progression of the blood, but brings about reflux toward the superficial network and the foot, due to postphlebitic valvular incompetence. The direction of the flow is reversed in the superficial veins, due partly to an incompetent ostial valve situated above.

On the right: relaxation phase.

♠ 2. The absence of plantar rest produces generalized reflux toward the foot.

♠ 1. Muscle relaxation no longer ensures efficient deep progression of the blood.

VS: superficial vein

VP: deep vein

P: perforating vein

SV: plantar veins

ADV: superficial dorsal venous arch

1: calf muscles

2: plantar rest

156

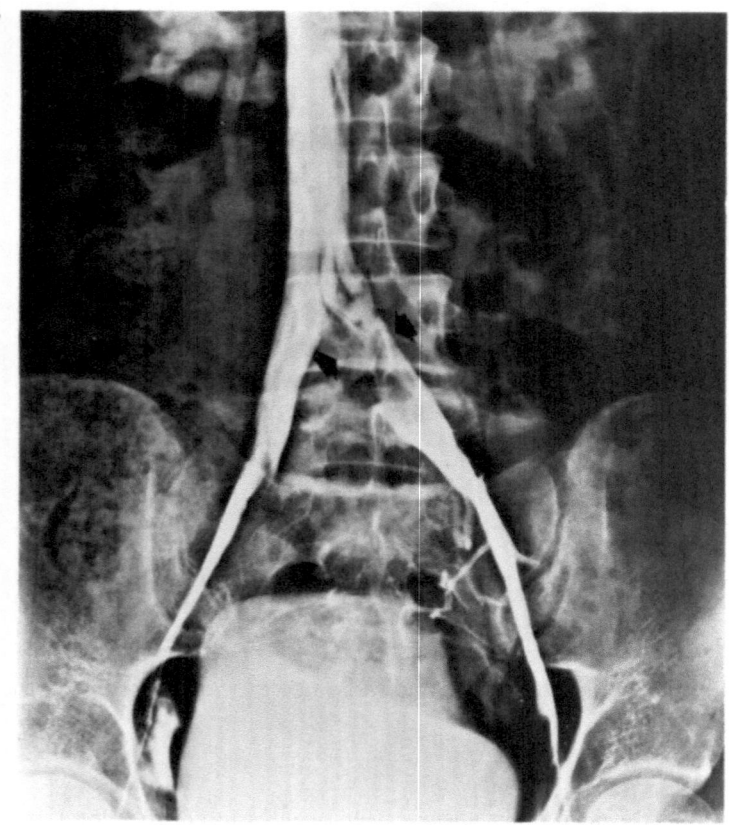

Fig. 228: Bifemoral percutaneous cavography. Cockett's syndrome of the left common iliac vein termination with fenestration ♦ ♦. The underlying venous pathway has a very small caliber and shows straticulate appearance, proof of ancient phlebitis, rather well recanalized.

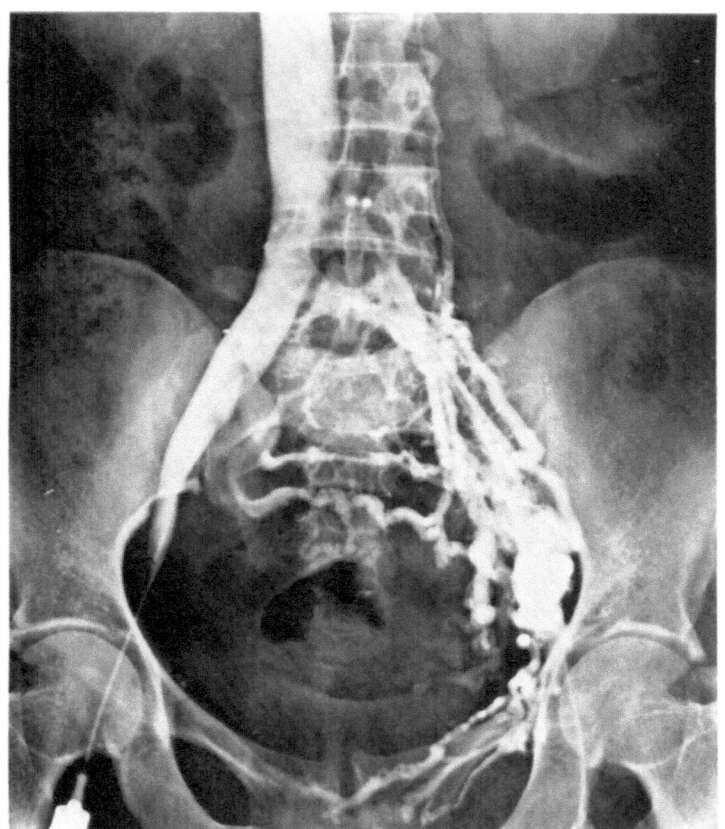

Fig. 229

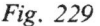

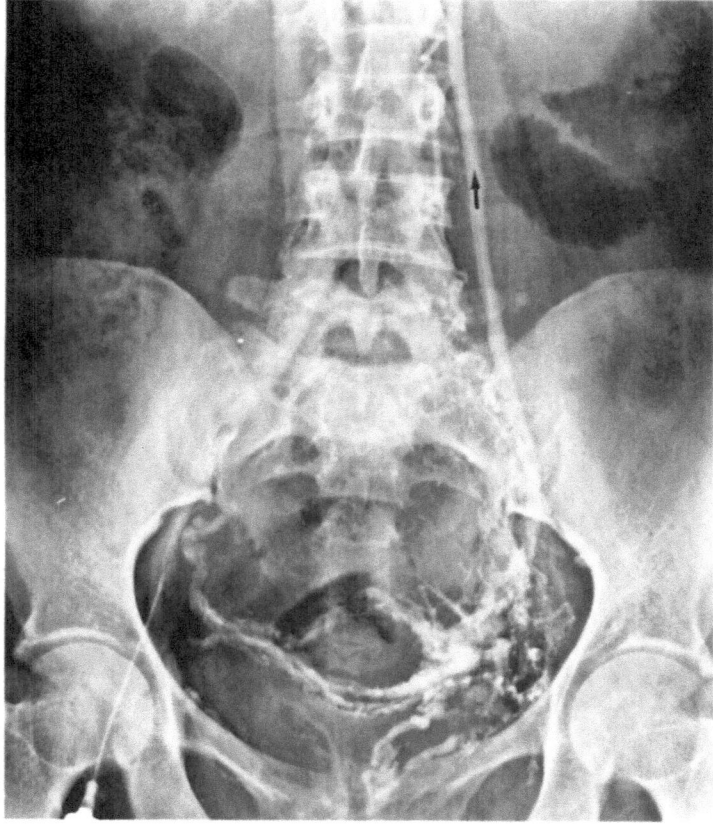

Fig. 230

Figs. 229 and 230: Chronic left iliac phlebitis. Bifemoral percutaneous cavography performed with two small neddle-catheters. Faint iliac recanalization. There are multiple homolateral collateral venous dilatations. Above all there is, on a late film (230), a collateral derivation through a left ovarian vein ↑ which drains toward the left renal vein.

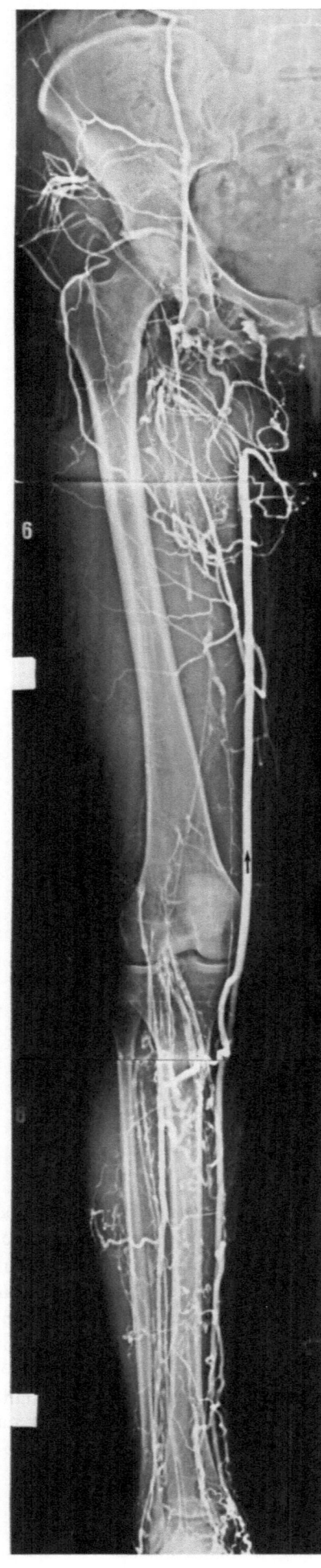

Fig. 231: Chronic phlebitis of the right lower limb. Segmental recanalization of the leg veins; collateral circulation mainly through the internal saphenous superficial system ↑. No filling of the deep venous system in the thigh. The internal saphenous proper is obliterated at the level of its termination. Superficial abdominal collateral circulation, proof of associated chronic iliac phlebitis.

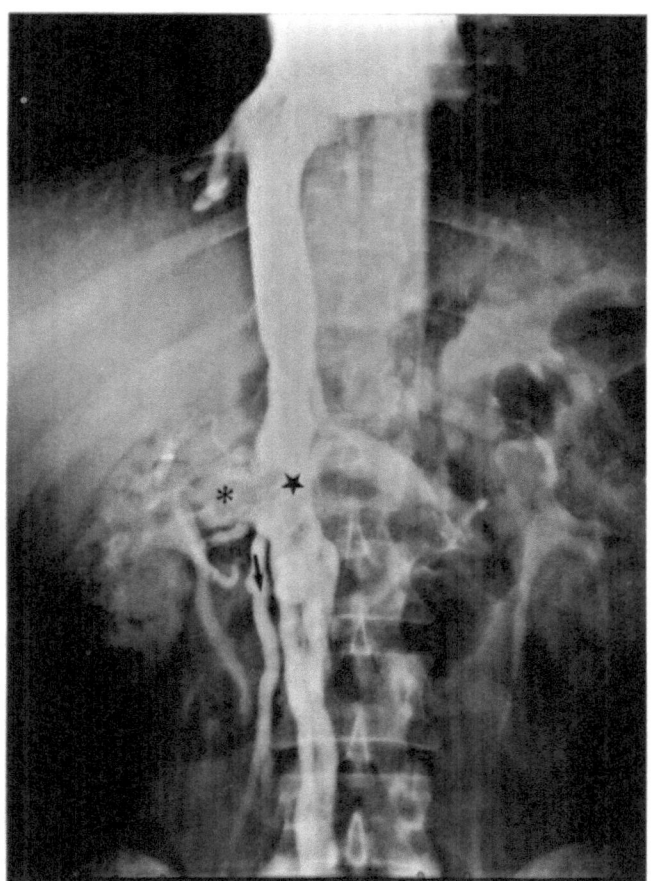

Fig. 232: Descending cavography by percutaneous brachial catheterization to demonstrate the upper level of ilioacaval phlebitic obliteration. Persistent obliteration of the infrarenal segment of the inferior vena cava which shows a lamellar and straticulate appearance. Thrombosis extends ★ to the interrenal segment of the inferior vena cava. There are also filling defects in the right renal vein ∗ and reflux † into a right spermatic vein.

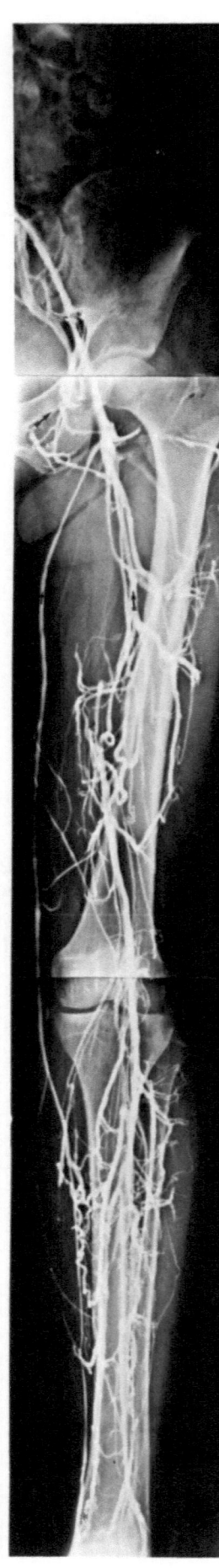

Fig. 233: Chronic phlebitis of the left lower limb. Rather good recanalization of the deep veins of the leg, some of which still have valves, namely the posterior tibial veins at the ankle ∗. Superficial femoral recanalization is almost non-existent and the collateral circulation is via the internal saphenous ↑ and the profunda femoris vein ↧. The left iliac vein seems to be of small caliber with collateral circulation via the obturator vein ↕ and the hypogastric system, proof of associated chronic iliac phlebitis.

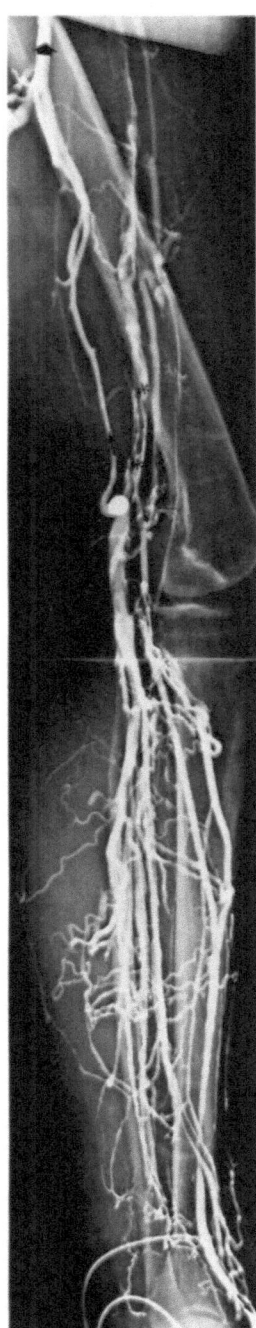

Fig. 234: Chronic phlebitis of the left lower limb. Lateral projection. Upstream injection into the internal saphenous vein at the ankle ⭡. Some of the deep veins of the leg are still patent. Significant reflux in the perforating veins of the leg. The popliteal vein is patent in its lower part, and then interrupted at the level of the femoro-popliteal pathway which shows a very marked straticulate appearance ✳. The collateral circulation is through a retro-adductor vein which drains into the profunda femoris vein ♠ at the upper part of the thigh. Note that the profunda femoris vein has a forward oblique course crossing the femoral shaft at the upper thigh.

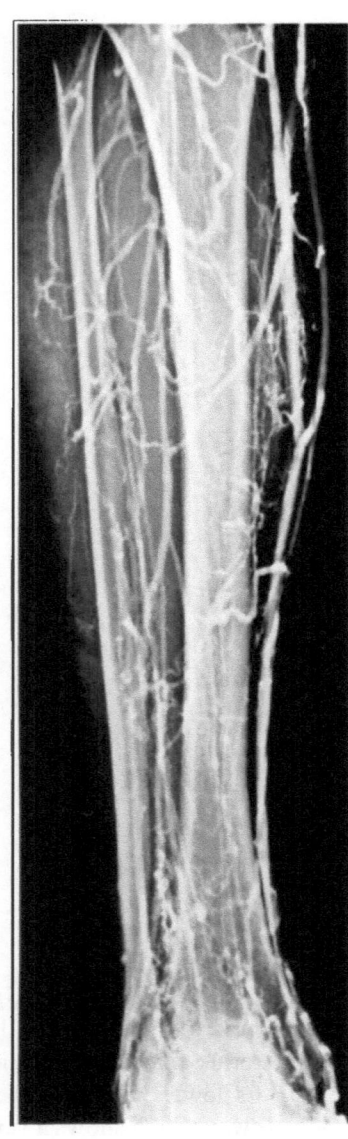

Fig. 235: Phlebography of the right lower limb. Centering on the leg. Chronic phlebitis with very poor recanalization of the deep venous system. Drainage is mainly via the superficial veins. Very marked post-phlebitic syndrome.

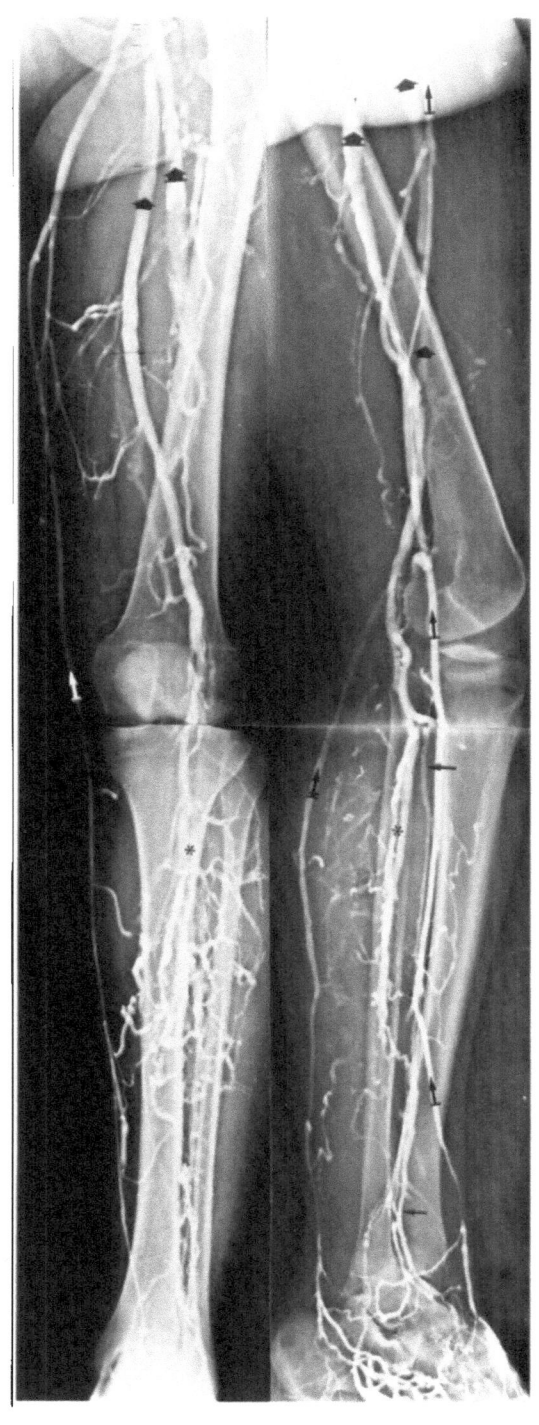

Fig. 236   Fig. 237

Fig. 236 and 237: Chronic phlebitis of the left lower limb. Frontal (236) and lateral (237) projection. Persistent obliteration of the part of the deep veins of the leg. Only the upper part of the peroneal veins * and the entire length of the anterior tibial vein ↑ seem to be patent. Collateral circulation through the internal saphenous vein ↕ and the external saphenous vein ↕ at the posterior aspect of the calf. The superficial femoral vein ● is rather well re-canalized but there is, however, marked opacification of the profunda femoris vein ♣. Note, as on the lateral view (237) the faint superficial femoral opacification, and the marked deep femoral ♠ drainage (postural variations influence the drainage of the venous flow). A case of chronic phlebitis with persistence of an important obliteration of the deep veins of the leg, and rather good femoro-popliteal recanalization.

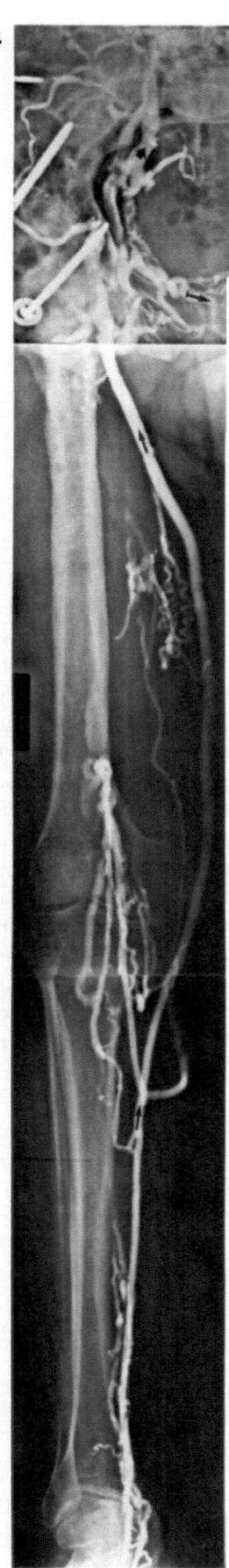

Fig. 238: Phlebography of the right lower limb with a non-pressurized injection. Chronic phlebitis. Almost non-existent recanalization of the deep venous system. Drainage occurs almost entirely through the internal saphenous vein ↑. Associated iliac phlebitis demonstrated by collateral circulation via the obturator vein draining into the hypogastric system ♠. and also via right to left suprapubic derivations ↑.

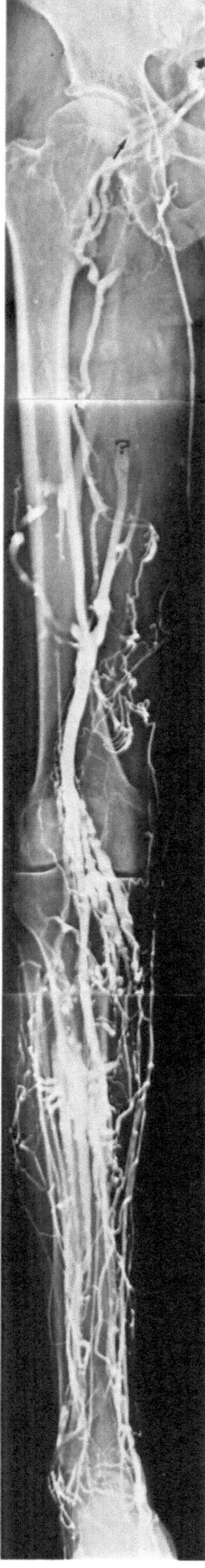

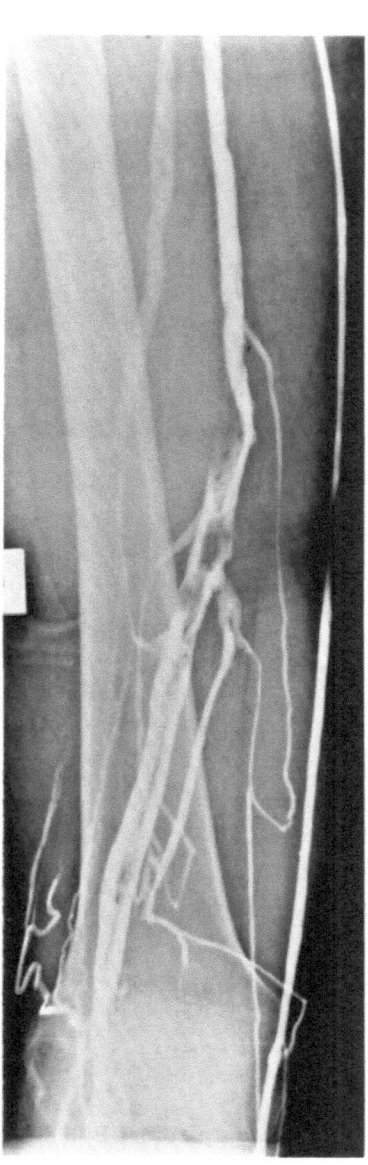

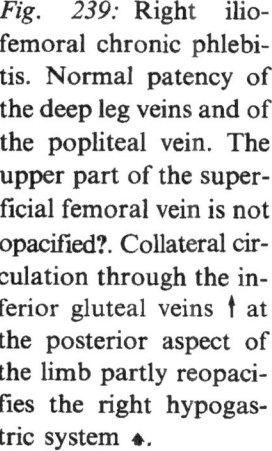

Fig. 239: Right iliofemoral chronic phlebitis. Normal patency of the deep leg veins and of the popliteal vein. The upper part of the superficial femoral vein is not opacified?. Collateral circulation through the inferior gluteal veins ↑ at the posterior aspect of the limb partly reopacifies the right hypogastric system ♠.

Fig. 240: Femoro-popliteal phlebitis treated by heparin for 1 month. Check-up. Partial recanalization of the superficial femoral vein, but persistent filling defects due to thrombi.

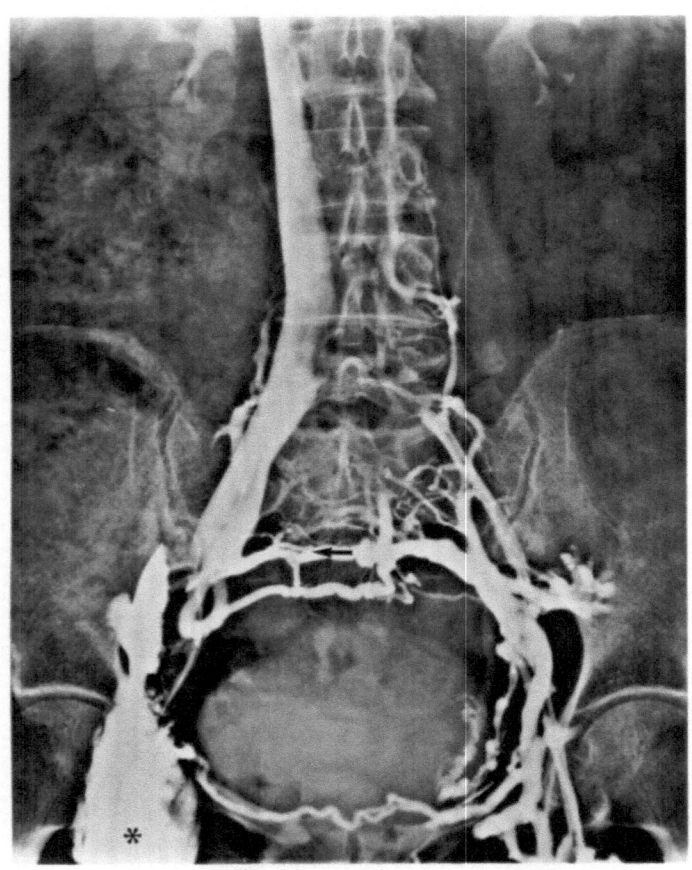

Fig. 241: Chronic left iliac phlebitis. Bifemoral percutaneous cavography. Extravasation of contrast medium on the right∗. On the left, the iliac system is faintly recanalized and has a straticulate appearance; there is significant left-to-right collateral circulation ↑.

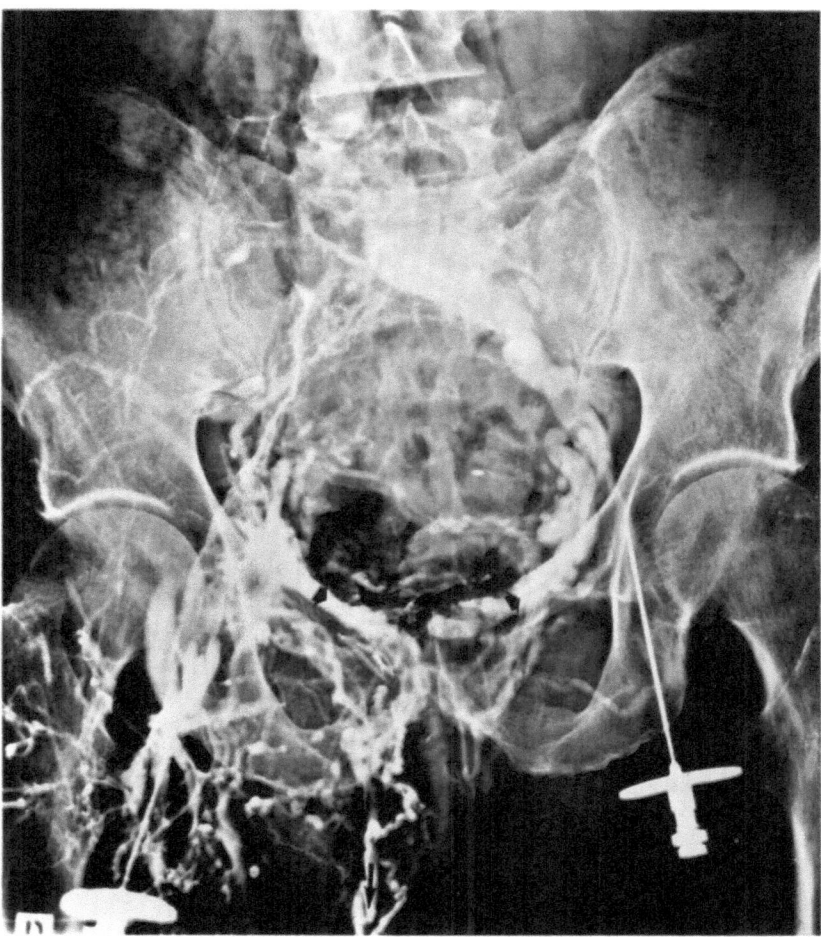

Fig. 242: Chronic right iliac phlebitis. Puncture into a thrombus on the right side reopacifies faintly the hypogastric axis through the obturator and inferior gluteal veins. Very marked downward reflux of the contrast medium. Note the right to left collateral circulation ● through the supra and retropubic area, with some varicosities ↑ on the penis and varicocele.

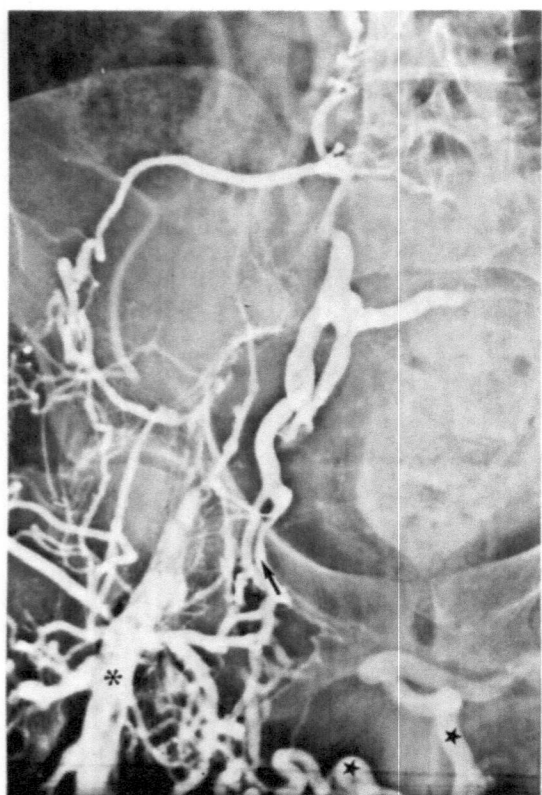

Fig. 243: Right chronic iliac phlebitis. Catheterization of a chronic obliteration of the femoral vein * Recanalization is almost non-existent and only the superficial and some obturator veins † drain the blood from the right side. Right-to-left derivation through prepubic superficial veins, probably vulvar varices ★.

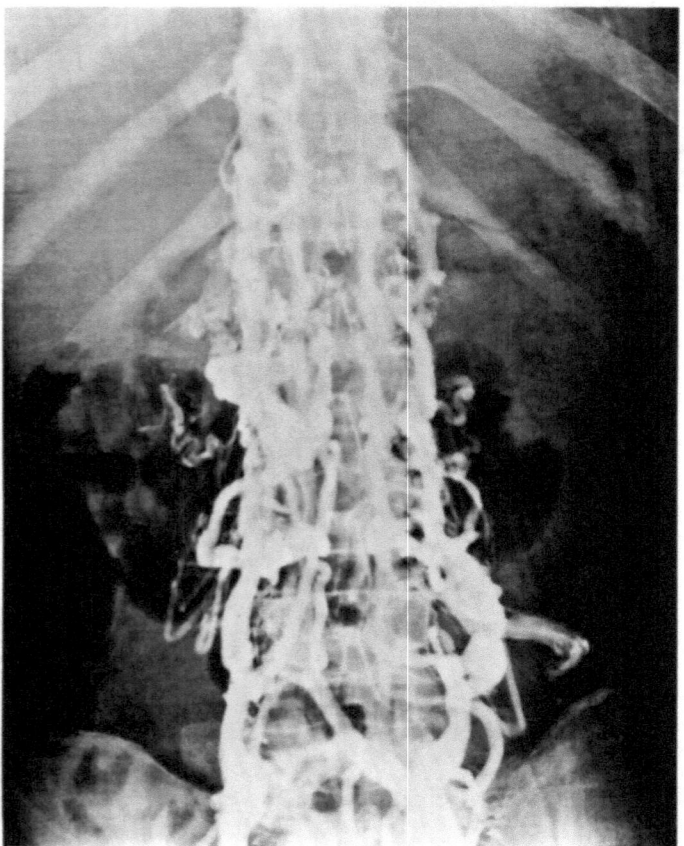

Fig. 244: Old bi-iliac and inferior caval phlebitic obliteration with collateral derivations mainly through the intra- and extraspinal plexuses.

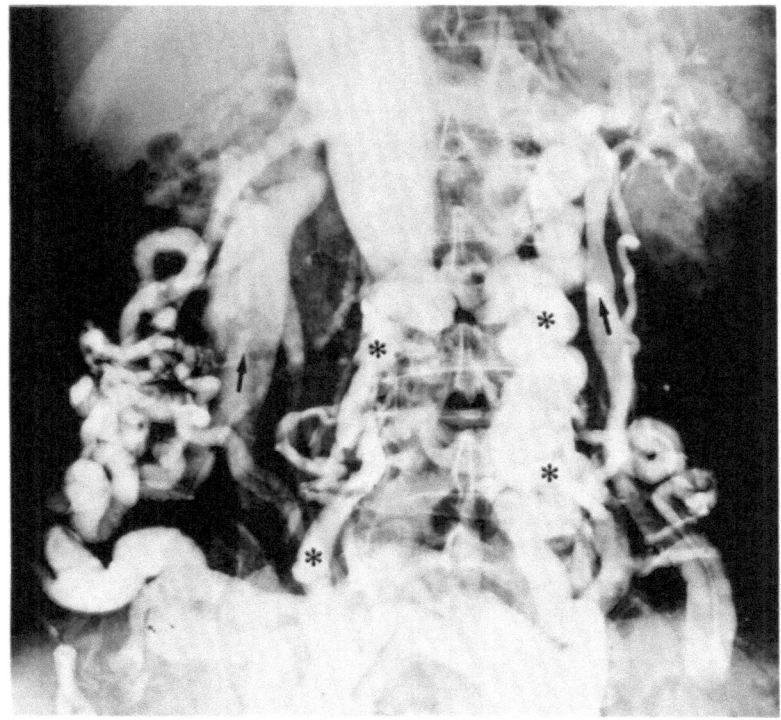

Fig. 245: Chronic phlebitis of the infrarenal segment of the inferior vena cava with very marked bilateral genital ↑ and lumbar ∗ collateral channels.

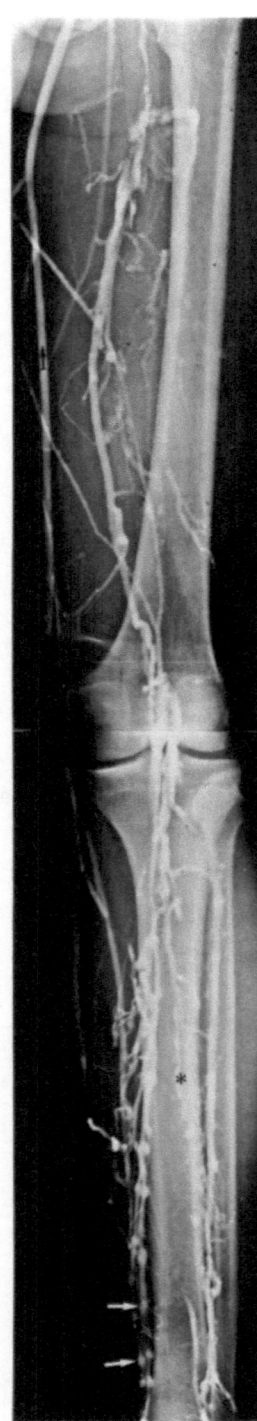

Fig. 246: Phlebography of the left lower limb. Chronic phlebitis for two months, threated by heparin. Some deep veins of the leg are still valvulated and have probably not been involved by the phlebitic process (namely the posterior tibial ↿ veins). The peroneal veins are opacified but show some filling defects ∗ . There is incomplete obstruction of the femoro-popliteal axis. The internal saphenous vein is opacified in its entire length, and functions always as collateral circulation ⇃. Poor results of anticoagulant treatment in chronic sural and femoro-popliteal phlebitis.

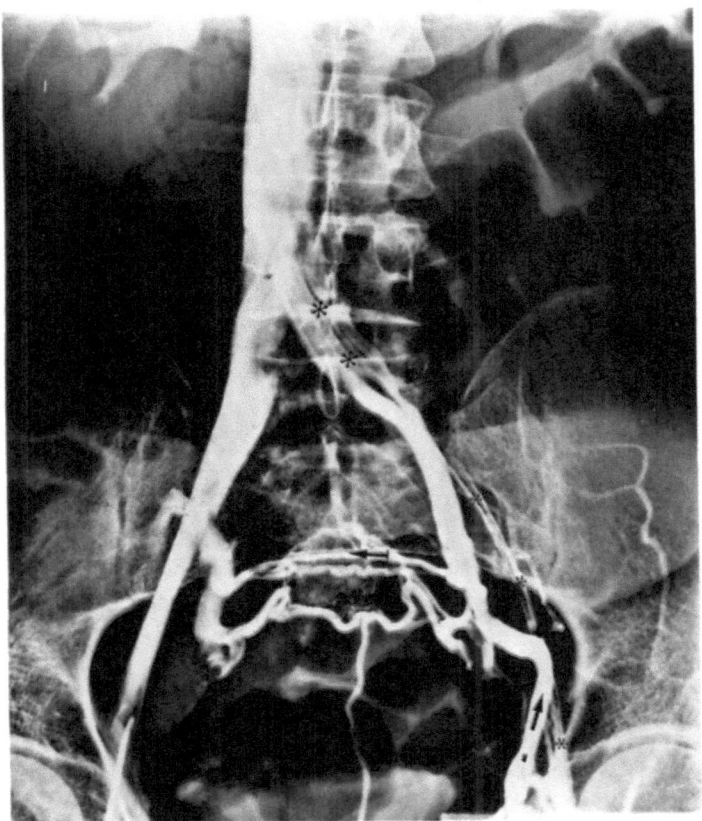

Fig. 247: Left iliac chronic phlebitis. Bifemoral percutaneous cavography. The left external iliac vein is hardly opacified; it shows a very marked fenestrated and straticulate appearance ∗ . The collateral circulation occurs through the left hypogastric vein ↿, and especially through the presacral plexuses, from left to right ⇃. The left common iliac vein is opacified but it shows the straticulate appearance of a thrombosis undergoing recanalization ∗∗ .

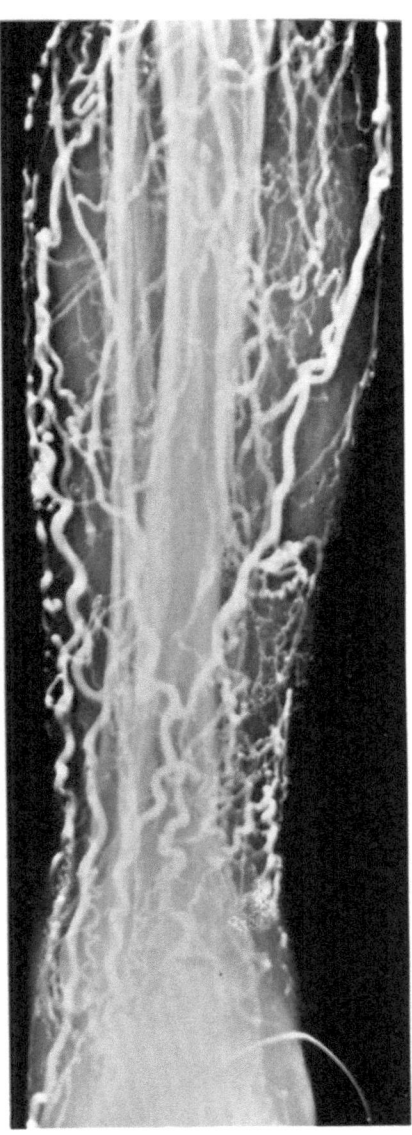

Fig. 248: Phlebogram of the right lower limb (centered on the leg). Sural phlebitis treated with heparin. Follow-up investigation 1 month later. No recanalization of the deep trunks; the collateral circulation is muscular and superficial. The patient complained of pain during the investigation.

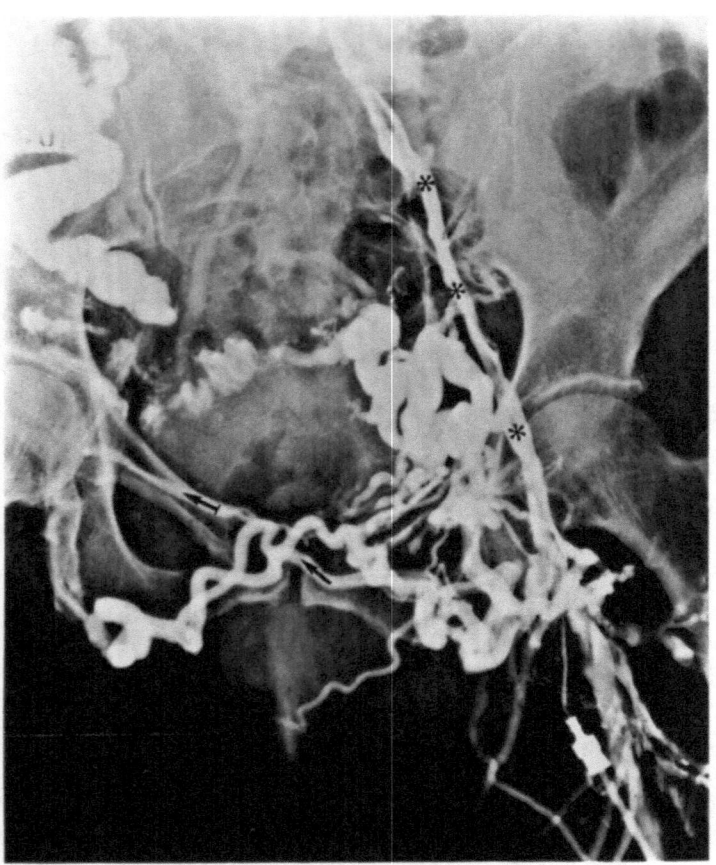

Fig. 249: Left iliac chronic phlebitis. Left femoral percutaneous catheterization. Very poor recanalization with lamellar appearance ∗ of the entire left iliac pathway. Contralateral derivation through retro ⭡ and suprapubic veins ⭣, from left to right.

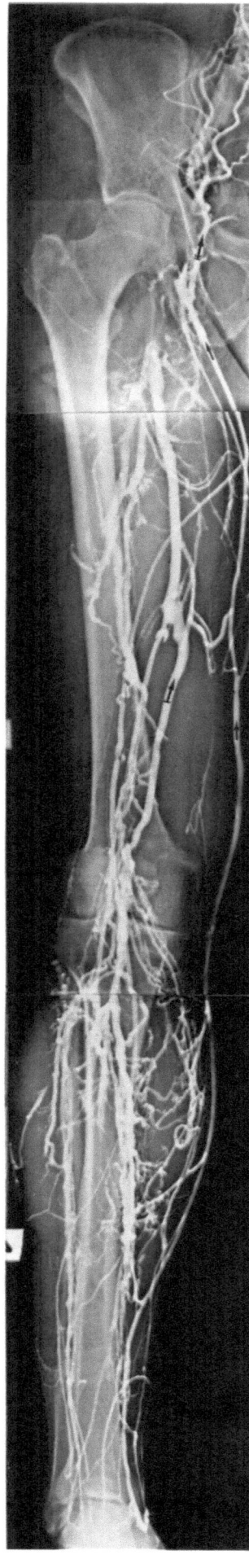

Fig. 250: Phlebography of the right lower limb with non-pressurized injection. 3 months' chronic phlebitis with occurrence of a thick leg. Recanalization of the deep veins is very fragmentary, and there is marked incompetence of the perforating veins of the leg. The internal saphenous system ↑ functions as collateral circulation. The popliteal and the superficial femoral vein are partly obliterated. Drainage is ensured by a retro-adductor vein ↕ and by venae comitantes anastomosed in a ladder-like manner along the course of the superficial femoral axis. The branches ↓ of the internal saphenous termination function as collateral pathway, proof of associated right external iliac phlebitis. Poor result of the anticoagulant treatment with occurrence of an early post-phlebitic syndrome.

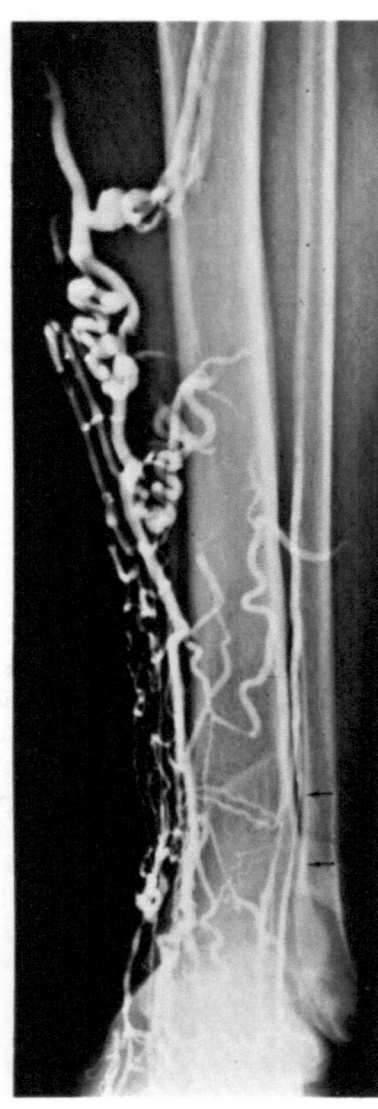

Fig. 251: Chronic sural phlebitis treated by heparin. Partial recanalization of the deep leg veins, namely of the anterior tibial veins which are seen in the intertibio-peroneal space at the lower part of the leg ↑↑. Huge post-phlebitic varices in the upper third of the leg fed by the perforating veins, of which some seem varicose.

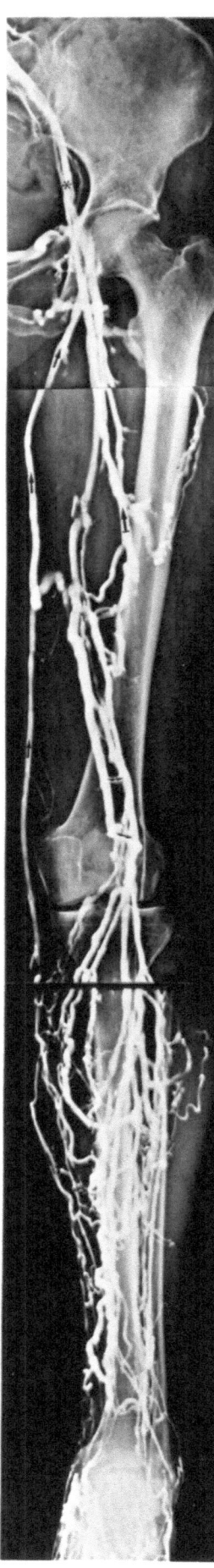

Fig. 252: Sural and ilio-femoro-popliteal chronic phlebitis. Partial recanalization of the deep veins of the leg which are valveless. Incompetence of the perforating veins in the leg with varices. Large internal saphenous vein ↑ has lost its valves. Note the opacification of venae comitantes ↓ at the level of the femoro-popliteal axis. Opacification of the profunda femoris vein ↥. "Lamellar" appearance ∗ of the iliac system with suprapubic collateral circulation. The radiologic features are those of chronic phlebitis treated by heparin, with fairly satisfactory recanalization of the deep system.

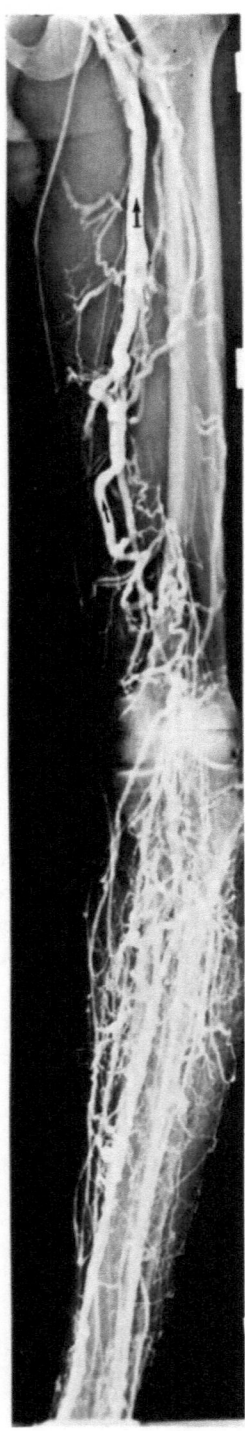

Fig. 253: Acute phase in chronic sural and femoro-popliteal phlebitis. The acute condition involves the leg veins. There is a very marked opacification of the venous network of the calf-muscle veins which intercommunicate in an arborizing pattern. The oblique projection shows the femoro-popliteal axis to be partly thrombosed and poorly recanalized. Circulation occurs mainly through the retro-adductor ↑ vein and then through the profunda femoris vein ↕ posterior to the femoral shaft.

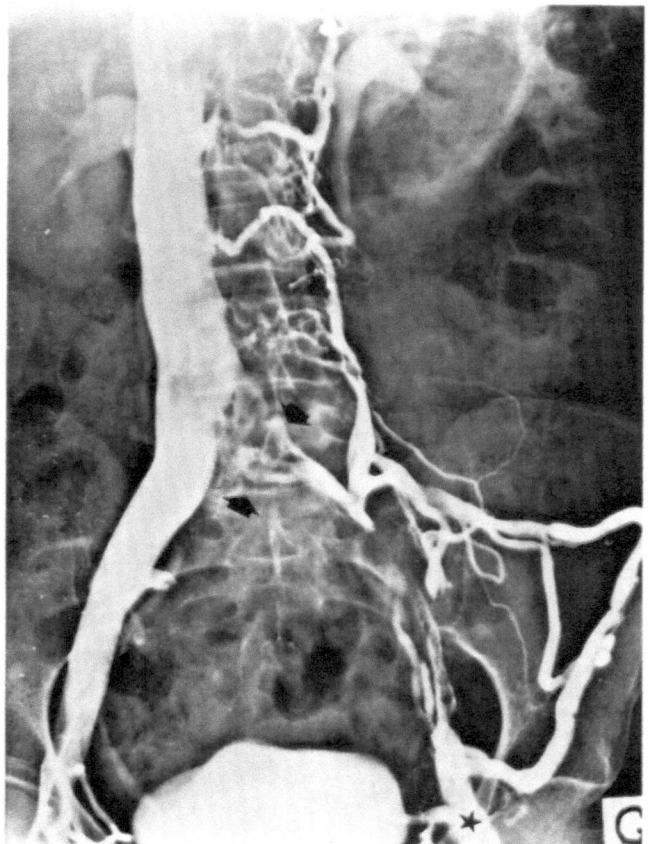

Fig. 255

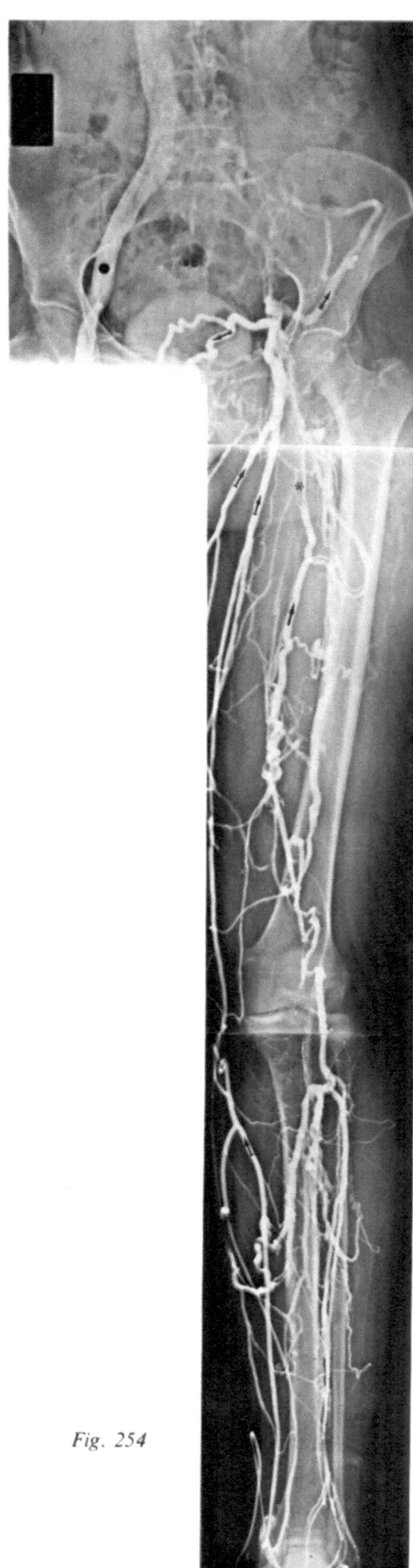

Fig. 254

Figs. 254 and 255.

254: Diffuse phlebitis in the entire left lower limb. Fairly good recanalization of the leg veins which remain, however, devoid of valves. The femoro-popliteal system is very poorly recanalized and collateral circulation is mainly via the profunda femoris vein ↑; there is a thrombus ∗ at the level of its opening into the common femoral vein. Therefore the internal saphenous vein ↕ ensures the major part of the collateral circulation of the left lower limb. Left iliac obliteration is witnessed by iliac ⬍ and suprapubic ↕ collateral circulation. The right system ● is opacified through this suprapubic circulation.

255: Bifemoral percutaneous cavography. On the left, the trocar ⋆ is within the ilio-femoral chronic thrombus. This cavography demonstrates the iliac pathway and gives evidence of a fenestrated aspect ➴ with numerous synechias of the left common iliac vein termination: Cockett's syndrome with underlying diffuse phlebitis in the chronic phase.

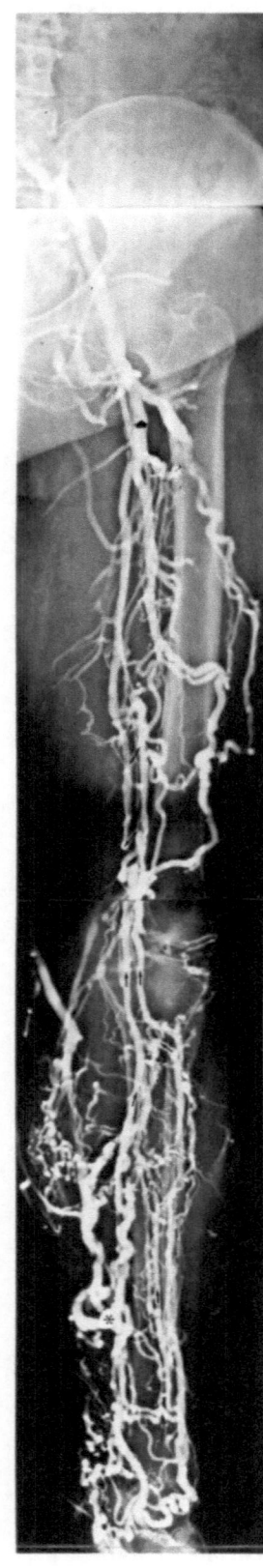

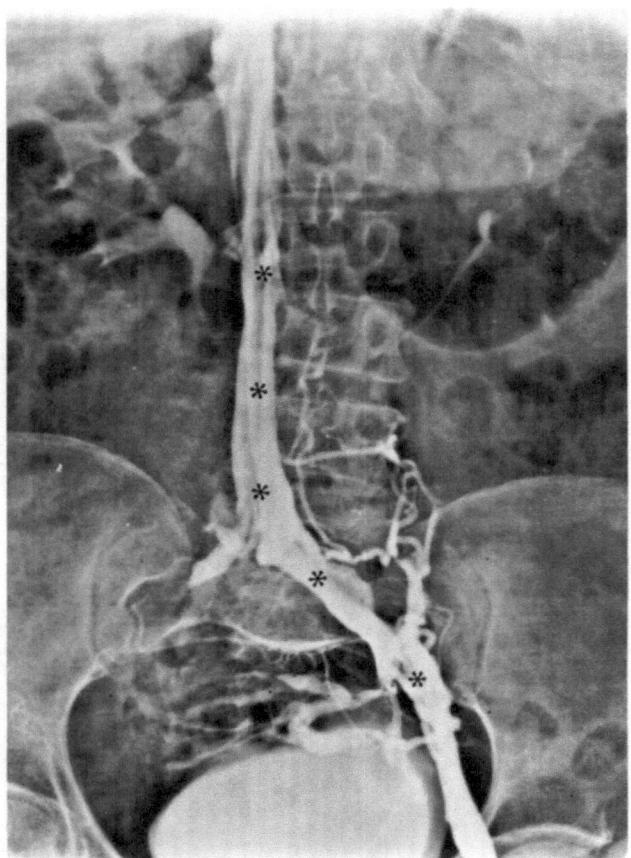

Fig. 257

Fig. 256

Figs. 256 and 257:

256: Diffuse chronic phlebitis of the entire left lower limb. Post-phlebitic varices of the leg. Relatively satisfactory recanalization of the deep veins of the leg which are avalvular ↑. At the level of the thigh, the venae comitantes with their ladder-like appearance ↓ have replaced the superficial femoral vein. The profunda femoris vein ▲ is opacified. Correct left ilio-femoral opacification.

257: Left unifemoral percutaneous ilio-cavography. Cavography shows that there is in fact a straticulate appearance* not only of the left iliac system but also of the infrarenal inferior vena cava *, proof of an associated ilio-caval involvement which was only poorly demonstrated by a non-pressurized venography. Importance of the cavography.

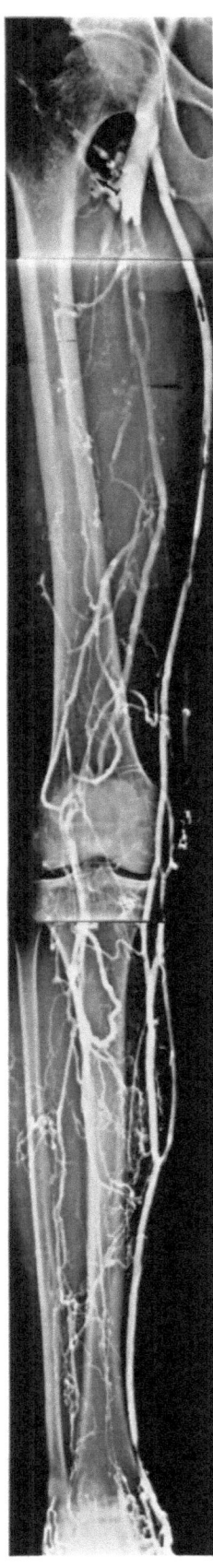

Fig. 258: Sural and femoro-popliteal chronic phlebitis of the right lower limb. Quasi non-existent recanalization of the deep system on the level of the leg as well as of the thigh. Collateral circulation is almost entirely ensured by the internal saphenous vein ↑, which is dilated and has no more valves. Right ilio-femoral patency with reflux into branches of the femoral neck ↑ up to the first valve. Venography of the lower limb with a large volume of contrast medium has the advantage of allowing demonstration of the ilio-femoral patency. Chronic phlebitis with poor recanalization of the deep system.

180

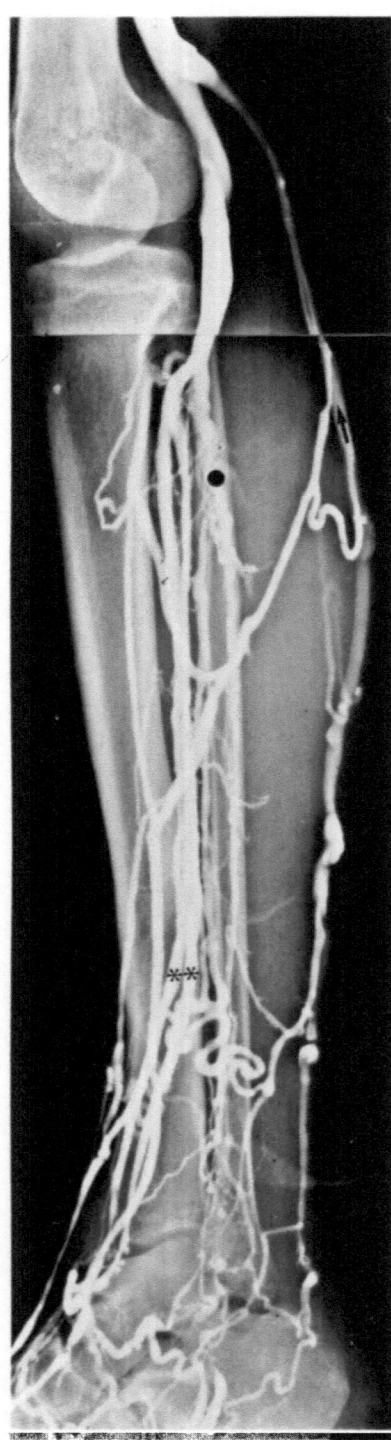

Fig. 259: Chronic sural phlebitis. Rather good recanalization of the anterior tibial veins ∗ (lateral projection) which are valveless. The posterior tibial veins ● have a straticulate appearance and very poor recanalization. Collateral circulation through the external saphenous vein ↑ at the posterior aspect of the leg; the external saphenous vein is becoming varicose. Note its rather high embouchment, well above the femoral condyles.

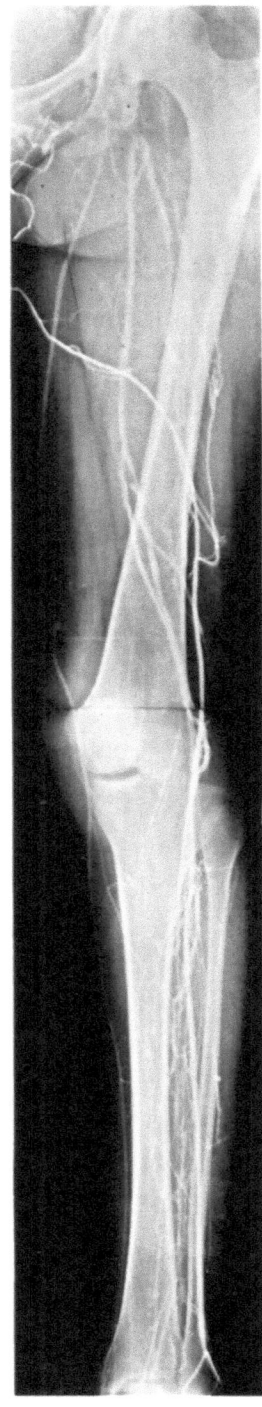

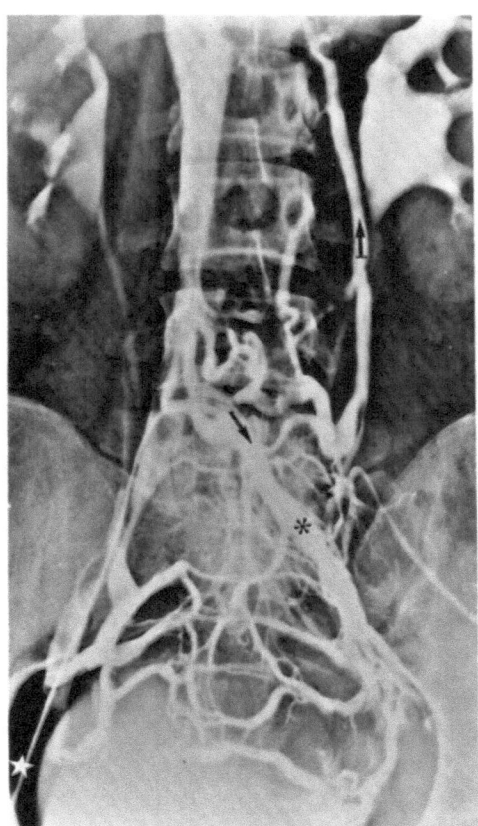

Fig. 261

Fig. 260

Figs. 260 and 261: Chronic phlebitis of the left lower limb.

260: Non-pressurized venography. No reopacification of the deep femoral system.

261: Contralateral iliocavography with the right * venous Seldinger technique: catheter tip in the left ↑ common iliac vein. Straticulate appearance of the left ∗ iliac venous system with fenestration and synechias on its termination: Cockett's syndrome with underlying chronic phlebitis with a hardly recanalized deep venous system. Note the anatomic variation with direct ending of a left ascending lumbar vein ↑ into the left renal vein. Patient with acute venous stasis, who developed, within 48 hours, ischemic phlebitis.

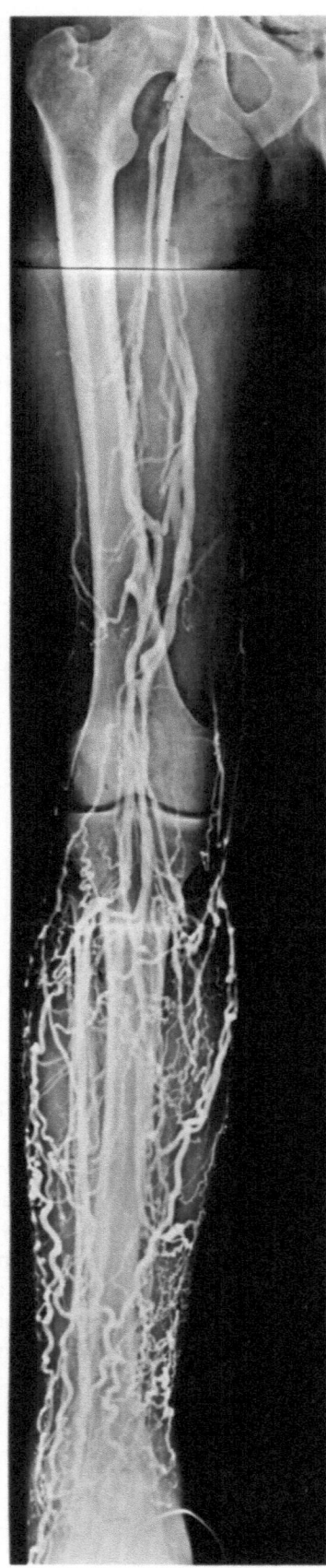

Fig. 262: Femoro-popliteal and sural chronic phlebitis. Quasi non-existent recanalization of the deep veins of the leg and development of a very marked varicose superficial circulation at the level of the leg. However, at the level of the thigh, the deep system is relatively well recanalized, and there is no varix. Disparity between the femoro-popliteal recanalization and the absence of recanalization of the deep leg veins accounts for the only sural location of post-phlebitic varices.

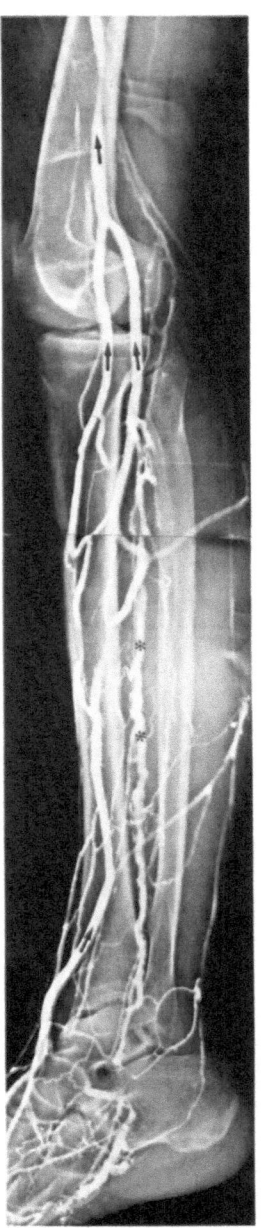

Fig. 264

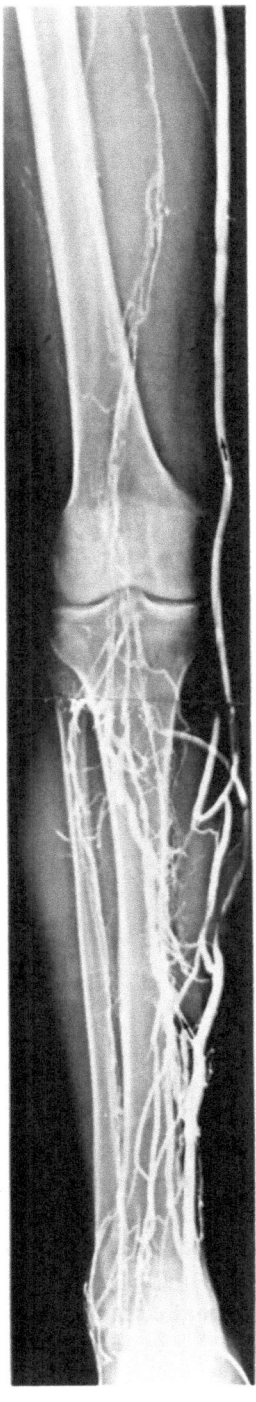

Fig. 263

Figs. 263 and 264: Chronic phlebitis of the left lower limb with involvement of the leg veins and of the femoro-popliteal vein. Importance of a biplane projection.

263: Frontal projection. Partial recanalization of the deep leg veins. This projection does not show the extent of recanalization of the deep leg veins. There is almost no femoro-popliteal recanalization, and the motor part of the remaining vein is occluded. Saphenous vein ↑.

264: Lateral projection. This projection demonstrates that recanalization of the leg veins is not as good as was thought, since only a part of the peroneal vein ✳✳ seems to be recanalized. Almost all leg veins which are seen on the frontal projection correspond in fact to branches of the internal saphenous vein which function as collateral circulation.

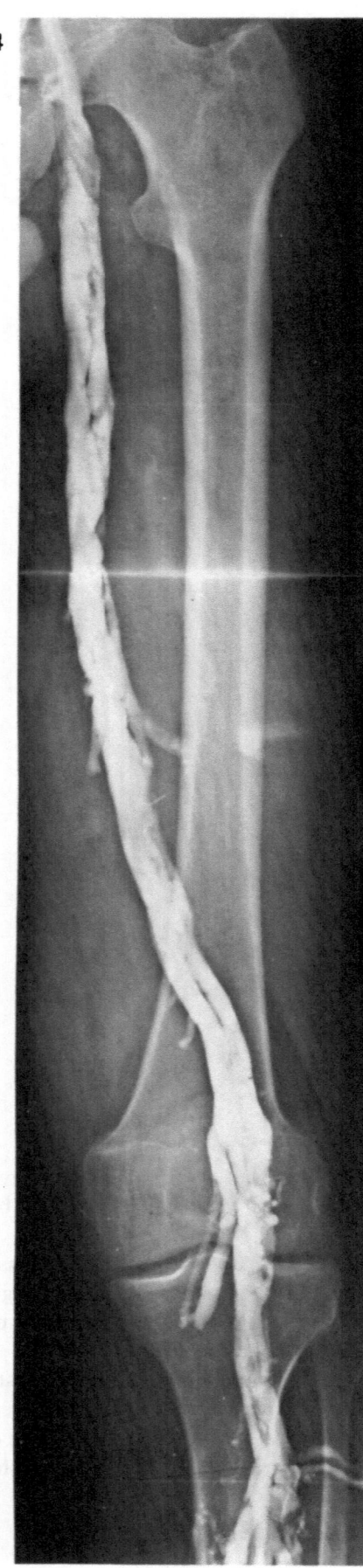

Fig. 265: Femoro-popliteal chronic phlebitis. Note the characteristic straticulate and irregular appearance of a chronic phlebitis in process of recanalization under heparin treatment. In this case there is no ladder-arranged anastomosis between the two femoral venous channels and it is very likely a matter of a recanalized superficial femoral vein, which is somewhat ectatic rather than of venae comitantes.

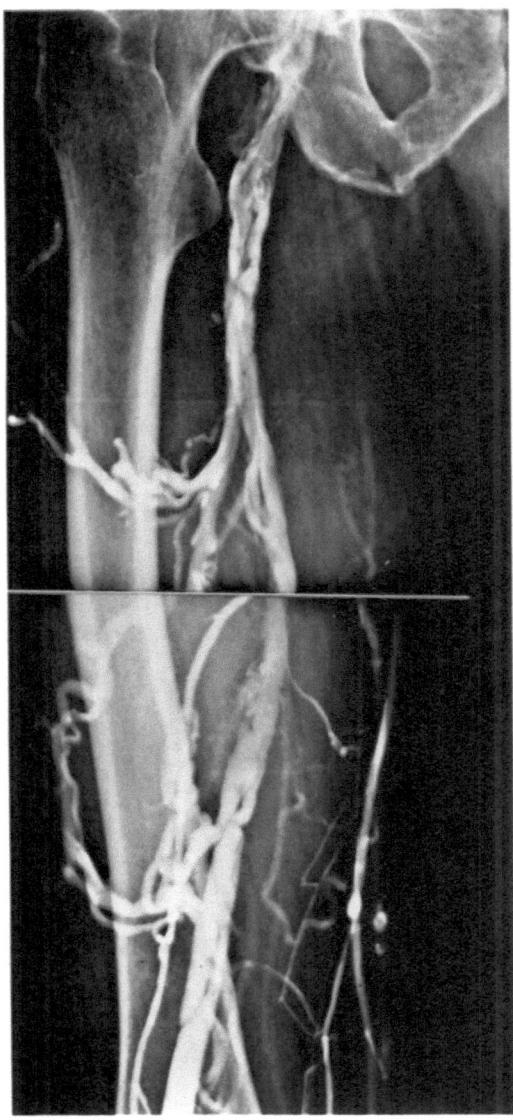

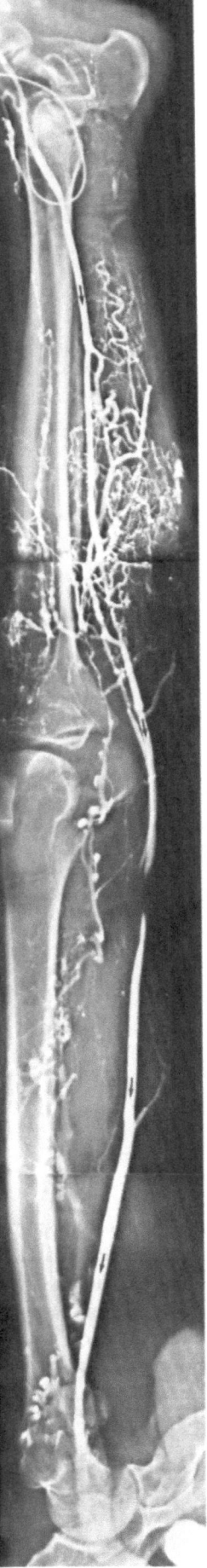

Fig. 266: Femoro-popliteal chronic phlebitis. Straticulate appearance of the superficial femoral system. Quite good recanalization of the femoro-popliteal system, under treatment by heparin.

Fig. 267: Chronic phlebitis of the left lower limb. Lateral projection. Phlebitis occurred one year earlier. Occurrence of a mass in the left calf. Suspicion of tumor of the soft parts. In this chronic phlebitis venography shows it to be, in fact, a venous "sponge" due to collateral circulation, with almost no recanalized deep system. The whole collateral circulation is through the calf muscle veins and the internal saphenous system ↑.

186

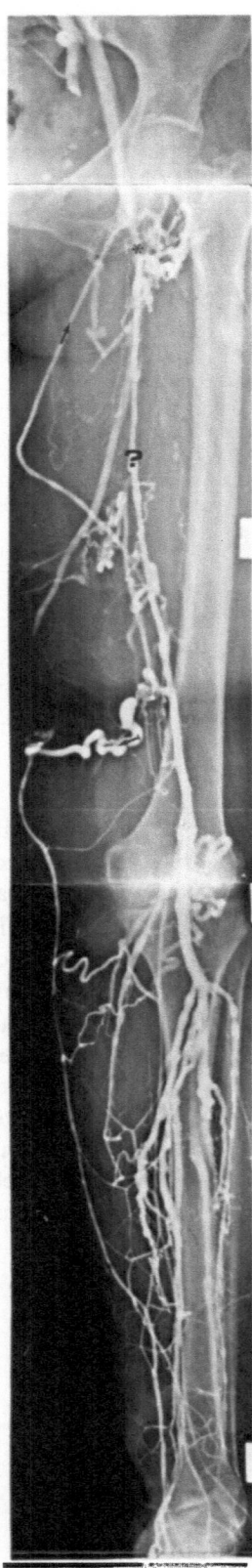

Fig. 268: Femoro-popliteal chronic phlebitis. All three deep veins of the leg seem to be patent and to have valves. From this frontal projection, only, it is difficult to give a name to the vein visualized on the thigh ? to drain the venous flow in the leg. Nevertheless, this drainage is inefficient in so far as the vein is cut off∗ below the common femoral vein, and, paradoxically, the venous drainage of the lower limb is mainly ensured by the superficial system. Note also that a large perforating vein is dilated at the Hunter's canal ⥯. The iliac vein is patent. In conlusion: chronic femoral phlebitis, inserted between two iliac and sural spared segments.

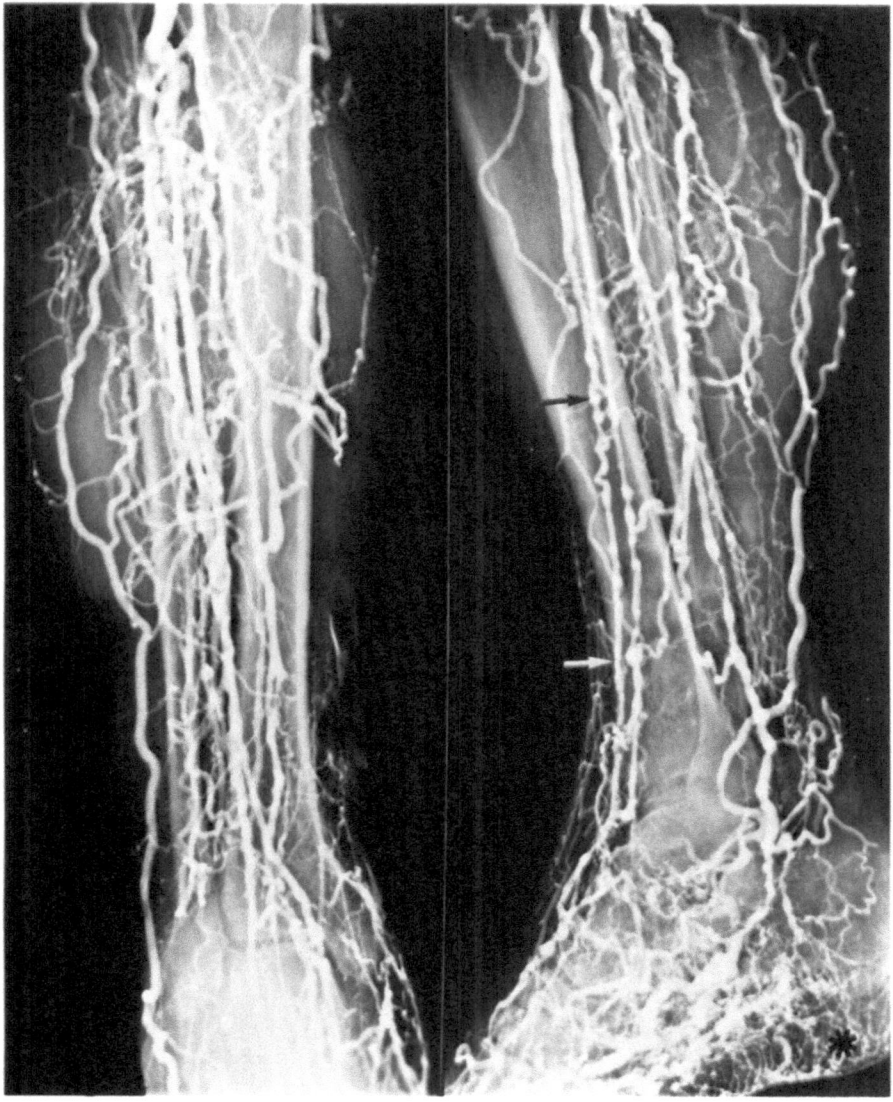

Fig. 269   Fig. 270

Figs. 269 and 270: Ancient sural phlebitis.
269: Frontal projection. Voluminous superficial derivation. From this one projection it is difficult to know whether there is complete recanalization of one or of several groups of deep leg veins.
270: Lateral projection demonstrating the anterior tibial ⭡ veins to be patent and valvulated. The phlebogram also includes the foot and shows obliteration of the plantar veins supplied by large derivations with reflux into the plantar venous system of the foot ∗.

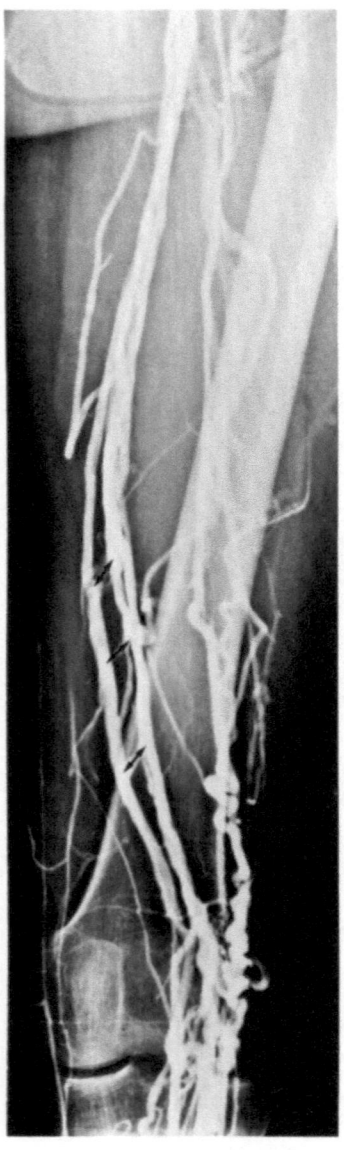

Fig. 271

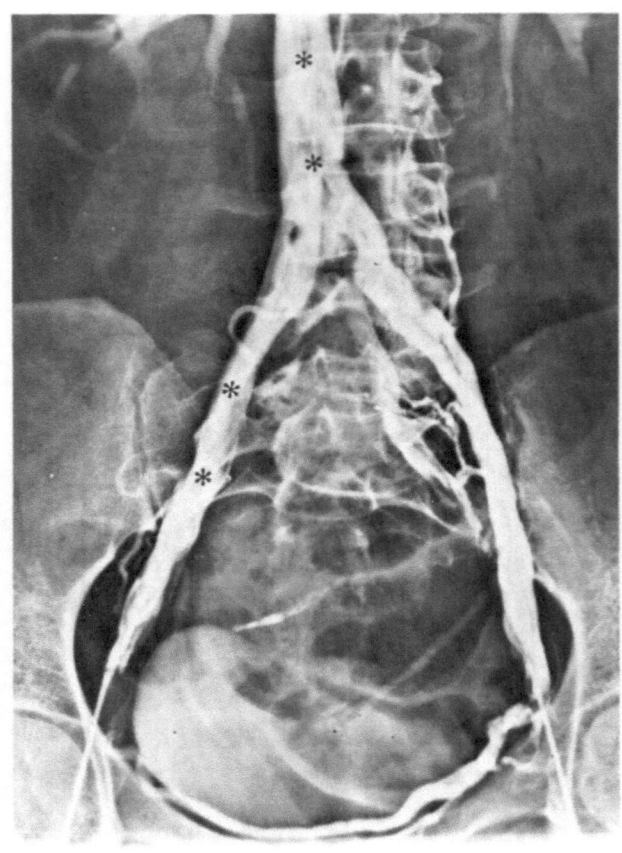

Fig. 272

Figs. 271 and 272: Chronic phlebitis of the left lower limb.
271: Film centered onto the thigh showing an ancient femoro-popliteal phlebitis with recanalization through venae comitantes ↕, anastomosed in a ladder-like fashion around the superficial femoral pedicle.
272: Bifemoral percutaneous ilio-cavography. This technique demonstrates the existence of an ancient chronic ilio-caval phlebitis with straticulate recanalization changes ∗∗. It also shows that the right iliac system is not normal (straticulate appearance ∗∗) and that there seems to be bilateral phlebitis, the right localization having passed undetected.

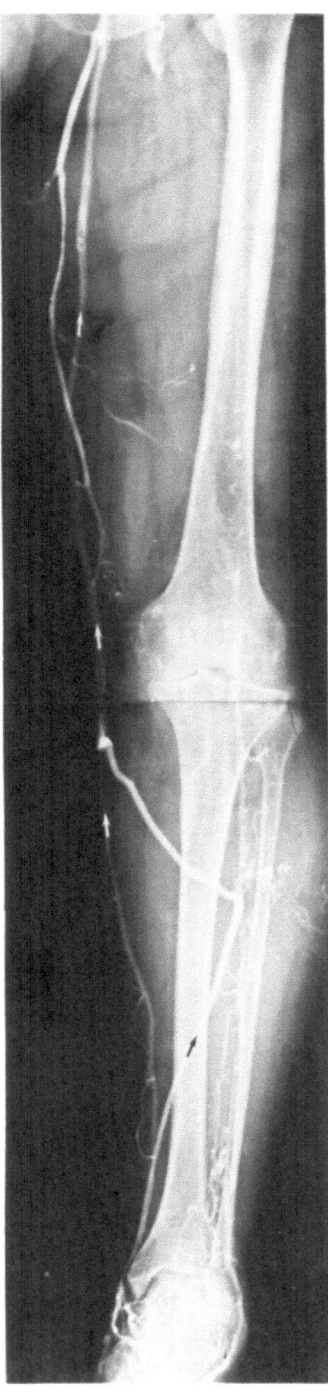

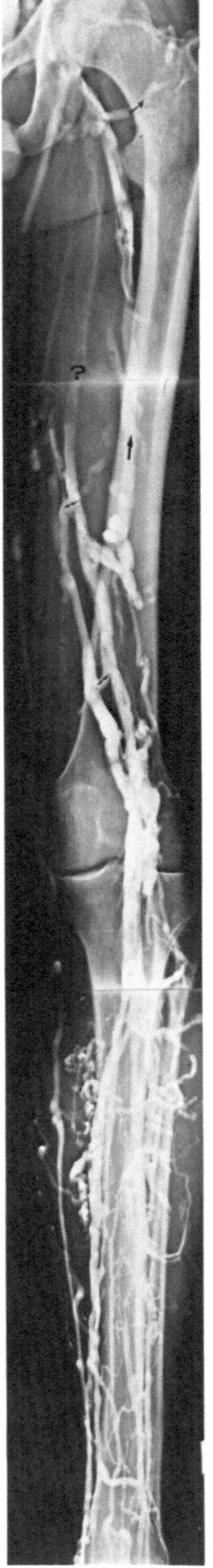

Fig. 273: Chronic phlebitis of the left lower limb. Patient had major clinical signs of chronic venous incompetence. No recanalization of the deep venous system. Circulation is ensured only by the internal saphenous system ↑.

Fig. 274: Chronic iliac phlebitis of the left lower limb. Sural and femoro-popliteal involvement. Partial recanalization of the deep veins of the leg. Straticulate appearance of the femoro-popliteal vein and opacification of the venae comitantes ↓ anastomosed in a ladder-like fashion. The injection rate is too low and there is some streaming in the upper part of the superficial femoral axis ?. Blood is partly drained due to the profunda femoris ↑ vein toward the common femoral vein. Note opacification of the femoral neck veins ↑.

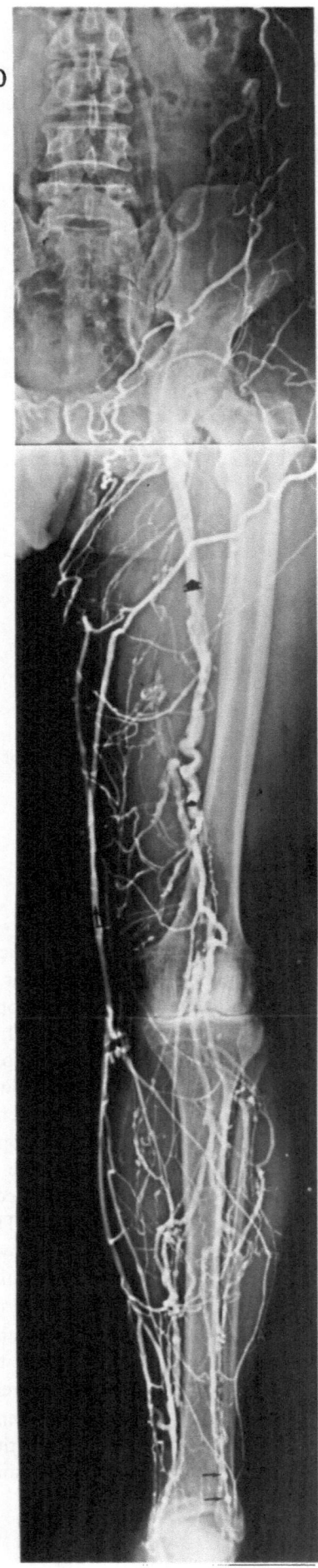

190

Fig. 275: Chronic phlebitis of the left lower limb. The anterior tibial veins ↑ which are seen on the external malleolus seem to be competent and valvulated in their lower part. Collateral circulation via the internal saphenous system ↕, though this is obliterated at the level of its termination. Opacification on the thigh occurs via a retro-adductor vein, and then via the profunda femoris ♠ vein, which is markedly enlarged. There is very faint opacification of the lift iliac vein and almost all blood is drained by superficial veins of the anterolateral abdominal wall. This type of collateral circulation is proof of associated and probably very long-standing obliteration of the inferior vena cava. This was confirmed by a descending cavography (not shown).

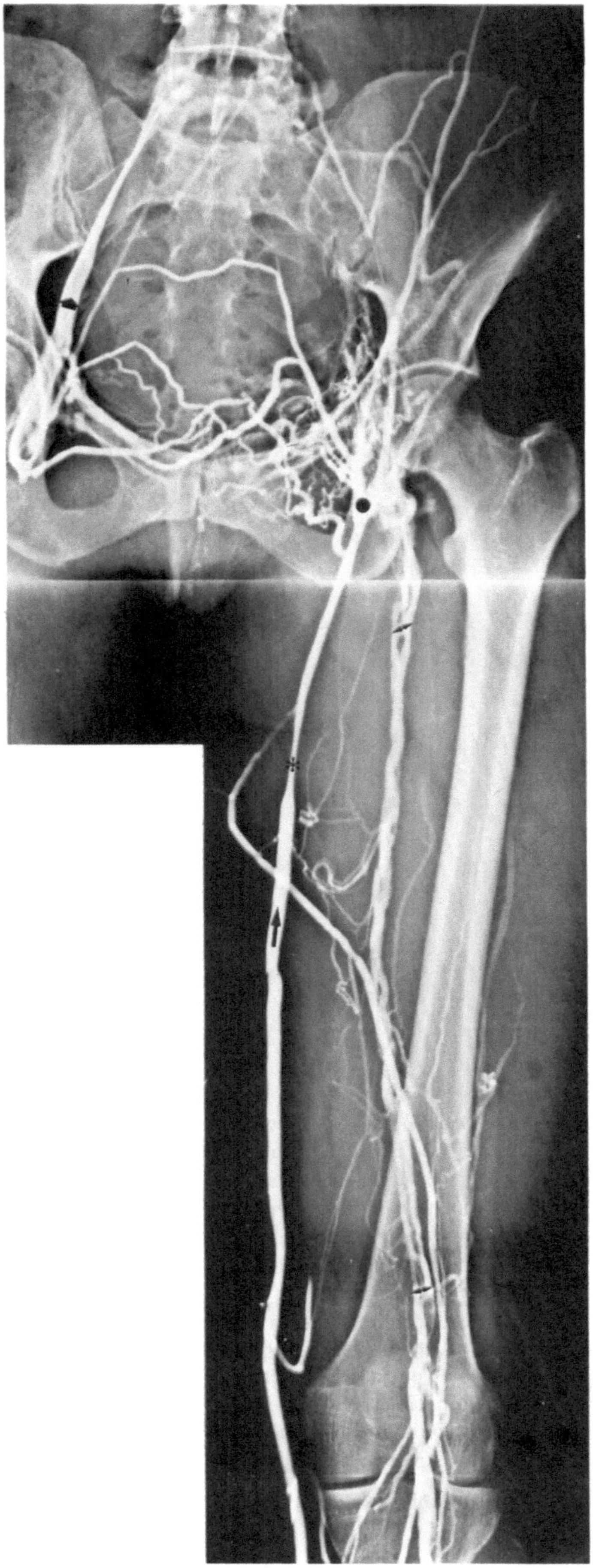

Fig. 276: Chronic phlebitis of the left lower limb, involving only the iliac and the femoro-popliteal segment. Collateral circulation through a large internal saphenous vein ↑ which is dilated, except for its upper part where it is narrowed * over 3 to 4 cm. Opacification of venae comitantes ↑ along the superficial femoral pedicle. The left iliac obliteration is demonstrated by the iliac and suprapubic opacification via branches of the termination of the left internal saphenous vein ●. Reopacification of the right iliac system ⬅.

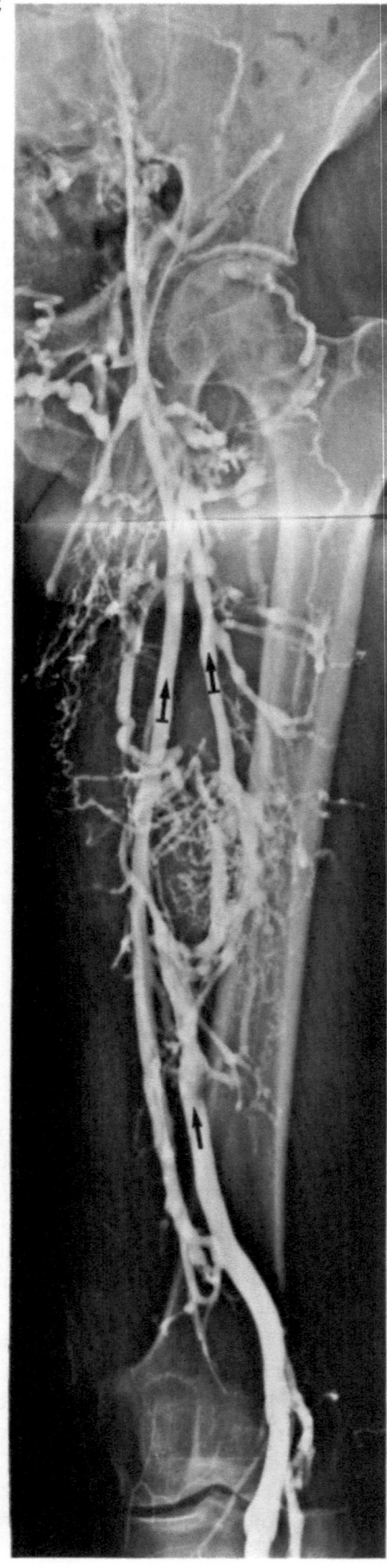

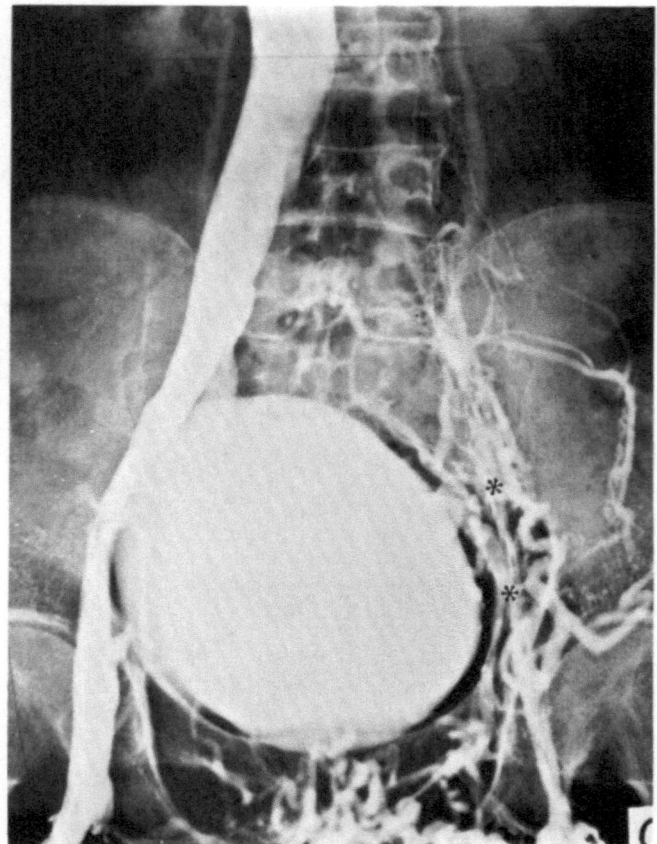

Fig. 278

Fig. 277

Figs. 277 and 278: Left ilio-femoro-popliteal chronic phlebitis.
277: Fairly good popliteal recanalization. Good recanalization of
the lower superficial femoral system ↑ though with marked collateral circulation through the profunda femoris vein ↑. Iliac
obliteration proved by the presence of suprapubic varices. Duplication of the profunda femoris vein ↑.

278: Bifemoral percutaneous cavography. Puncture into a chronic
thrombus of the left femoral vein. The iliac system is very
moderately recanalized. The left iliac route is straticulate * and
there is no opacification of the left common iliac vein.
The iliac phlebitis is not recanalized, whereas the femoro-popliteal
phlebitis undergoes a much better recanalization.

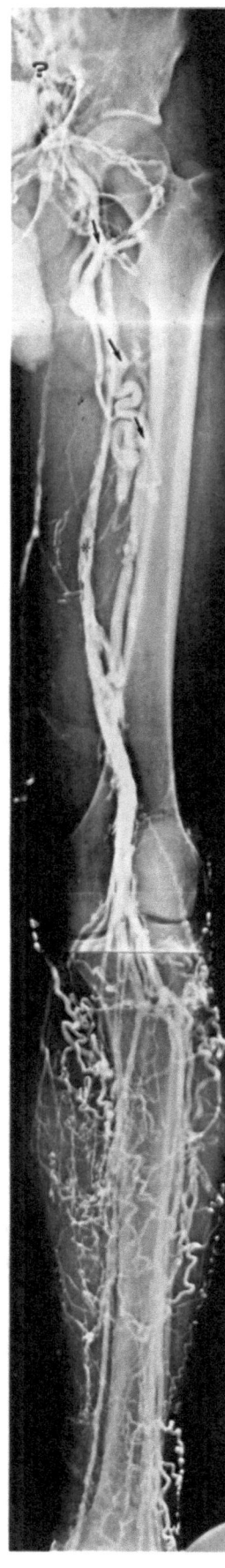

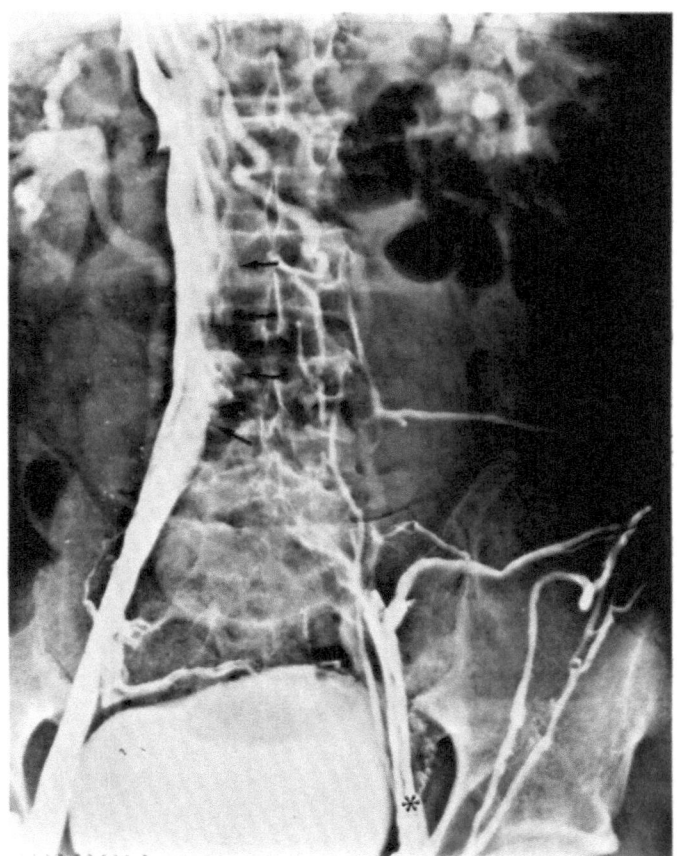

Fig. 280

Fig. 279

Figs. 279 and 280: Diffuse chronic phlebitis extending from the left iliac venous confluence to the deep veins of the lower limbs.

279: No recanalization of the deep leg veins. Very marked and slightly varicose superficial network. Straticulate appearance of the femoro-popliteal axis ∗. Note the existence of varicose dilatations ↑ at the upper and posterior third of the thigh, branched on the internal saphenous system ↑; they are seen on this projection to "falsely" take the place of the profunda femoris vein. Very faint left iliac opacification ?.

280: Bifemoral percutaneous cavography. Catheterization of a left femoral chronic thrombus. Straticulate appearance of the left external iliac vein ∗. No filling of the left common iliac vein. The irregular appearance of the infrarenal inferior vena cava is probably related to phlebitic obliteration undergoing recanalization; in fact, the radiolucent structures seen along its left aspect cannot be due to the left iliac flow ↑↑↑, since this is obliterated: it is thus a matter of ilio-caval chronic phlebitis undergoing recanalization.

Note, as in most of the cases demonstrated in this chapter, the very significant predominance of phlebites involving the left lower limb.

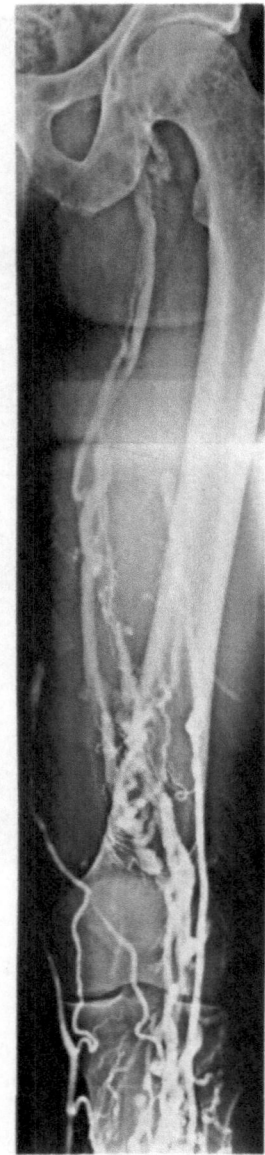

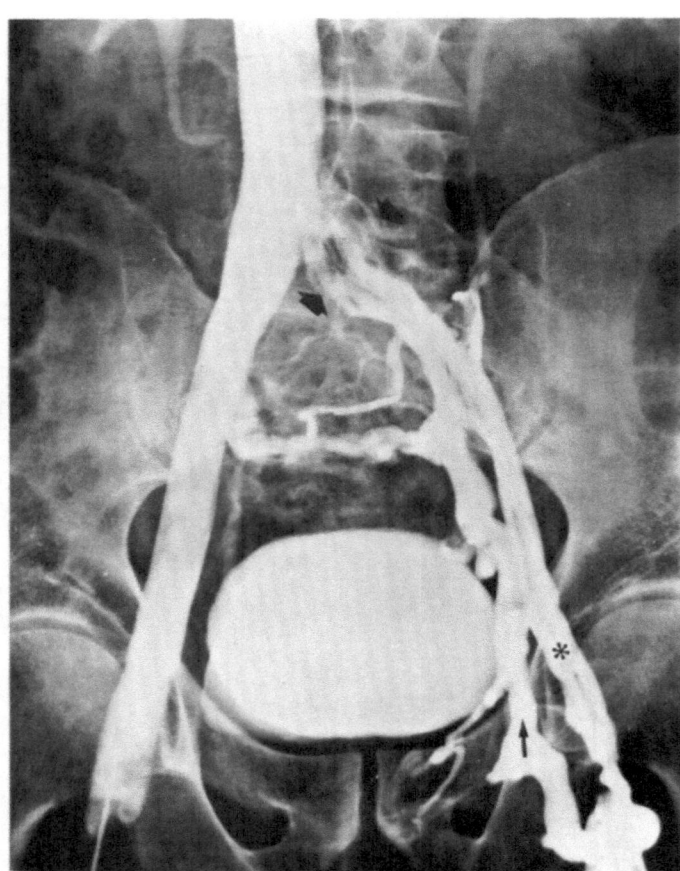

Fig. 282

Fig. 281

Figs. 281 and 282: Ilio-femoro-sural chronic phlebitis of the left lower limb.

281: Venogram of the left lower limb. Pooling of contrast medium in the post-phlebitic varices of the leg. In spite of a high rate injection of 100 ml of contrast, there is very faint opacification of the recanalized superficial femoral vein, due to stagnation in the varices of the leg.

282: Bifemoral percutaneous cavography. Rather low left femoral catheterization. Opacification of a gross obturator vein ↑ and of the straticulate * left iliofemoral system. Cockett's syndrome with fenestration, synechia and flattening of the termination of the left common iliac vein ◆◆.

Because of the presence of post-phlebitic varices of the leg, and without cavography, it would have been quite impossible to diagnose phlebitis of the common iliac vein with downward progression of the thrombosis.

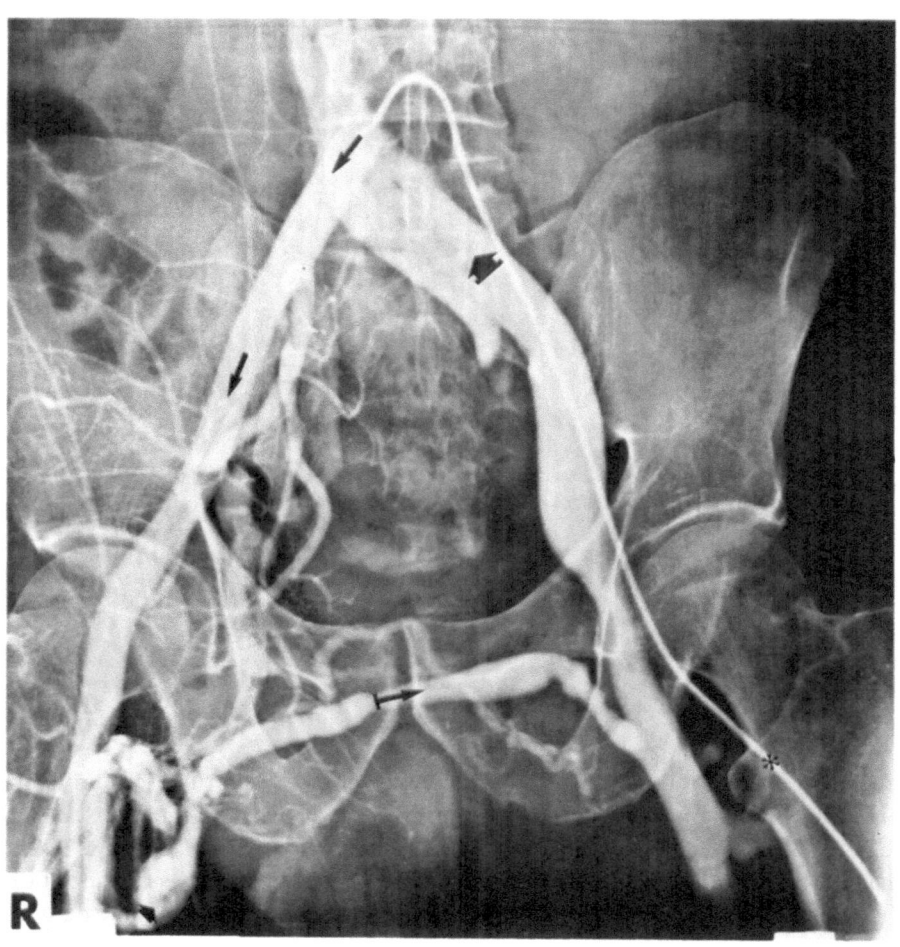

Fig. 283: Right iliac chronic phlebitis treated by arterialization (Palma's operation, see diagram in Fig. 284C). Control of this operation by a downstream right iliac arteriography ↑. Left femoral Seldinger ∗. Successive opacification of the right iliac artery ↑, then of the arteriovenous fistula in the right Scarpa's triangle ●, of the internal saphenous vein transposed ↕ in the retropubic area, and finally of the left iliac venous system ♠, thus decompressing the right iliac chronic phlebitis.

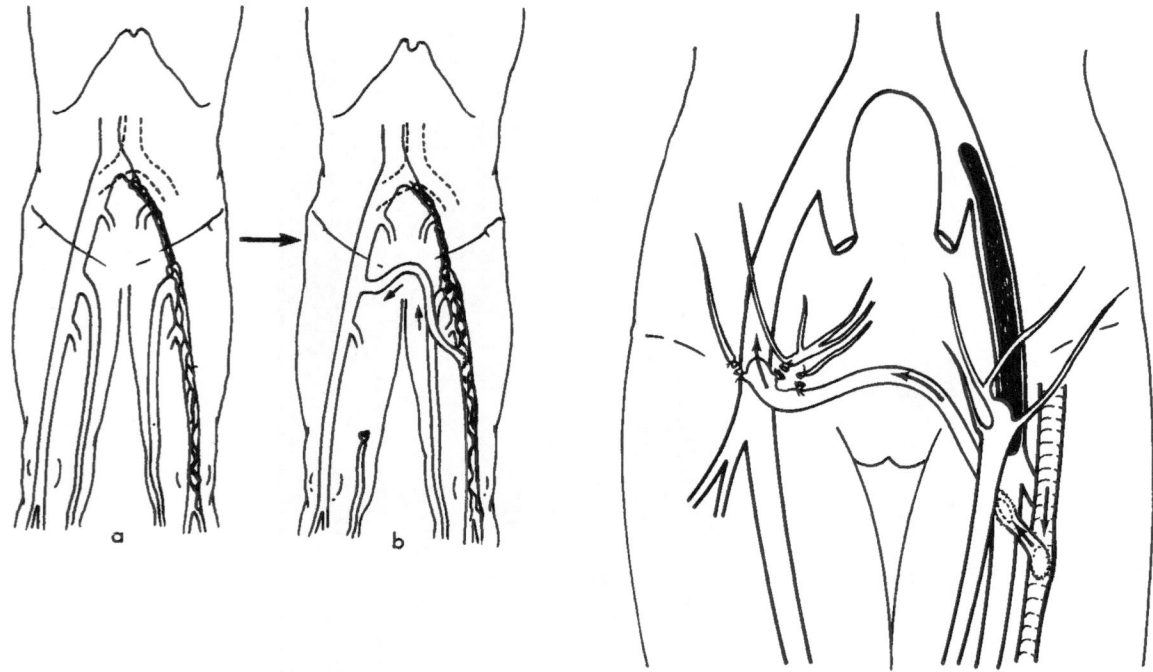

Figs. 284A, B and C: Surgery in ilio-femoral chronic venous incompetence. A: Pattern of left ilio-femoral diffuse chronic phlebitis. B: So-called Palma operation with transposition of the right internal saphenous branched onto the left femoral venous pathway. (Redrawn from H. Dodd and F.B. Cockett, p. 242, fig. 16.19.) C: So-called Palma operation with arterialization associated to internal saphenous transposition; a transient arteriovenous fistula keeps the venous flow patent. In this latter case it is a matter of isolated left iliac obliteration.

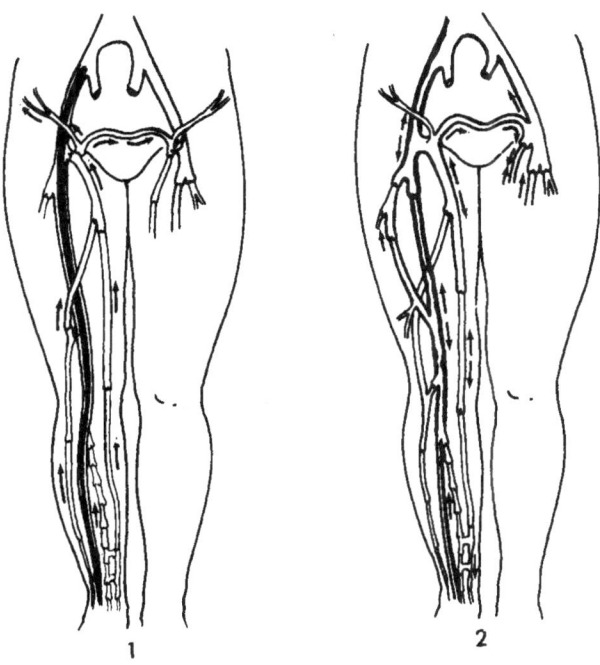

Figs. 285, 1 and 2:

285,1: Diagram showing extended obliteration of the ilio-femoral segment. The communicating veins derive the blood in the superficial network. The internal saphenous vein drains the whole blood of the lower limb, and the branches of its termination function in the upstream direction.

285,2: Appearance of chronic phlebitis undergoing recanalization changes in the deep system. Note that the valves are destroyed in the superficial network and in the deep veins, thus allowing bidirectional flow.

Chapter 8

VARICES AND VENOGRAPHY

Figures 286–304

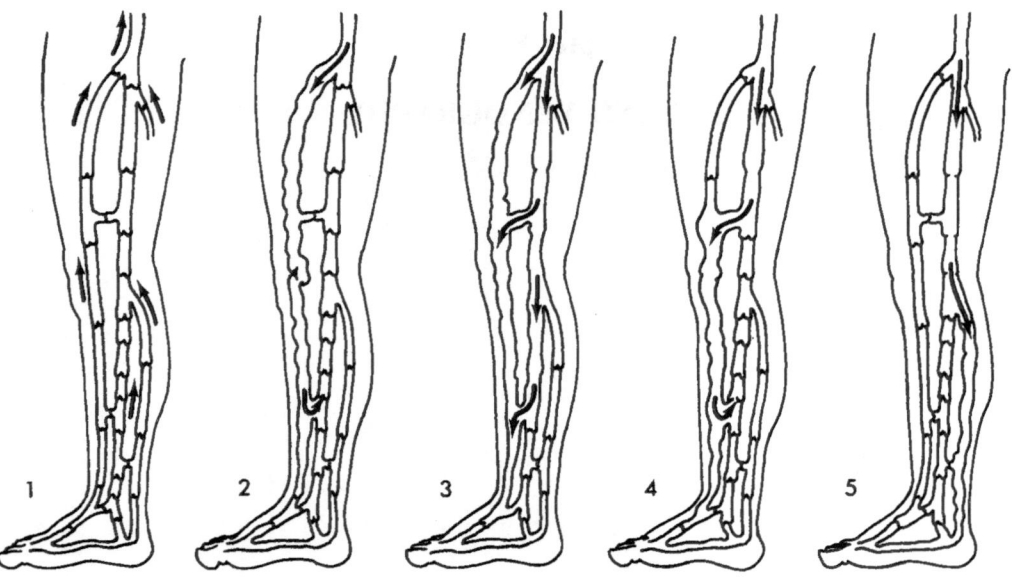

Fig. 286: Diagram showing the main types of varices.

1: Normal venous flow.

2: Varices by isolated ostial incompetence of the valve of the internal saphenous vein.

3: Varices with a triple mechanism. i) Femoro-popliteal post-phlebitic acquired destruction of valves; ii) ostial incompetence of the termination of the internal saphenous vein; iii) incompetence of the perforating veins at the thigh and at the leg.

4: Varices with a double mechanism. i) Post-phlebitic acquired femoral incompetence of valves; ii) incompetence of a perforating vein at the thigh.

5: Varices with a double mechanism. i) External saphenous varices by ostial incompetence of the external saphenous termination; ii) post-phlebitic acquired valvular incompetence of the deep femoro-popliteal system.

Essential varicose veins coexist with normal deep venous trunks. The other varices associate extended deterioration of the superficial and of the deep venous system, the latter being most often post-phlebitic and much more rarely congenital. This latter condition does not correspond exactly to varices but rather to a global chronic insufficiency of the entire deep and superficial venous system. The theoretical distinction of two types of varices does not always correspond to the reality which may be much more complex.

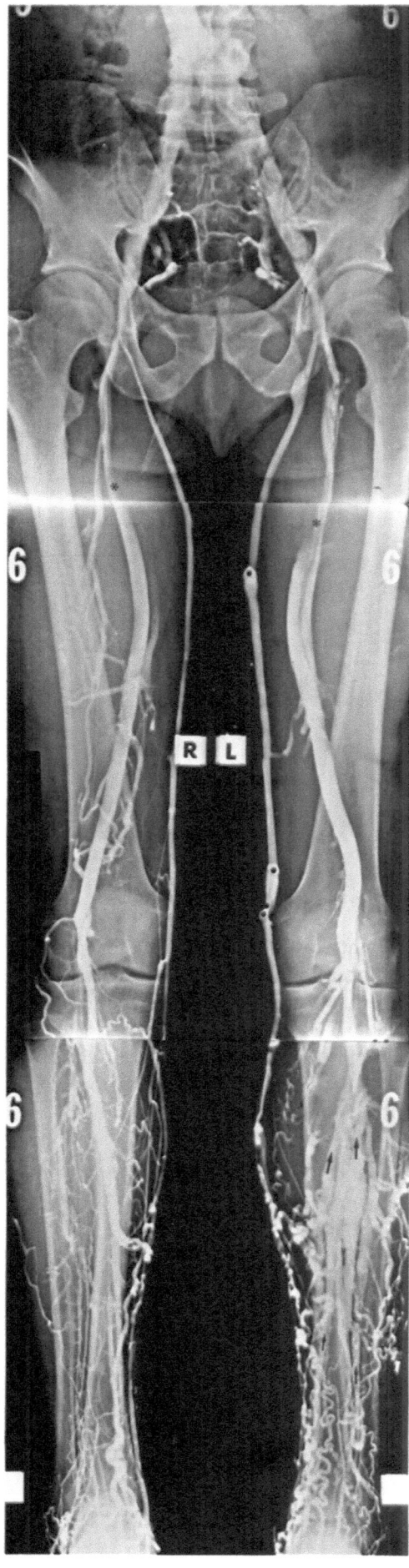

Fig. 287: Bilateral venography with non-pressurized injection. Female presenting with bilateral essential varices. Note the artefact occurring very frequently with this bilateral technique when only 100 ml of contrast materal are injected: Dilution flow ✱ with false stenosis of the upper part of both superficial femoral veins. Varices of the leg on both sides. On the left, good opacification of the deep trunks ↑ rules out post-phlebitic sequelae at this level. On the right, the opacification is very fragmentary: is it a matter of a technical artefact or of an old phlebitis of the right leg? Note the enlarged appearance of the left internal saphenous vein with pseudo-ectasis ● which could lead to suspected ostial incompetence of the termination, without the utilized technique confirming it. Only a dynamic phlebogram in the vertical position suggests ostial incompetence of the internal saphenous vein termination.

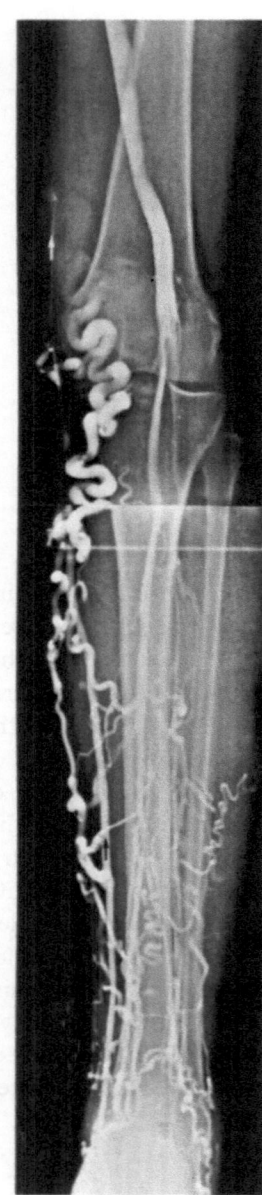

Fig. 288: Venography of the right lower limb with a non-pressurized injection. Partial filling of the deep veins of the leg. Varicose veins of the leg and of the thigh branched on the internal saphenous system. The internal saphenous vein proper is not dilated ↑ and one can consider that incompetence of the perforators of the leg plays a predominant part in the origin of these varices. Inadequate study of the deep venous system of the leg.

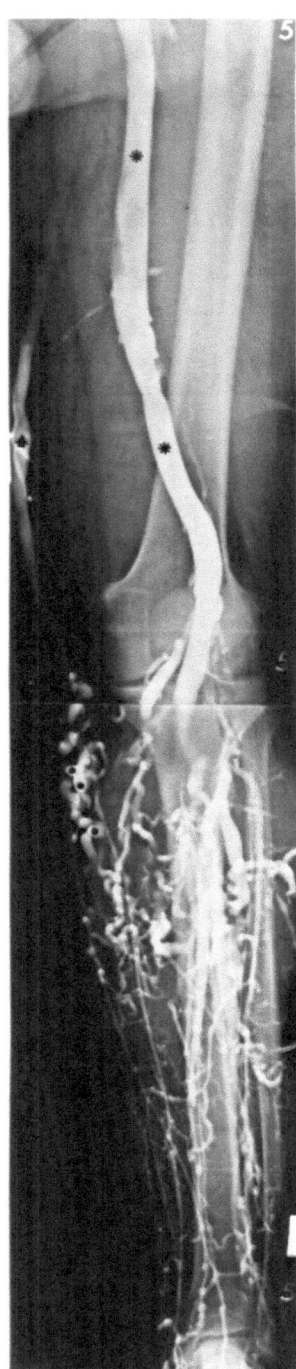

Fig. 289: Phlebography of the left lower limb with a non-pressurized injection. Partial opacification of the deep veins of the leg. Varicose internal saphenous vein ● with dilatation of the internal saphenous vein ♠. Reflux into the perforating veins at the leg. Pseudo-ectatic appearance of the femoropopliteal vein ∗ with poorly visible valves. A phlebography performed in the supine position does not affirm the presence of acquired or congenital incompetence of the valves. Retrograde femoral phlebography (not shown) rules out any valvular incompetence of the deep venous trunks and shows ostial incompetence of the internal saphenous vein termination.

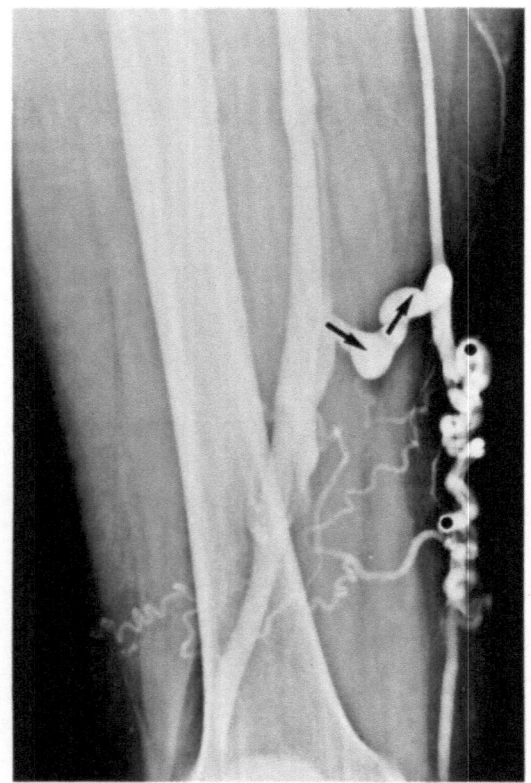

Fig. 290: Pre-varicose stage. Reflux into the still tubular internal saphenous vein through the perforating veins of the knee ↑ from the femoro-popliteal axis. Small varices ● localized to the lower third of thigh. Note the ectatic appearance of the incompetent perforating vein at the knee.

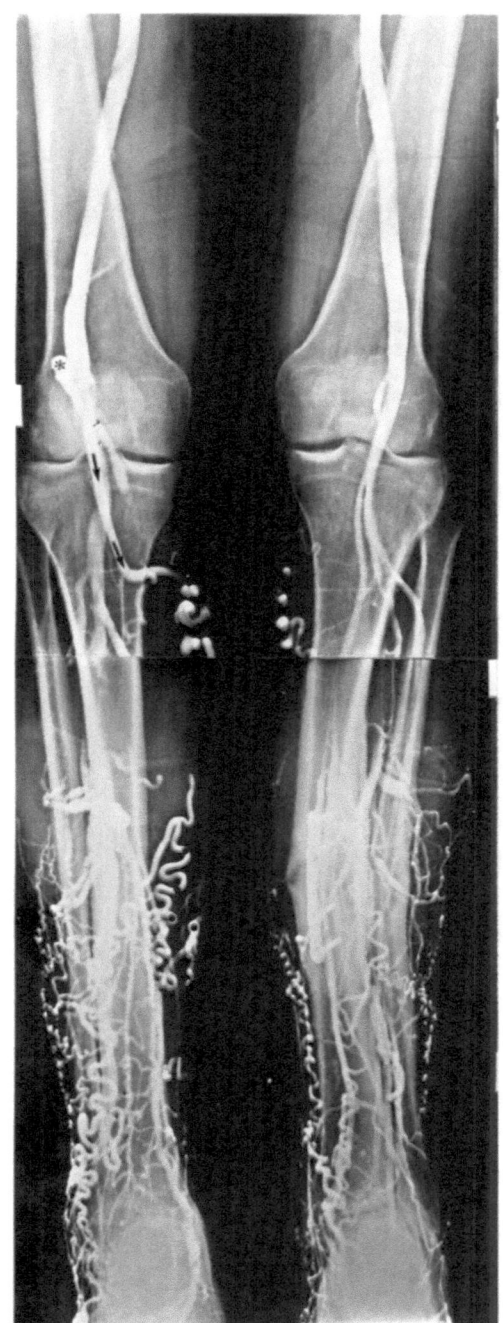

Fig. 291: Bilateral phlebography with free flow injection in a patient with so-called essential varices. In fact, old fracture of the left leg with post-phlebitic varices and incomplete obstruction of the deep veins of the left leg. On this frontal projection the varices of the right leg seem to be located on the internal aspect of the leg •. A lateral view will show that they are in fact branched on the external ↑ saphenous vein. Interest of the phlebography: it shows on the left side post-phlebitic varices due to post-traumatic phlebitis, and on the right the presence of varices localized to the external saphenous vein due to ostial incompetence of the external saphenous termination *.

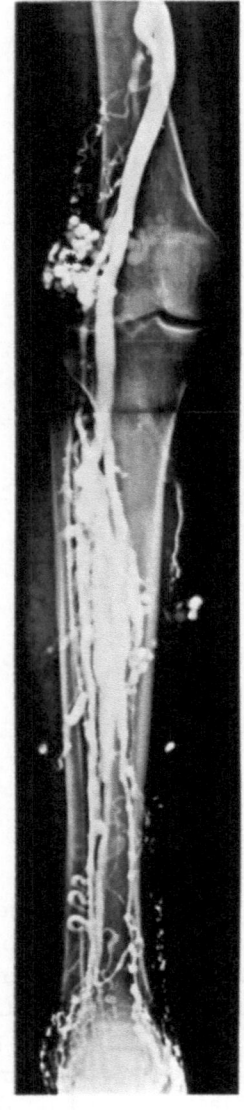

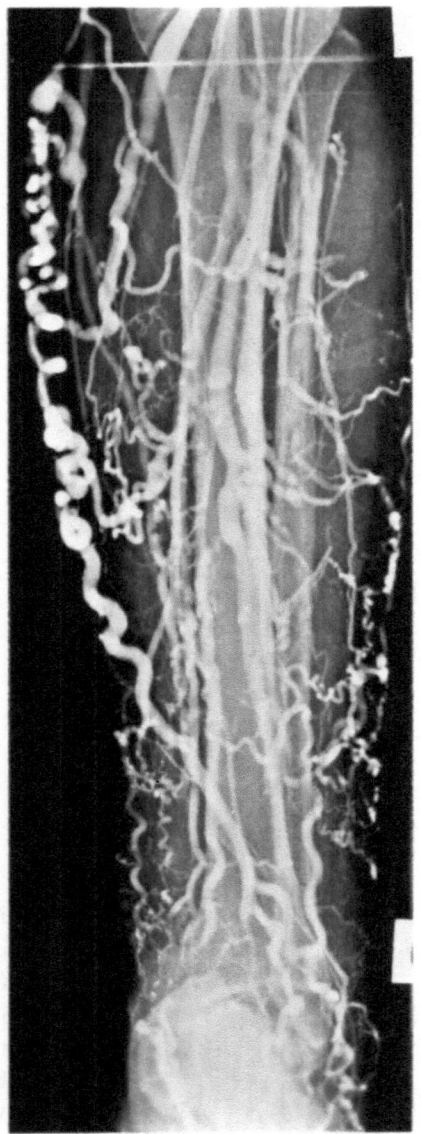

Fig. 293

Fig. 292: Patient who underwent a phlebography of the right lower limb for suspicion of a tumor of the soft tissues in the popliteal space. In fact, it is a voluminous bunch of varices branched on the external saphenous vein * with some discrete varicose veins on the leg, and specially on the ankle.

Figs. 293 and 294:
293: Varicose veins on the leg: frontal projection. On this simple projection it is quite impossible to locate the saphenous system which feeds the varices.
294: (lateral view): the varices are mainly varices of the external ↑ saphenous vein, at the posterior aspect of the thigh. Interest of biplane phlebographic projections for the topographic study of varicose veins.

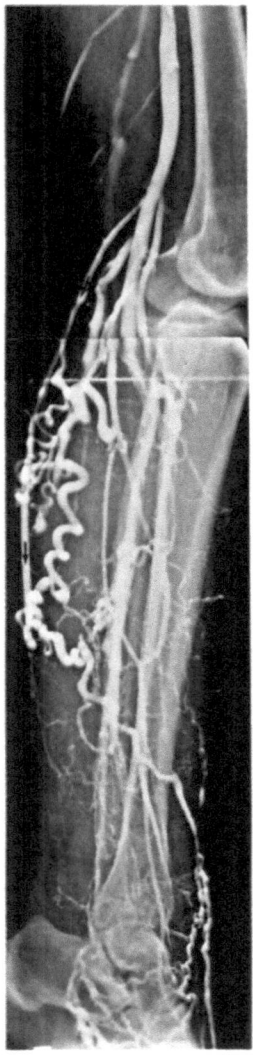

Fig. 294

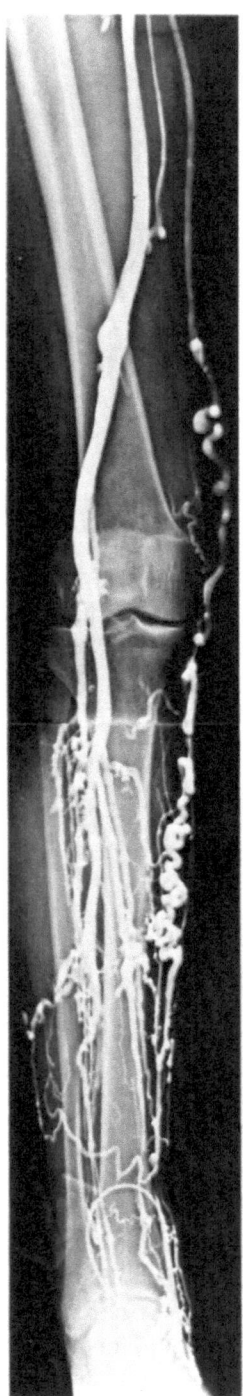

Fig. 295: Phlebography of the right lower limb with a free flow injection. Competence of the entire deep venous system. Internal saphenous varices on the leg and thigh (lower third). Above, the internal saphenous vein is not enlarged but no valve is demonstrated: It is thus probably a matter of saphenous valvular incompetence without any enlargement in its upper part, with, in addition, some incompetent perforating veins in the right leg.

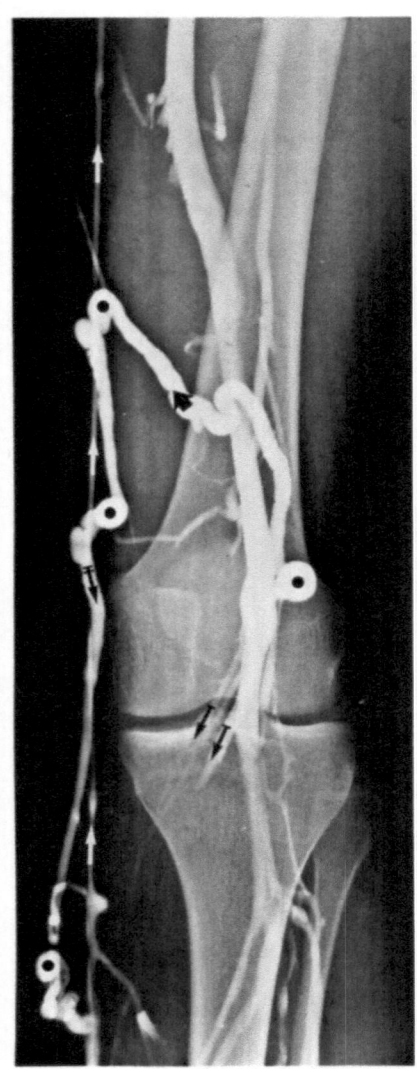

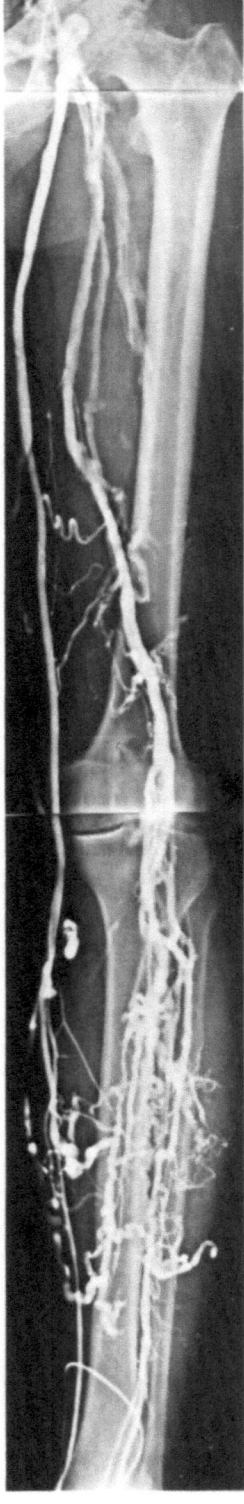

Fig. 296: Phlebography of the left lower limb with a free flow injection. Reflux into the internal gastrocnemial veins ⬆. Varicose dilatation of a superficial anastomosis between the external and the internal saphenous system. Thus, it is not a dilated perforating vein, but a reflux, due to incompetence of the external saphenous vein termination, via a superficial anastomosis ◆ toward the internal saphenous vein which remains very slender ⬆. In the present case, the reflux is slightly descending ⬇, but it may also, through the vein of Giacomini, be ascending toward the internal saphenous vein in the upper thigh.

Fig. 297: Recent varicose veins of the left leg, thought to be essential varices. Phlebography of the left lower limb by free flow injection. This patient was shown to have entirely unknown chronic phlebitis with partial recanalization of the deep femoro-popliteal system, and partial obstruction of the deep veins of the leg. Slight enlargement of the internal saphenous vein with gross varicose veins on the leg. Interest of phlebography in sequelae of clinically unknown phlebitis.

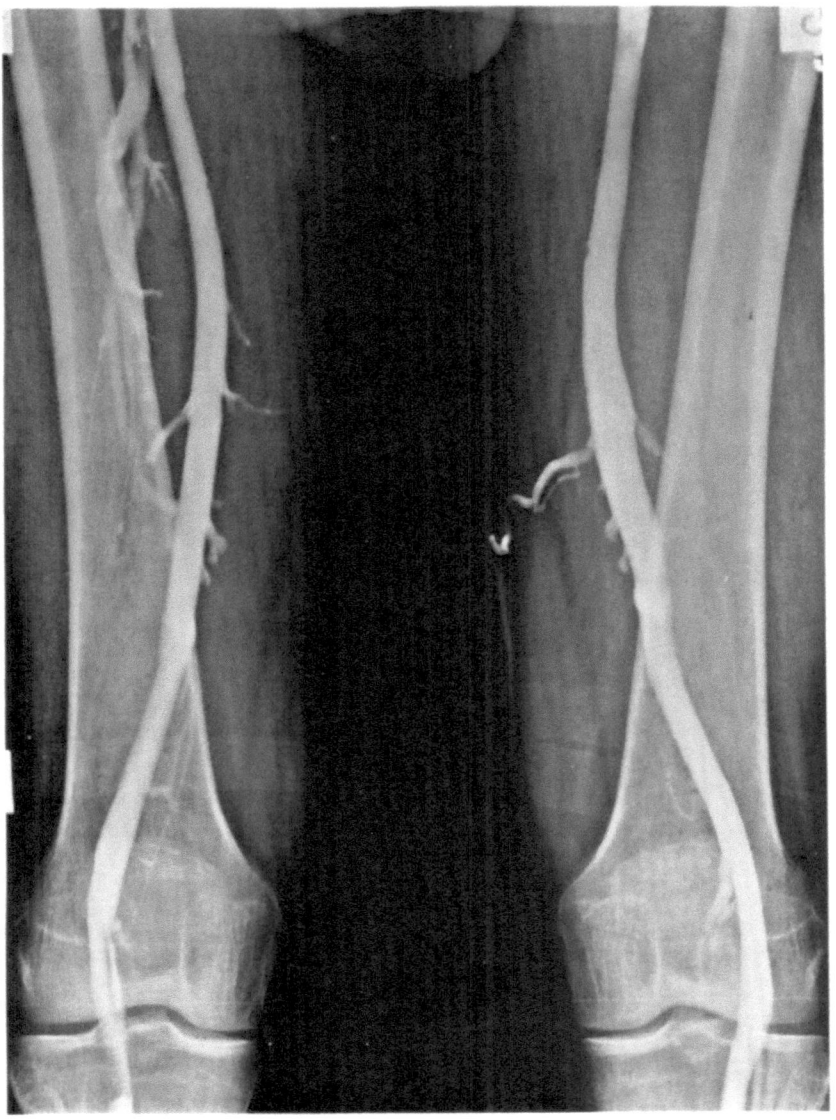

Fig. 298

Figs. 298 and 299: Importance of phlebography in the vertical position.

298: Bilateral phlebography with a free flow injection, carried out in the supine position. Normal appearance.

299 (see p. 210): Same patient in the vertical position, biplane frontal and lateral projection. Note the ostial incompetence of the saphenous vein ↑, and its ectatic∗ enlargement in the upper third of the thigh. Interest of the vertical position to demonstrate ostial incompetence while providing satisfactory data about the deep venous system.

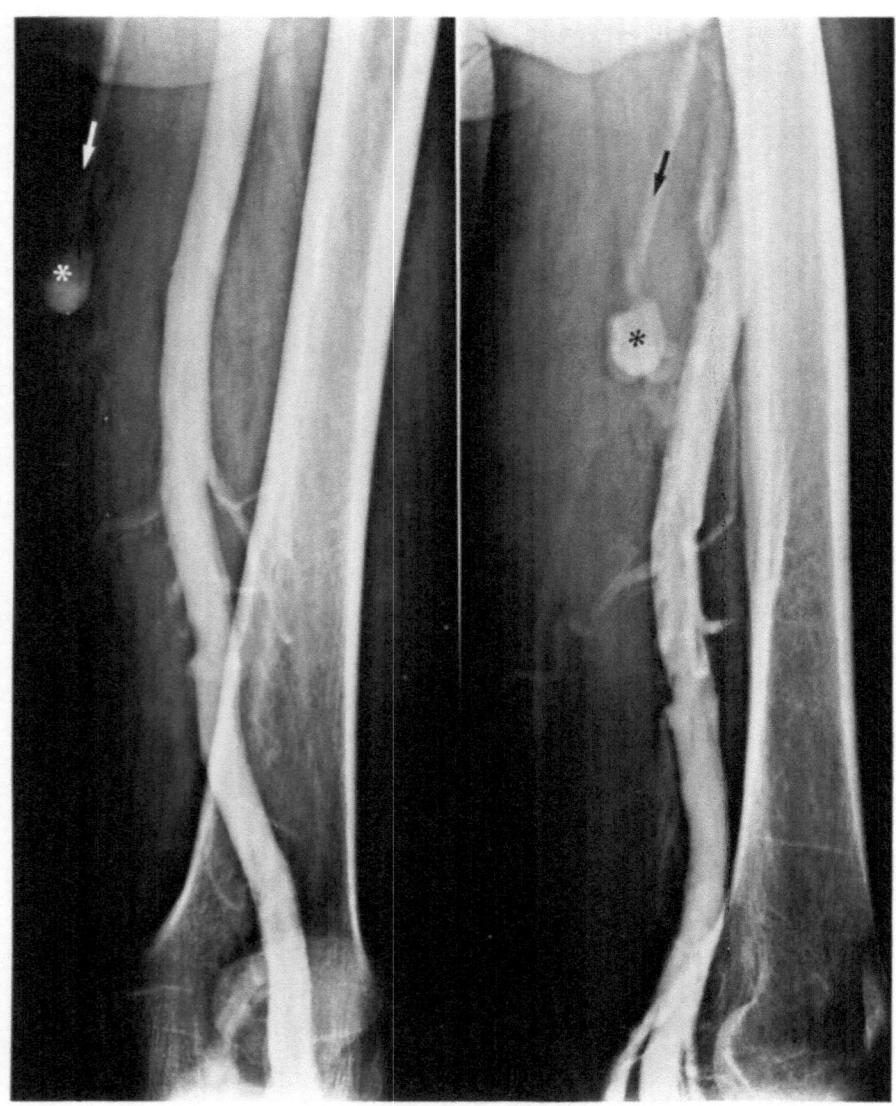

Fig. 299

299: Same patient as in Fig. 298 (see p. 209), in the vertical position, biplane frontal and lateral projection. Note the ostial incompetence of the saphenous vein ↑, and its ectatic * enlargement in the upper third of the thigh. Interest of the vertical position to demonstrate ostial incompetence while providing satisfactory data about the deep venous system.

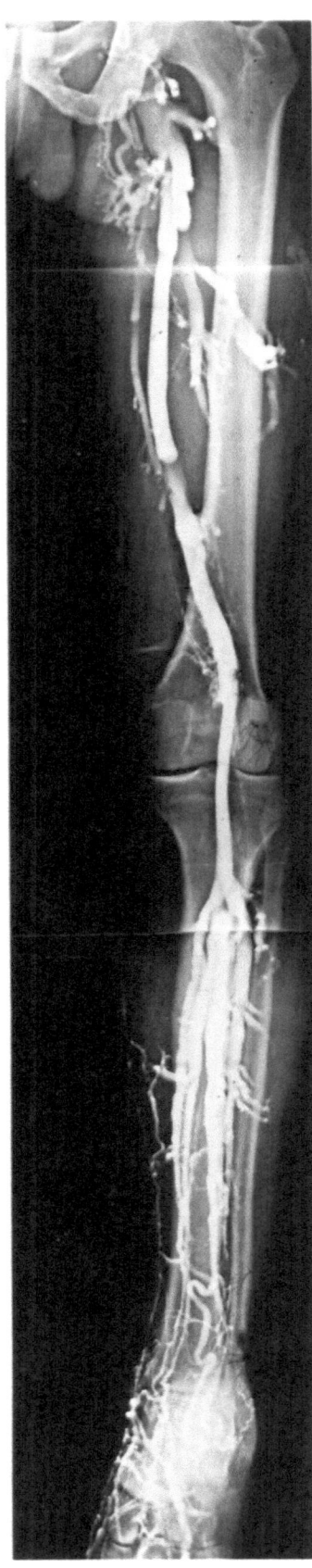

Fig. 300

Figs. 300, 301, 302, 303 and 304: Patient presenting with a thick leg on the left.

300: Phlebography of the left lower limb performed with a free flow injection demonstrates the perfect patency of the deep venous trunks.

301 (see p. 212): Phlebography in the vertical position: early phase, film centered on the thigh showing patent deep venous trunks. Small collateral channel ↑ medial to the superficial femoral vein.

302 (see p. 213): Later phase of the same phlebography in the vertical position. Significant ostial incompetence ← of the internal saphenous termination.

303 (see p. 213): Better visualization of the anomalies already shown in Fig. 302. Note the ectatic enlargement 4 cm below the internal saphenous termination *.

304 (see p. 213): Lateral projection of the leg in the vertical position showing marked incompetence of the perforating veins of the leg ↑ and ostial incompetence of the internal saphenous termination.

Man aged 50 with a thick leg due to essential varices, presenting at once incompetence of the internal saphenous vein and of the perforating veins of the leg on the left leg. On the right side, this patient had varices without thick leg.

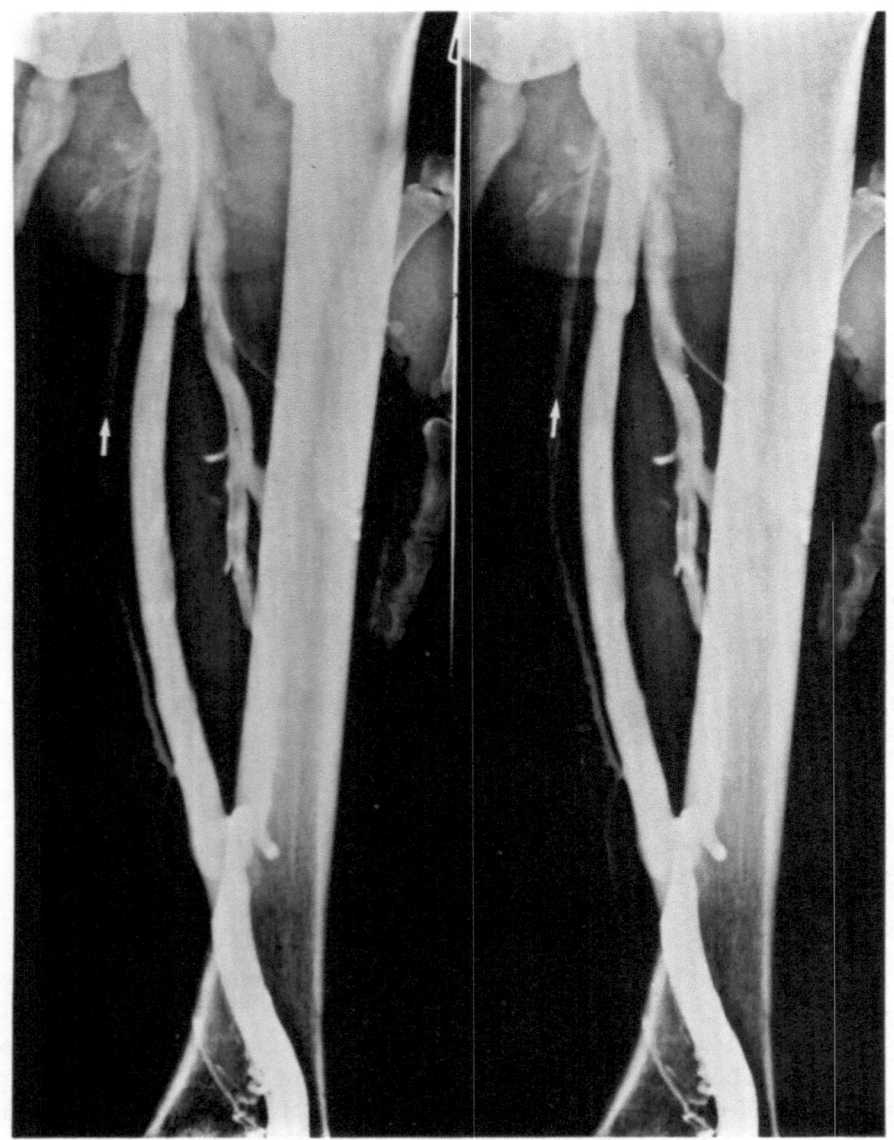

Fig. 301

301 (see also legend on p. 211): Phlebography in the vertical position: early phase, film centered on the thigh showing patent deep venous trunks. Small collateral channel ↑ medial to the superficial femoral vein.

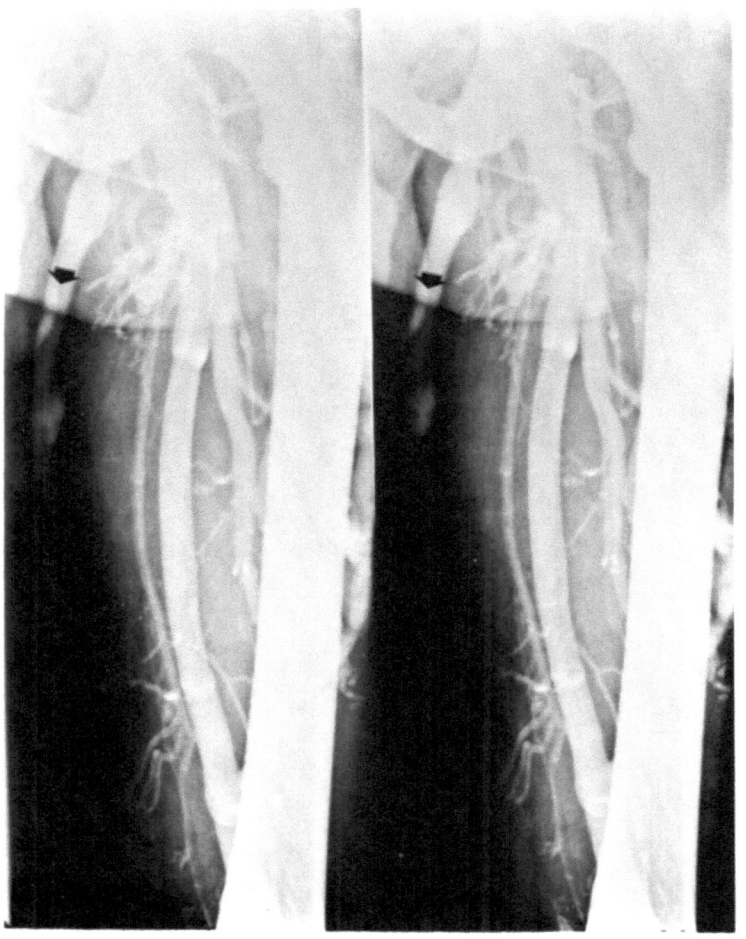

Fig. 302

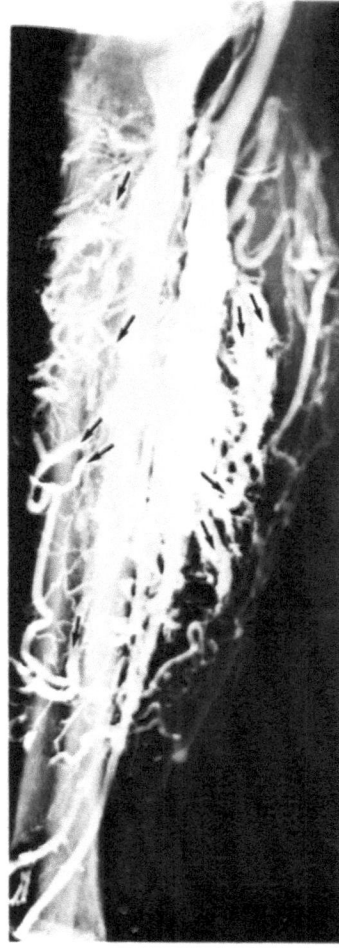

Fig. 304

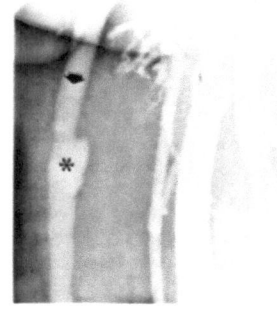

Fig. 303

302: Later phase of the same phlebography in the vertical position. Significant ostial incompetence ➴ of the internal saphenous termination.
303: Better visualization of the anomalies already shown in Fig. 302. Note the ectatic enlargement 4 cm below the internal saphenous termination ∗.
304: Lateral projection of the leg in the vertical position showing marked incompetence of the perforating veins of the leg ⭡ and ostial incompetence of the internal saphenous termination.
(See p. 211 for more information.)

Chapter 9

RECURRENT VARICOSE VEINS. OPERATIVE TREATMENT OF VARICOSE VEINS

Figures 305–316

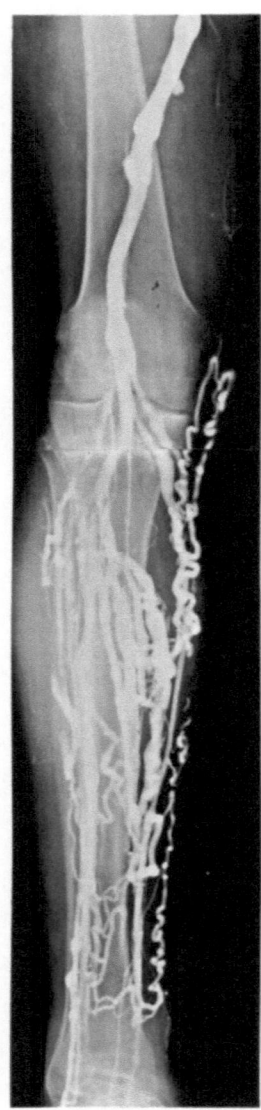

Fig. 305: Patient who underwent operative removal of the terminal segment of the internal saphenous vein and stripping of this vein. Recurrent varicose veins of the leg due to incompetent perforating veins at this level. The operative technique did not include ligation of all these perforating veins. Internal saphenous stripping is however perfect.

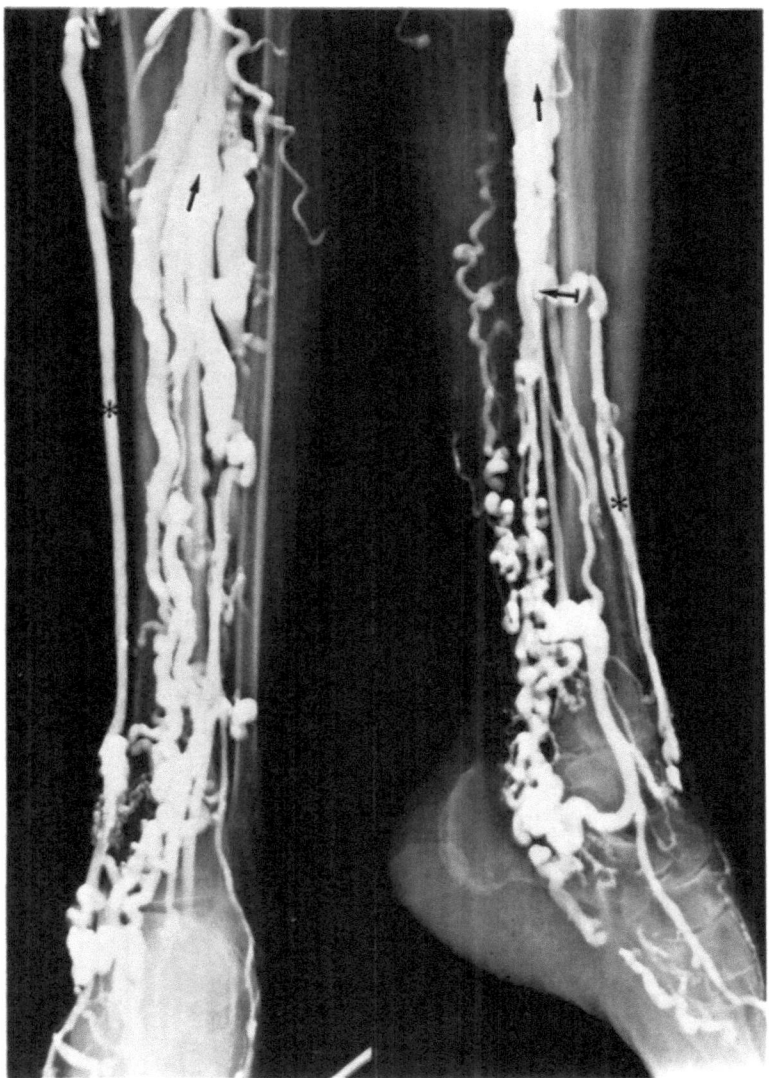

Fig. 306   *Fig. 307*

Figs. 306 and 307: Varices of the legs involving predominantly the left internal supra-malleolar area. Patient who has already been operated on for varices: no operative report in the files.

306: Frontal phlebogram of the left lower limb performed with a free flow injection of contrast medium. *307:* same patient, lateral view. The internal saphenous vein∗ has certainly not been stripped in so far as it is easily visible on the frontal projection. The varices are well displayed on the lateral view; they are branched on the internal saphenous vein, but also on the perforating veins of the deep system. Note the opacification of the anterior tibial veins, well visualized anteriorly, which are drained by an uncommon anastomosis ⇂ directly into the peroneal ↿ veins. The latter show the usual fusiform enlargement (well displayed in Fig. 306).

In conclusion: Internal saphenous stripping seems very improbable. Incompetence of some perforating veins above the ankle, which would deserve ligation on the occasion of internal saphenous stripping.

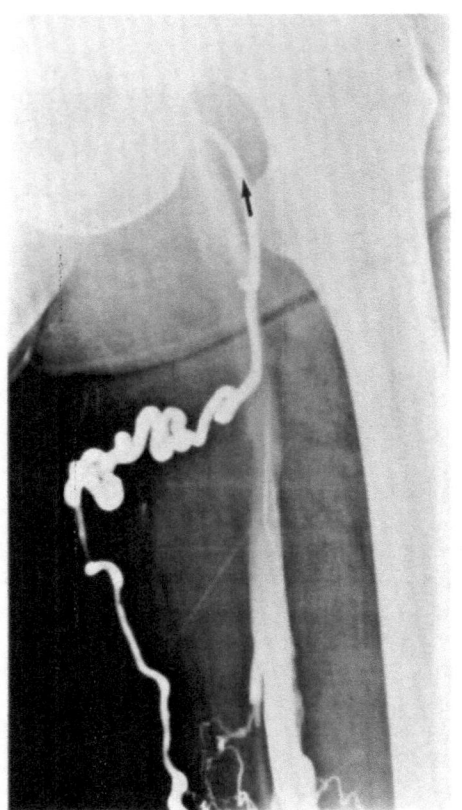

Fig. 309

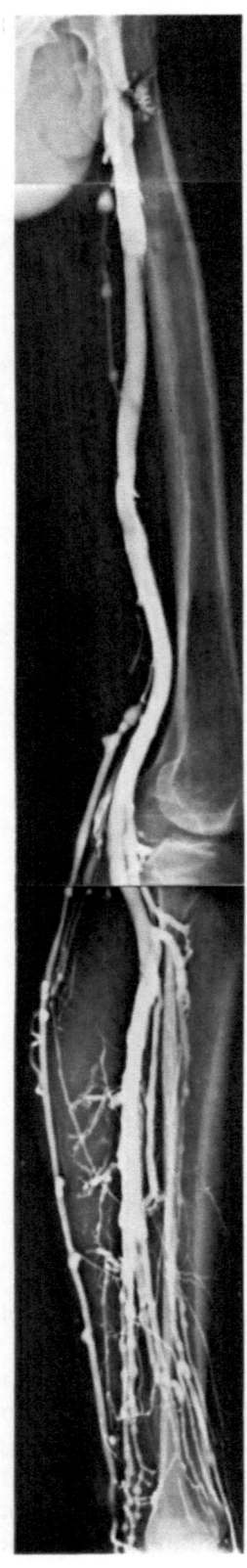

Fig. 308

Figs. 308 and 309: Appearance of varices at the internal aspect of the thigh in a patient who had stripping 5 years earlier.

308: Venography of the left lower limb with a free flow injection. Semi-lateral projection. Patency of the deep venous network. The internal saphenous vein is not opacified. No incompetent perforating vein feeding the varicose network on the thigh.

309: Varicography by direct cannulation of the varices on the thigh. The drainage of the varicose system occurs at the level of the Scarpa's triangle, probably at the level of a branch ↑ of the internal saphenous termination which has either not been ligated or has an ectopic embouchment. Interest of direct varicography in cases where deep venography failed to demonstrate the varicose network.

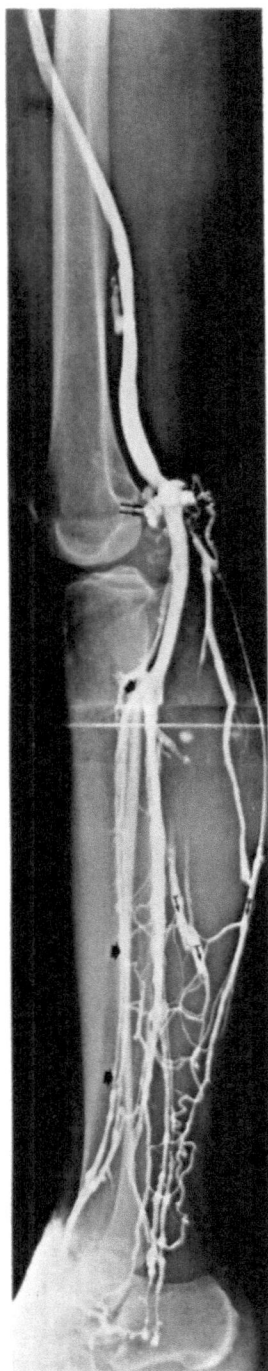

Fig. 310: Varicose veins which have appeared during pregnancy. Stripping of the internal and of the external saphenous vein of the left lower limb had been performed two years earlier.

Venography of the left lower limb with a free flow injection of the contrast medium. Lateral projection. The deep leg veins are competent and the anterior tibial veins are readily visible ♠. A residual ↑↑ bunch of varices is demonstrated at the termination of the external saphenous vein which has not been entirely ligated, as there is still a branch on the posterior part of the calf ↨. Note the reflux into the muscle veins ↑ which feeds a discrete small superficial varicose network on the lower part of the leg.

220

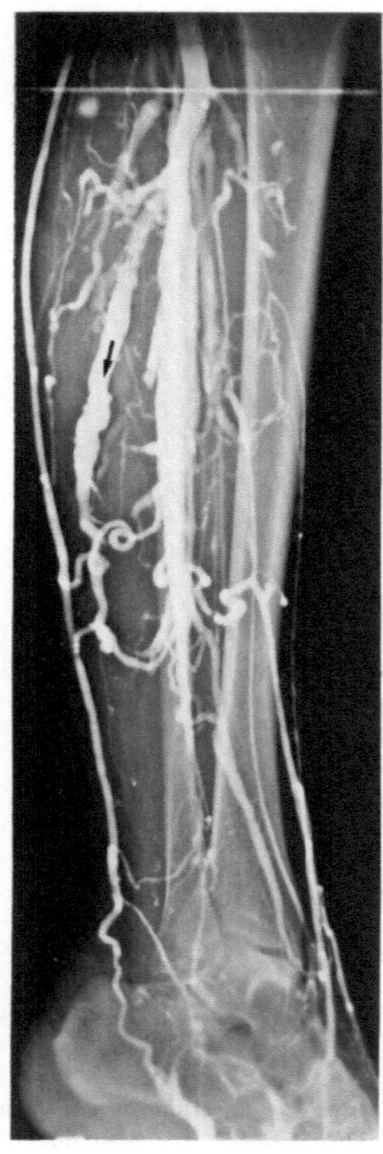

Fig. 311

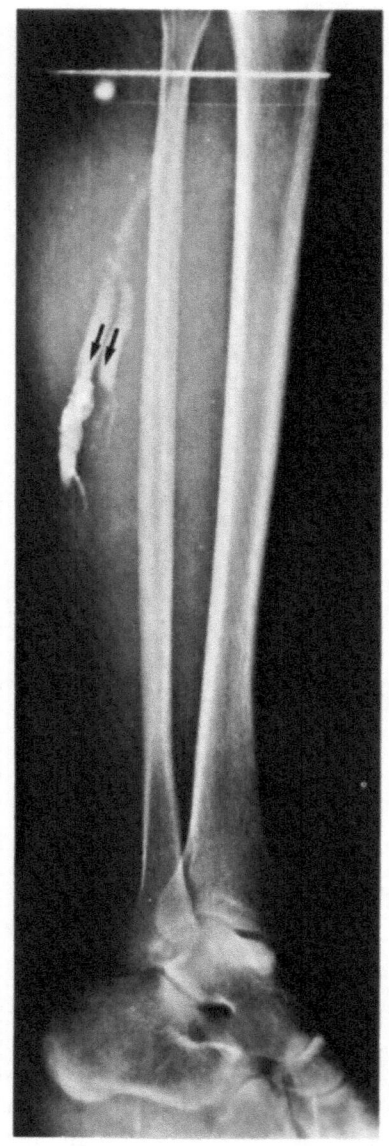

Fig. 312

Figs. 311 and 312: Lateral venogram of the left lower limb.

311: Patency of the deep trunks. Incompetent internal gastrocnemial veins ↑ with downward reflux.

312: Stagnation of contrast medium in these incompetent muscle veins ↑↑.

This is a rather uncommon example of (moderate) varices of the leg fed by valvular incompetence of the muscle veins (internal gastrocnemial).

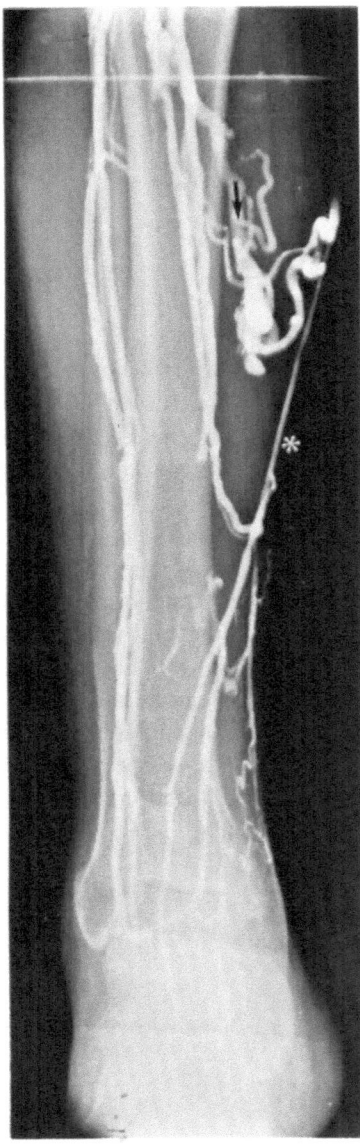

Fig. 313

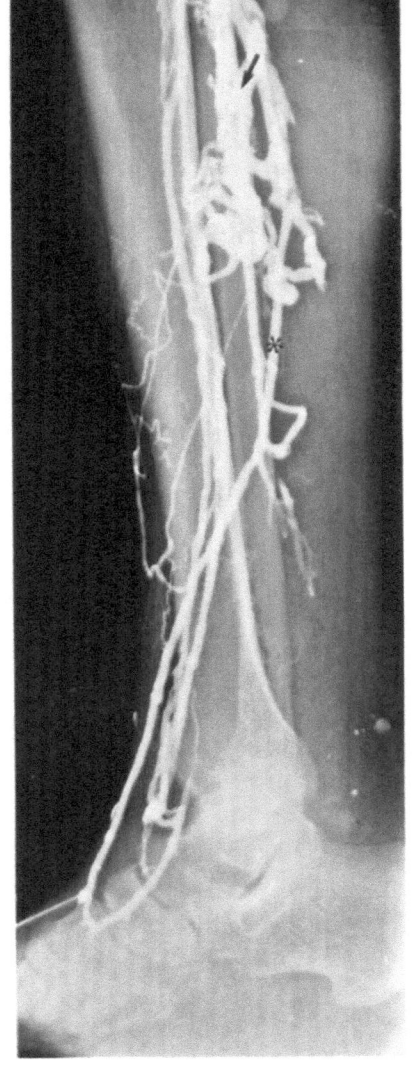

Fig. 314

Figs. 313 and 314: Venogram of the left lower limb. Frontal and lateral views. Stripping of the internal saphenous vein. Reappearance of varices on the posterior part of the leg. The varicose bunch is fed by a large incompetent perforating vein ↑ which is branched onto the posterior tibial venous system, and on a very thin residue of the internal saphenous vein ✱ which has not been stripped.

222

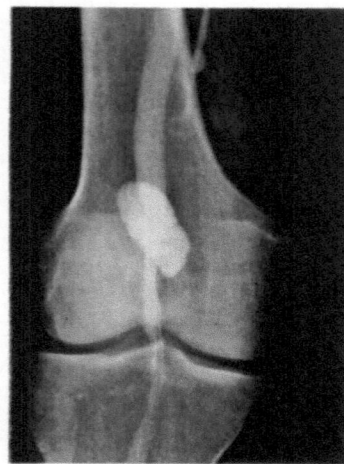

Fig. 315: Occurrence of a large isolated varicose enlargement of the ampular type, in the popliteal space. Patient who had stripping of the internal and of the external saphenous vein. There is a varicose dilatation of the origin of the external saphenous vein, too distally ligated.

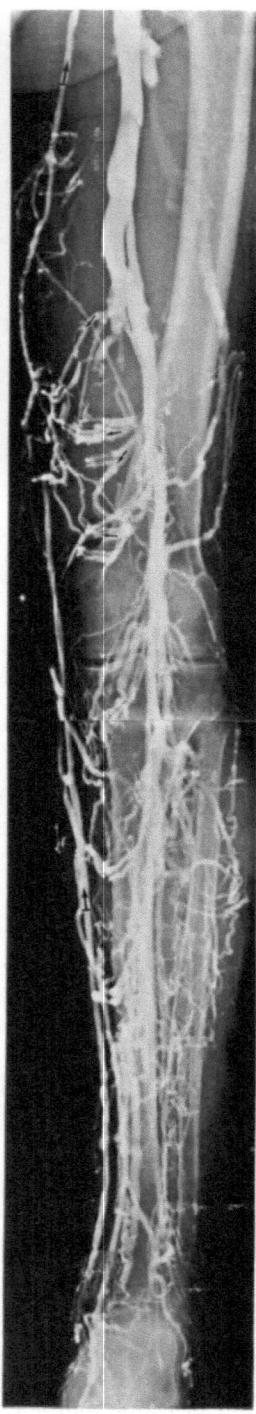

Fig. 316: Recurrence of varices following stripping of the internal saphenous vein of the left lower limb. Phlebography with free flow injection of contrast medium. Marked collateral circulation at the level of the leg, proof of obliteration of a part of the deep leg veins. Numerous incompetent perforating veins in the thigh ↑. Opacification of a branch of the internal saphenous system ↑ which has not been stripped and drains into the internal saphenous termination. Conclusion: Incomplete internal saphenous stripping associated with incompetence of the perforating veins of the leg and especially of the thigh and with partial obliteration, which has probably passed undetected, of a part of the deep veins of the leg.

Chapter 10

ACQUIRED AND CONGENITAL VALVULAR INCOMPETENCE. FEMORAL AND POPLITEAL RETROGRADE VENOGRAPHY

Figures 317–331

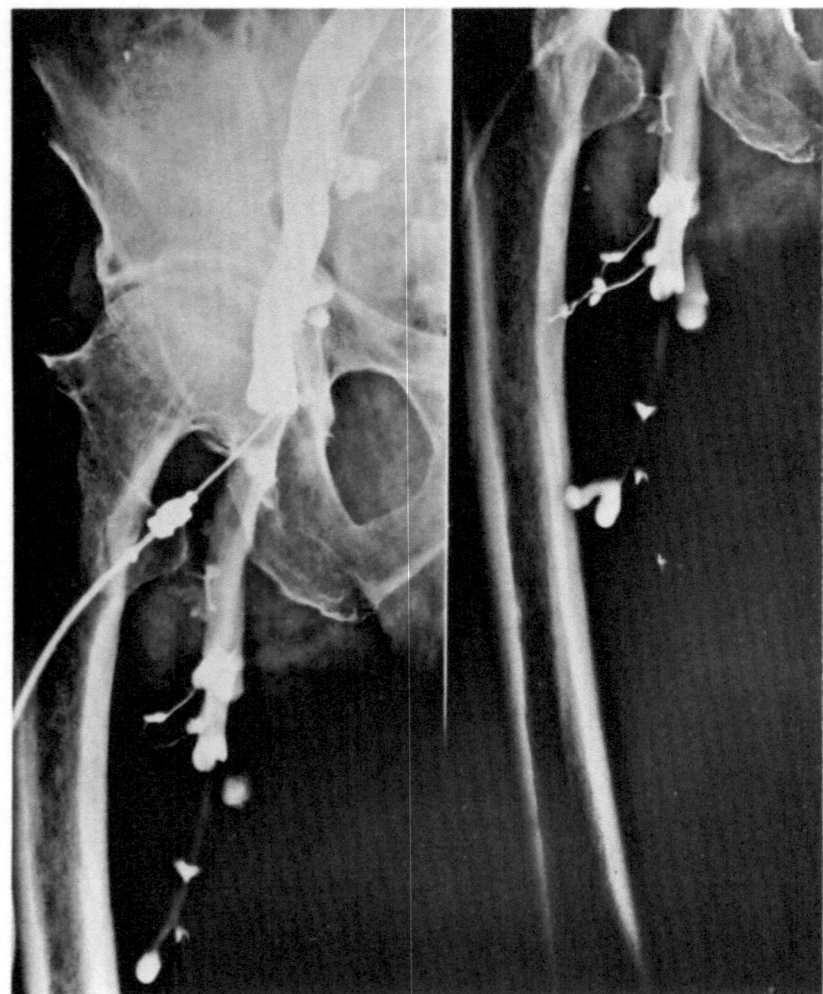

Fig. 317: Normal retrograde femoral phlebography (in the upright position). The onset of the injection is made while a Valsalva maneuver is performed, and corresponds to the dynamic phase of phlebography. The second film (right side of the figure) corresponds to the relaxation phase when the patient takes a deep breath. Note that Valsalva maneuver distends the femoral and the iliac veins. Normally, the reflux should not descend further than the first or the second valve of the common femoral vein (about 2 to 3 cm below the inguinal ligament). There always exists in the normal condition a slight reflux into the first superficial femoral valves, and sometimes in the deep femoral valves. The valve pockets with their "pigeon-nests" images are shown clearly during the relaxation phase.

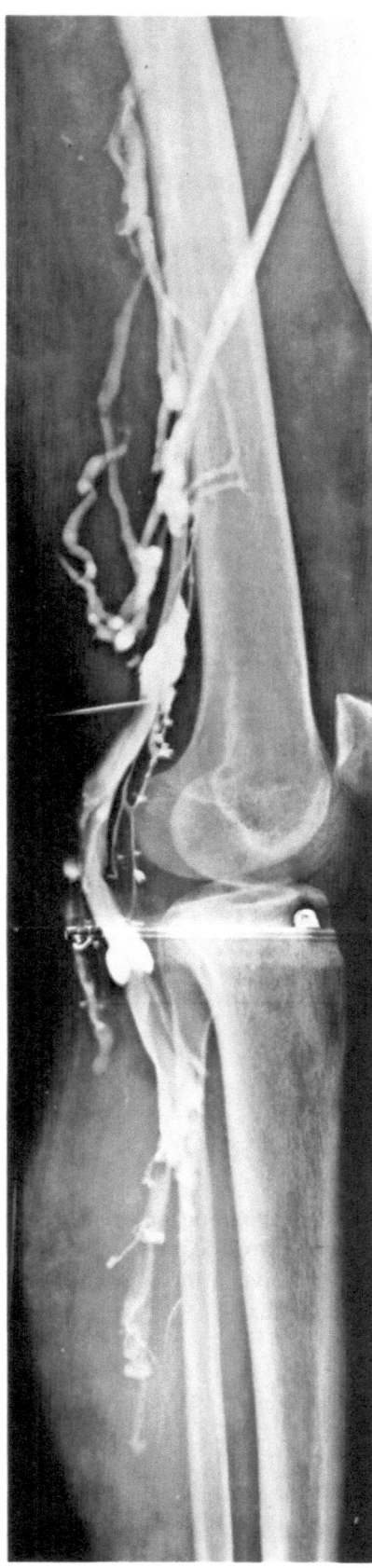

Fig. 318: Normal popliteal retrograde phlebography (vertical position). The normal reflux is not beyond the upper part of the deep veins of the leg. The muscle collaterals, namely the internal gastrocnemial veins, must not be opacified. This technique for investigation of valvular incompetence may also be useful for the exploration of the femoro-popliteal and iliac system when one cannot catheterize a dorsal vein of the foot.

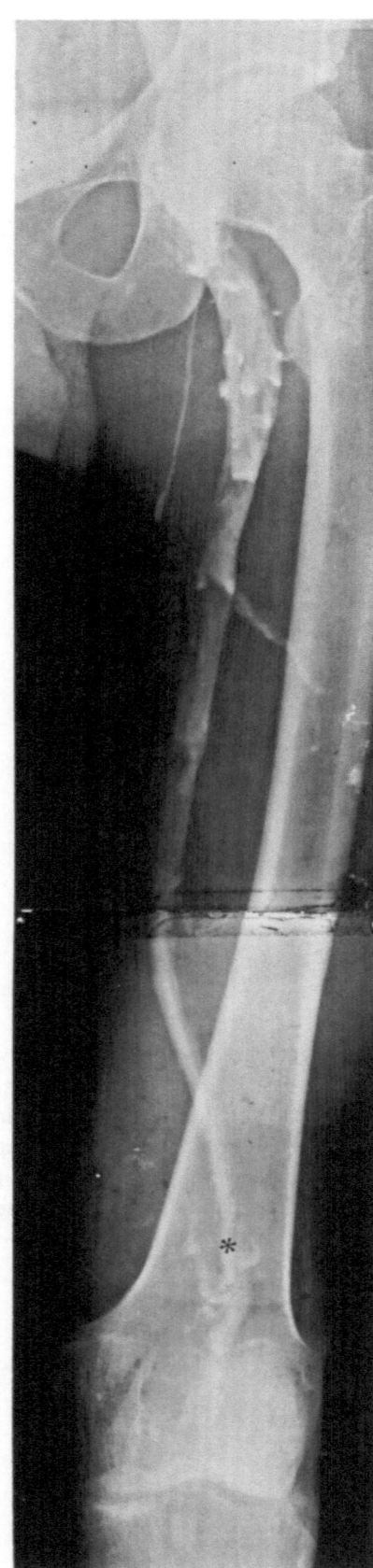

Fig. 319: Femoral retrograde phlebography in a patient presenting with varicose veins of the leg. Reflux of contrast medium as far as the popliteal vein∗, witnessing valvular incompetence of the deep veins. No internal saphenous reflux.

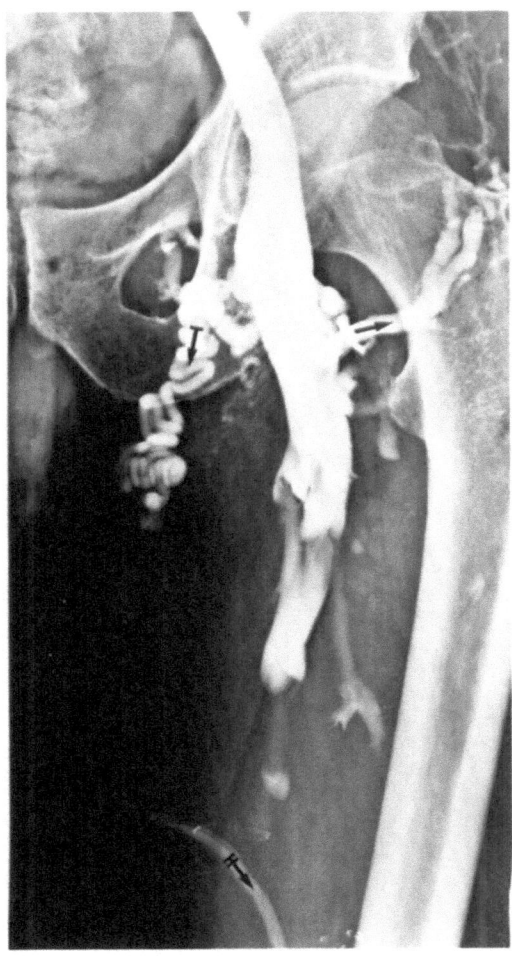

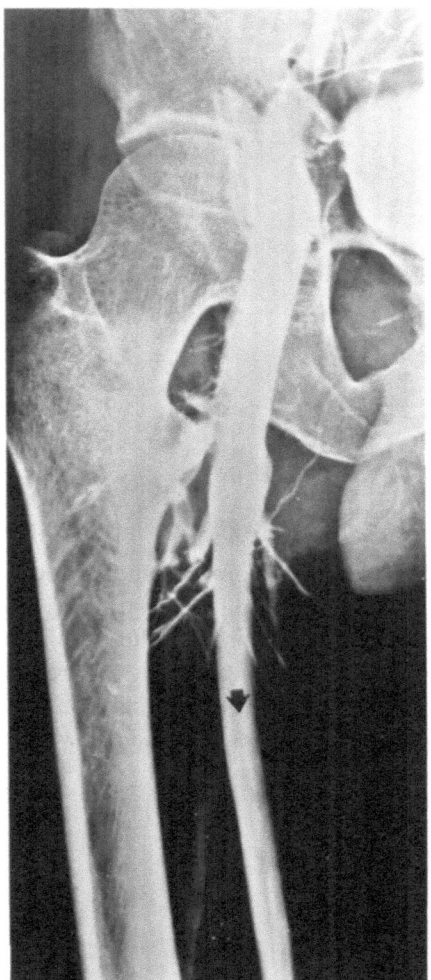

Fig. 320: Femoral retrograde phlebography for recurrence of varicose veins after stripping of the internal saphenous vein and operative removal of its termination. Normal appearance of the reflux in the deep veins with opacification of the circumflex veins of the femoral neck ↑. Reflux into a varicose ↑ internal saphenous stump with opacification of a branch of the internal saphenous system which has not been stripped; on the lower part of the film: opacification of a posterior vein of the thigh which should be the vein of Giacomini ↓.

Fig. 321: Retrograde femoral phlebography. Patient operated upon varices by stripping and removal of the terminal segment. Total valvular incompetence of the superficial femoral vein with reflux as far as the popliteal space ◆.

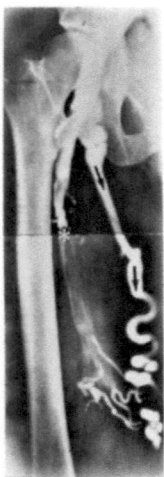

Fig. 322: Retrograde femoral phlebography. Recurrence of varicose veins following stripping of the internal saphenous vein. Normal reflux as far as the first valves of the deep veins ∗. Contrariwise, marked reflux into a branch of the internal saphenous system which is very dilated and varicose, and had not undergone stripping ↑.

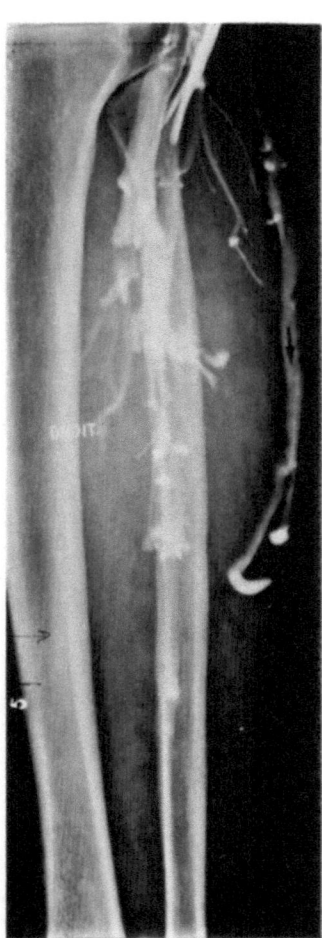

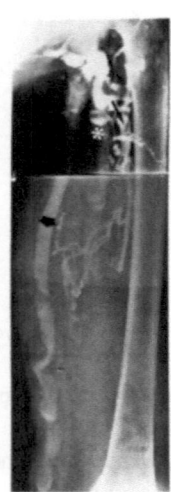

Fig. 324: Retrograde popliteal phlebography. Normal continence of the deep veins of the leg. Incompetence of the terminal segment of the external ↑ saphenous vein which is opacified as far as the lower third of the leg.

Fig. 323: Retrograde femoral phlebography. Global and massive reflux into the internal saphenous vein ●. Associated reflux into the profunda femoris vein ↑. Normal continence of the superficial femoral vein ∗.

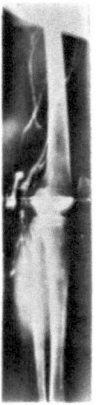

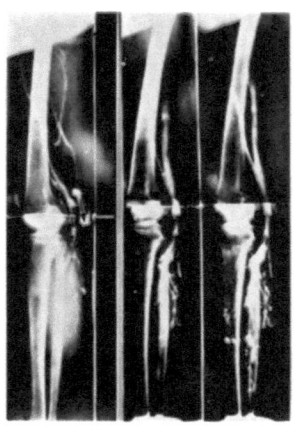

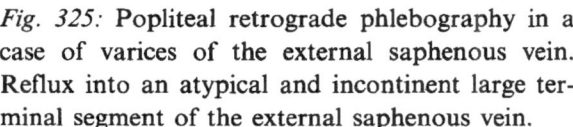

a   b   c

Fig. 325: Popliteal retrograde phlebography in a case of varices of the external saphenous vein. Reflux into an atypical and incontinent large terminal segment of the external saphenous vein.

Fig. 327: Popliteal descending phlebography for varices of the lower third of the leg, belonging to the external saphenous territory. a) Atypical, long and incontinent ↑ terminal segment of the external saphenous vein, responsible for varices in the popliteal space. b) and c) Reflux into the deep veins of the leg by valvular incompetence.

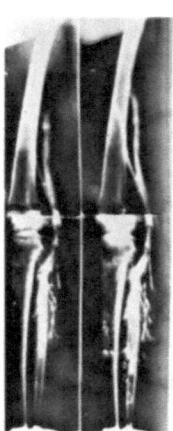

Fig. 326: Popliteal descending phlebography in a case with varicose leg veins. Reflux into the deep veins with valvular incompetence.

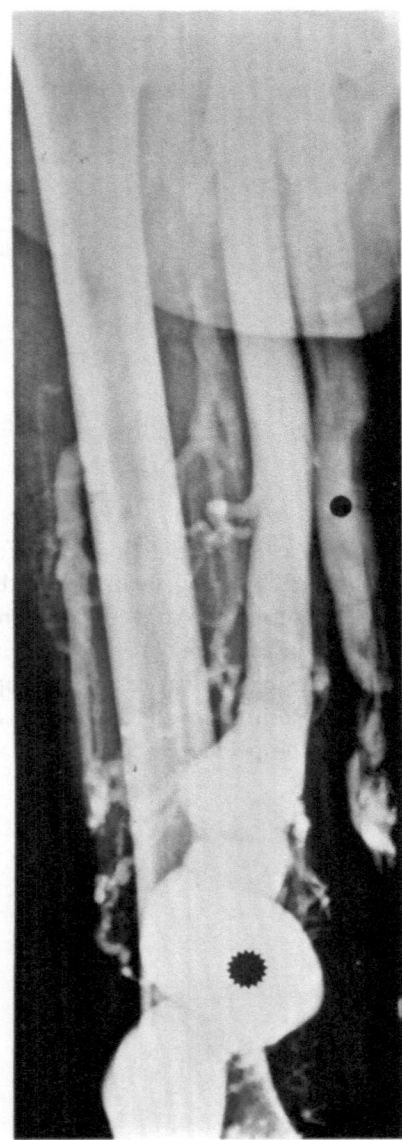

Fig. 328

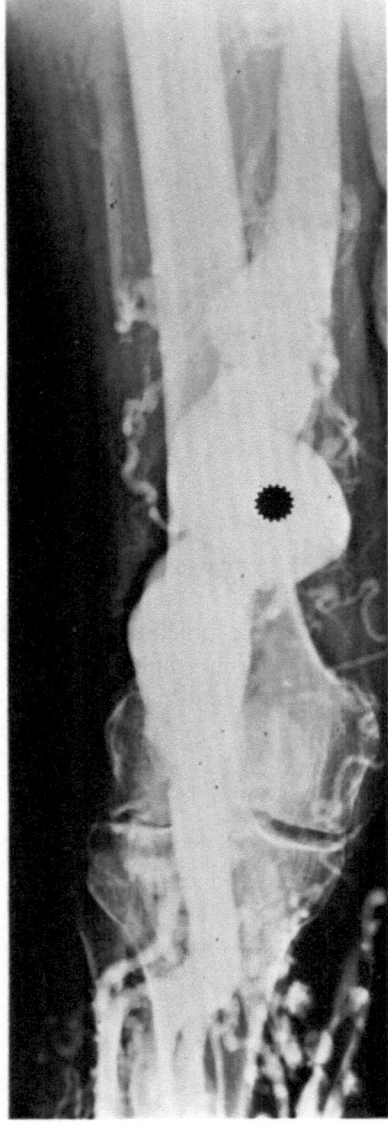

Fig. 329

Figs. 328 and 329: Phlebography of the right lower limb with a free flow injection of contrast medium, performed in the vertical position. The patient presents huge varices and a gross venous ampulla in the upper part ● of the popliteal space. Thick leg. Complete avalvulation of the femoro-popliteal deep venous system. Note the ectatic appearance of the internal saphenous vein ● on the medial aspect of the thigh. No history of phlebitis: congenital valvular incompetence of the deep venous trunks.

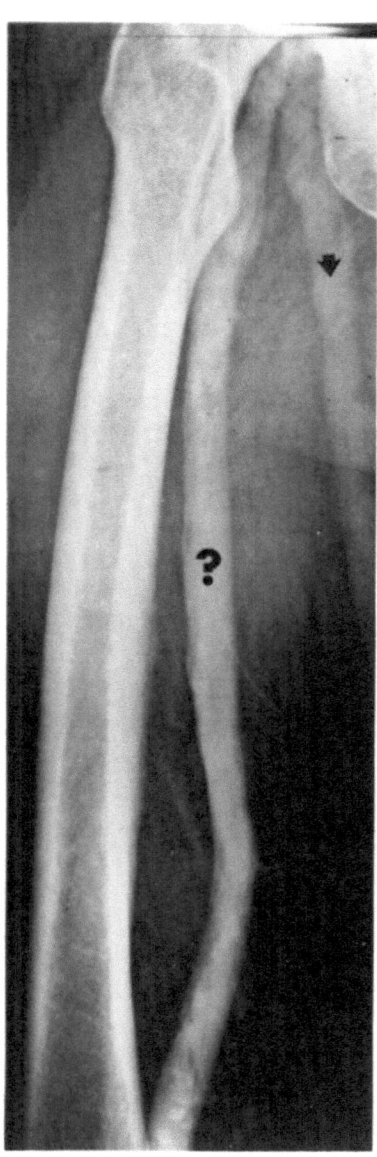

Fig. 330: Phlebography of the right lower limb performed in the vertical position. Thick leg with varices of the leg. Complete absence of valves in the femoro-popliteal veins?. Note reflux into the terminal segment of the internal saphenous vein ♠ which is also dilated. No history of phlebitis: congenital absence of valves in the deep venous sytem, associated with ostial incompetence of the saphenous terminal segment.

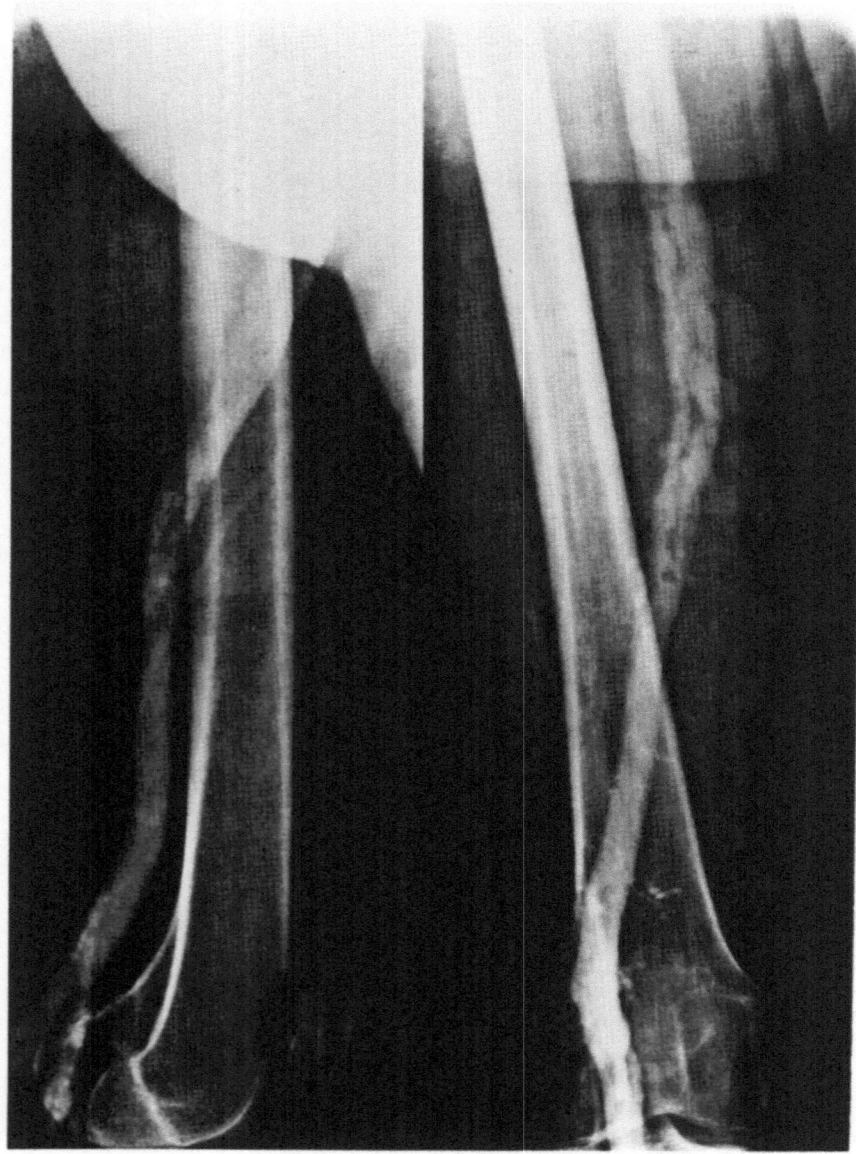

Fig. 331: Phlebography of the right lower limb with a free flow injection of contrast medium, performed in the vertical position. Lateral and frontal view. Straticulate appearance of the femoro-popliteal vein which is dilated. Disappearance of any valvular structure. Acquired, post-phlebitic valvular incompetence.

Chapter 11

EXTRINSIC COMPRESSION OF THE VEINS OF THE LOWER LIMB AND THE ILIAC VEINS. COCKETT'S SYNDROME

Figures 332–374

234

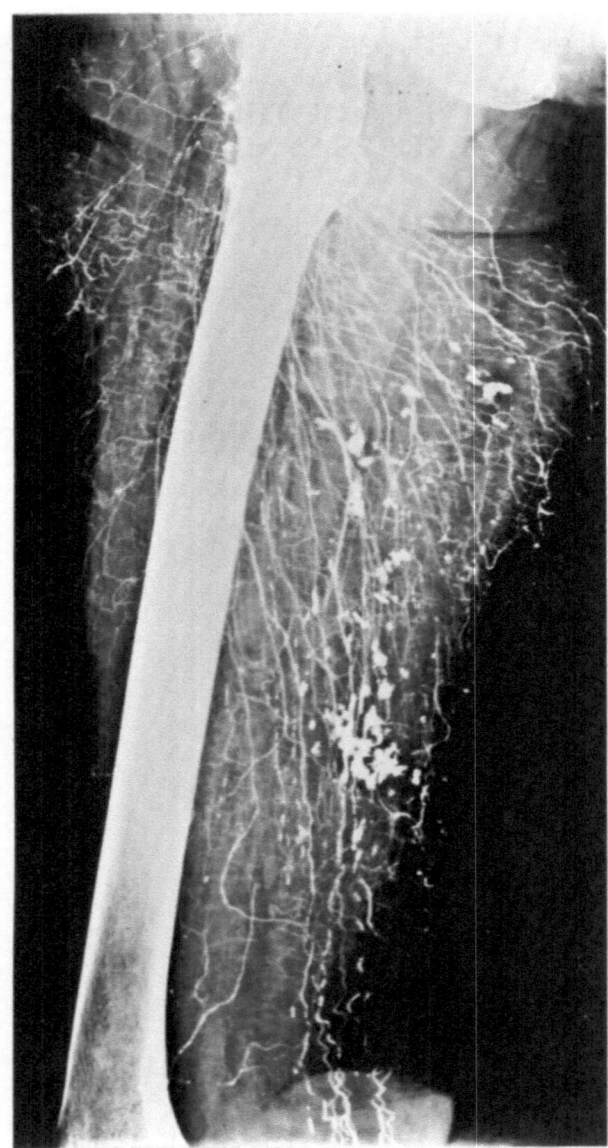

Fig. 332

Figs. 332, 333 and 334: Thick leg by lymphatic and right ilio-crural blockage. Hodgkin's disease.

332: Lymphography of the right lower limb. Lymphatic obstruction at the level of the inguinal lymph nodes with dermal back-flow into the superficial lymphatics in the thigh; extra-vasation of contrast medium.

333: Phlebography of the right lower limb with a free flow injection of the contrast. "Flake-like" stop at the level of the common femoral vein∗ and significant collateral circulation at the level of the abdomen, as well as through the obturator vein into the hypogastric system ↑.

334: Left unifemoral cavography. Arciform imprint on the right aspect of the infrarenal ♠ segment of the inferior vena cava, associated with beginning uretro-hydronephrosis on the right.

Hodgkin disease with right crural lympho-venous obstruction and retroperitoneal lymph node involvement, and extrinsic compression of the inferior vena cava.

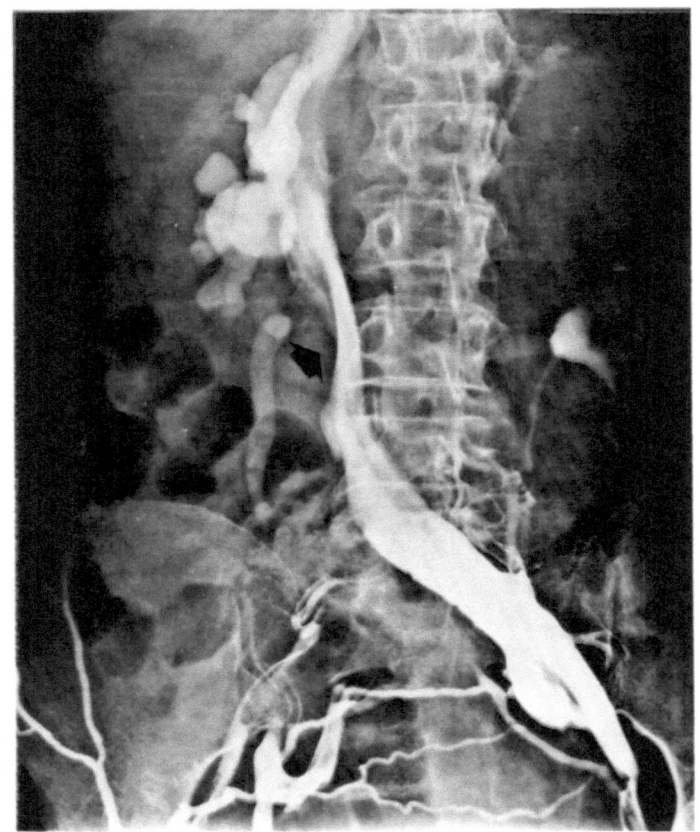

Fig. 334

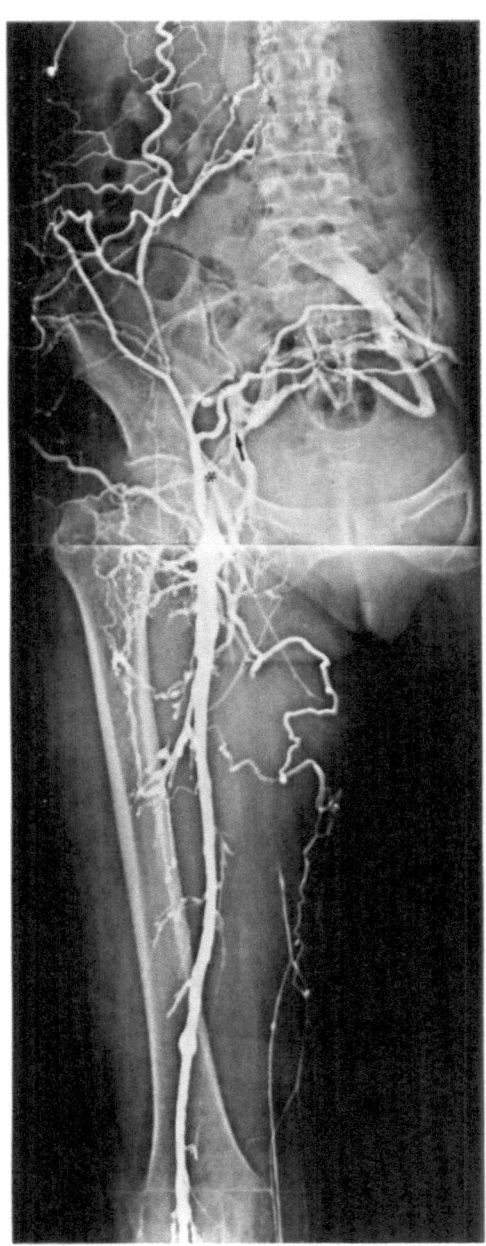

Fig. 333

236

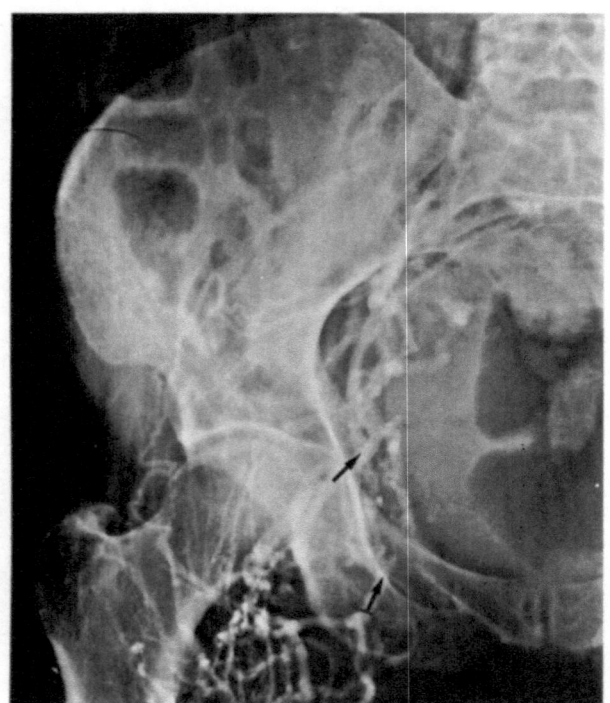

Fig. 335

Fig. 336

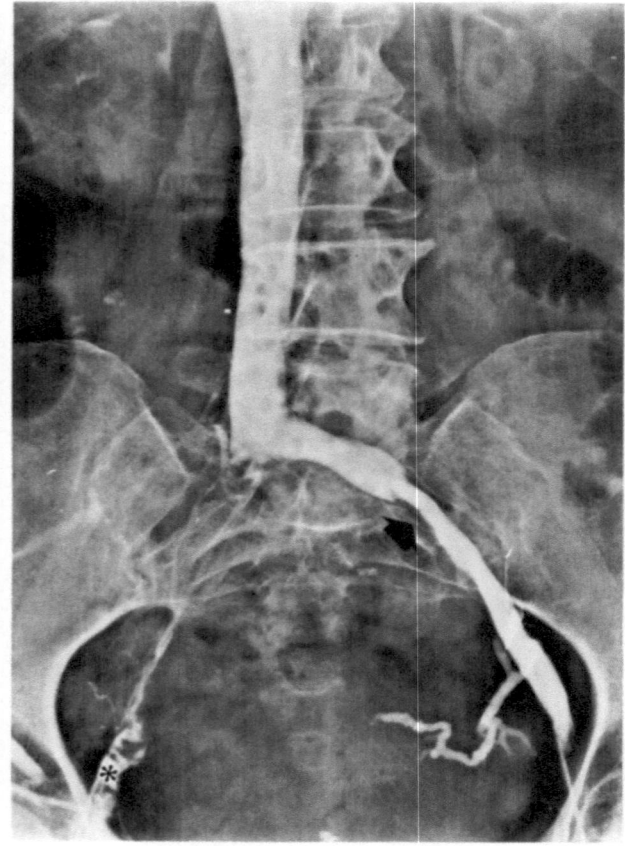

Figs. 335 and 336: Apparently trivial right iliac phlebitis.

335: Phlebography of the right lower limb performed with a free flow injection of contrast medium. Centering onto the pelvis. Diffuse obliteration of all veins of the lower limb and of the ilio-femoral vein and drainage through the inferior gluteal ↑ and obturator ↑ veins into the right hypogastric system.

336: Systematic bifemoral percutaneous cavography. Catheterization into a thrombus on the right *. On the left, the entire external iliac system ◄ seems to be ensheathed. This appearance corresponds to pelvic neoplastic fibrosis in this female who presents a very advanced carcinoma of the cervix uteri.

Interest of cavography to demonstrate the secondary character of the right ilio-femoral thrombosis in the case of a pelvic carcinosis.

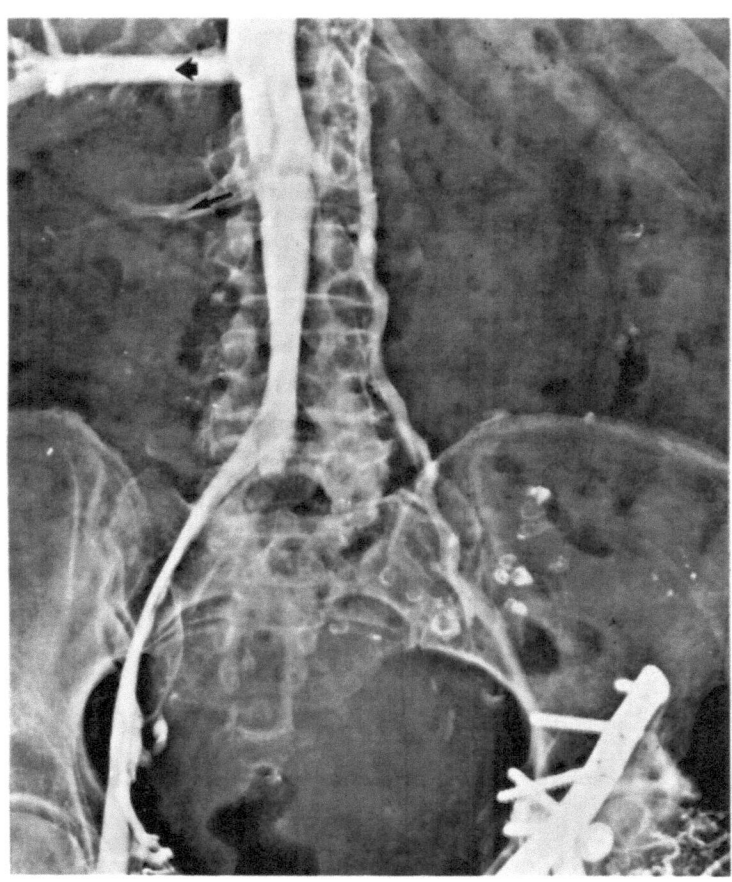

Fig. 337: Edema of both lower limbs. Amount of urea: 0.80 g/l. Bifemoral percutaneous cavography. On the left, superficial catheterization of a branch of the internal saphenous vein with almost complete obstruction of the left iliac system. On the right, filiform, stenosed and ensheathed appearance of the entire iliac vein. The infrarenal segment of the inferior vena cava shows a fibrotic concentric narrowing. No secretion of the two kidneys. Reflux into the right renal vein ⭡ and in a large accessory ♣ suprahepatic vein. Retroperitoneal and pelvic fibrosis of malignant origin: carcinoma of the cervix uteri. Left ilio-femoral obliteration, probably related to cotyloid osteo-synthesis.

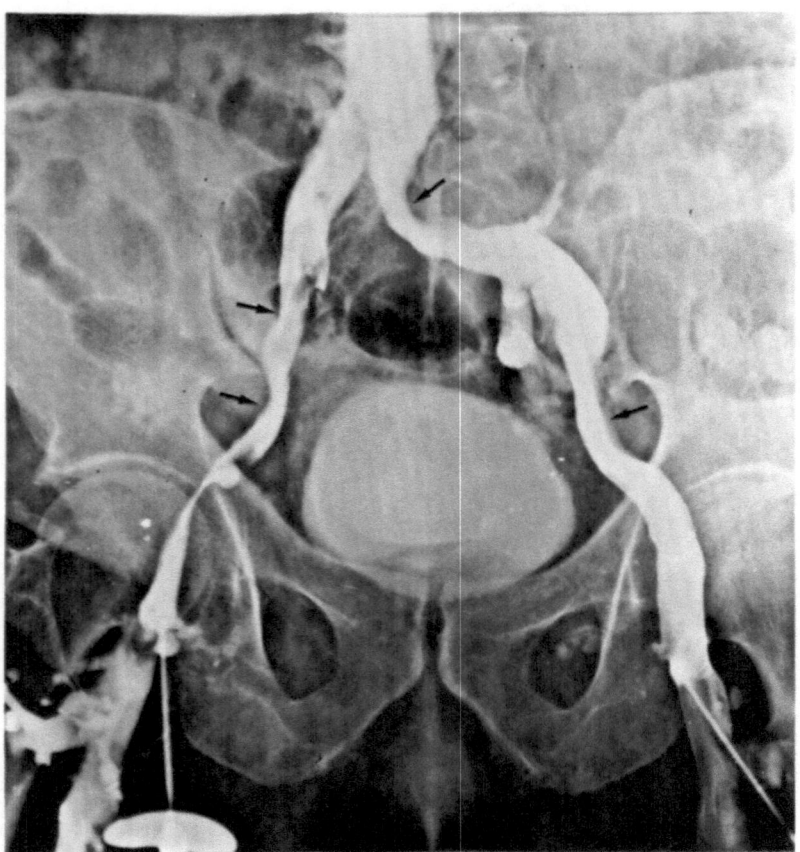

Fig. 338

Figs. 338 and 339:

338: Bifemoral percutaneous cavography. Images of multiple arciform ↑ extrinsic compression of both iliac pathways, clearly predominant on the right side. The right iliac system is quasi-stenosed to 90%, above the inguinal ligament. Marked deep and superficial femoral back flow on the right. Patient with a carcinoma of the prostata.

339: Phlebography with a non-pressurized injection of the right lower limb performed 2 weeks later for appearance of a thick right leg. The right ilio-femoral stenosis has not reached the stage of complete obstruction at the level of the common femoral vein.

Note the moderate collateral circulation.

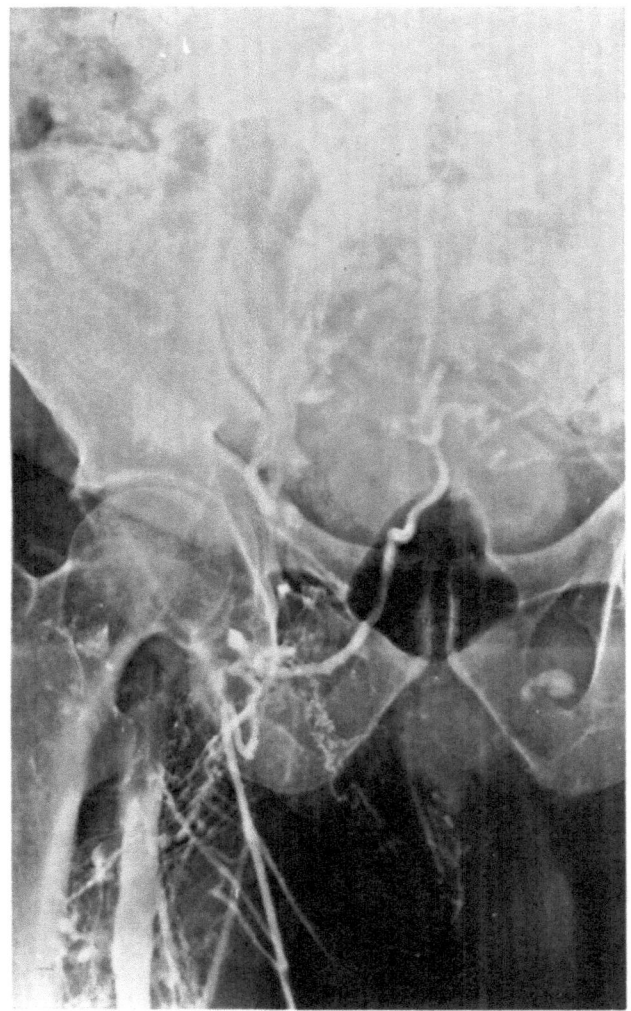

Fig. 339

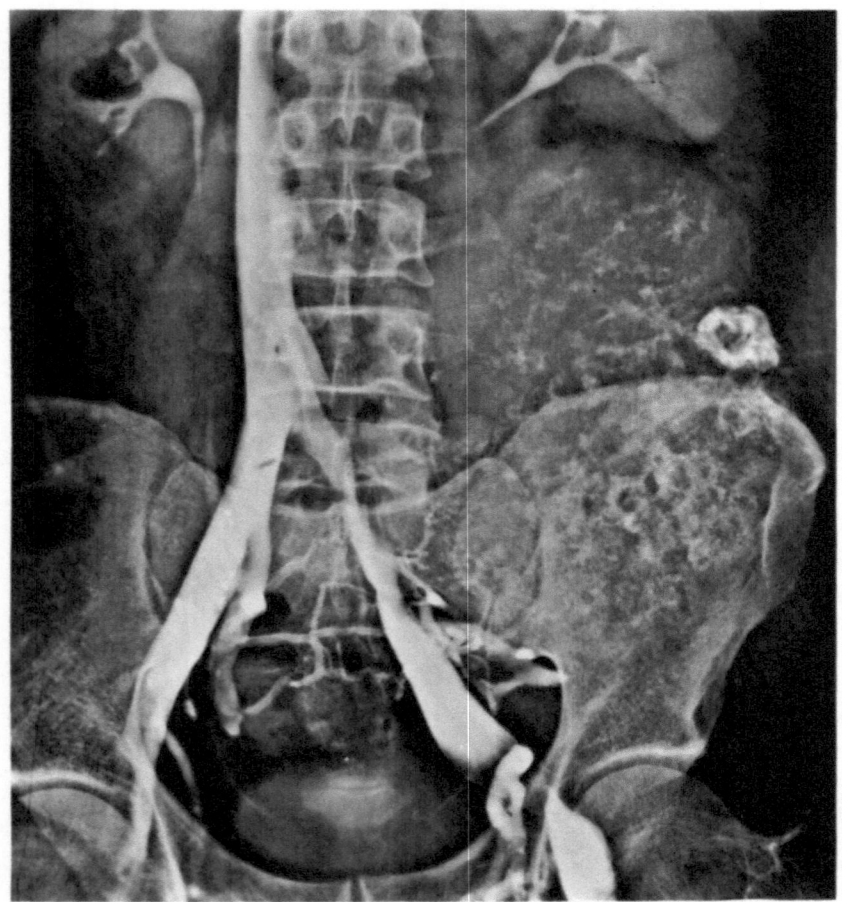

Fig. 340: Bifemoral percutaneous cavography. Slight extravasation on the left. Displacement and stenosis of the left iliac route. Raised left kidney. Chondrosarcoma of the upper portion of the left ilium with multiple calcifications.

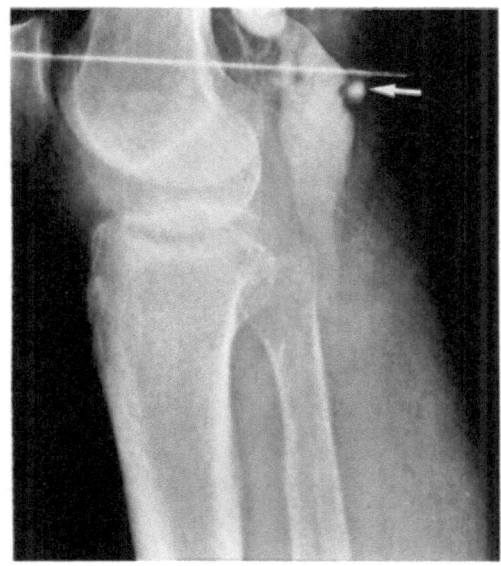

Fig. 341

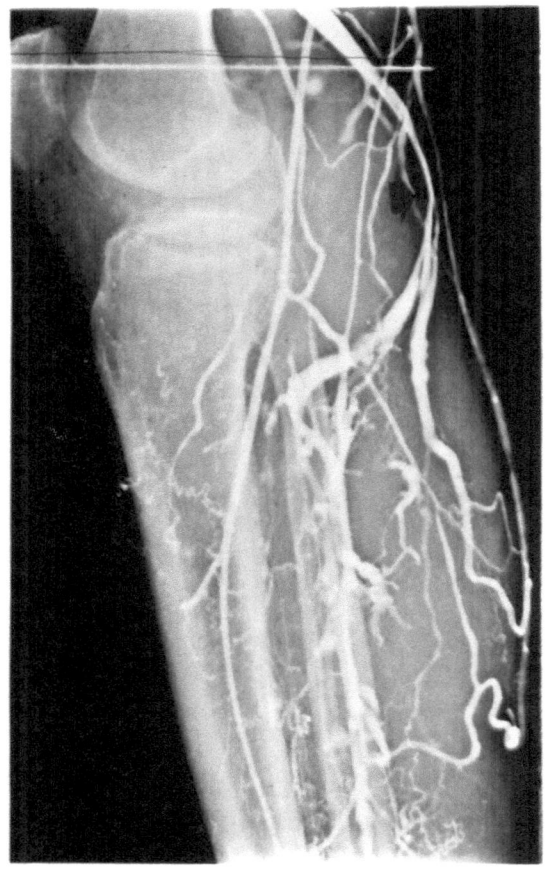

Fig. 342

Figs. 341 and 342: Ruptured popliteal arterial aneurysm.

341: Arteriography of the right lower limb. Lateral projection. Small sacciform aneurysm with a ball-like image on the posterior aspect, showing fissuration. The greater part of the aneurysm is not opacified and is located in the posterior part of the popliteal space.

342: Patient with a thick leg associated to this popliteal arterial aneurysm. Lateral view of the phlebogram of the right lower limb. Thick leg accounted for by the compression of the popliteal vein by the aneurysmal fissure. Note the disproportion between the aneurysmal opacification on the arteriogram and the popliteal ⁀ venous compression, due to non-opacification of the aneurysmal sac. Rare example of a thick leg of venous origin by compression from an artery.

242

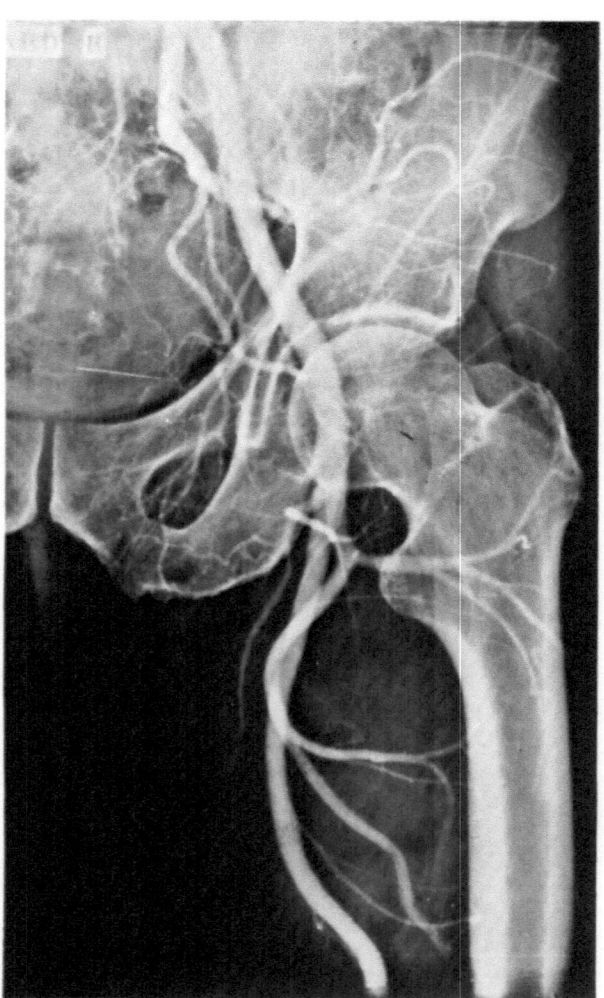

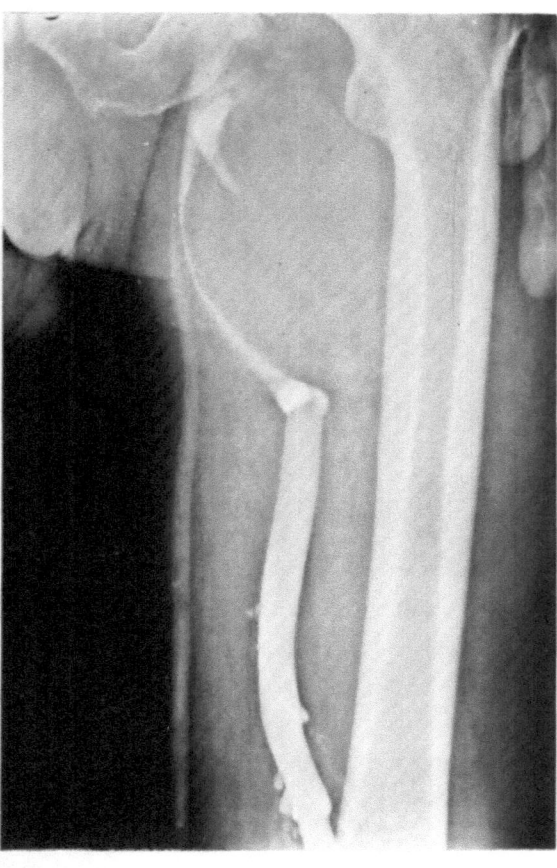

Fig. 344

Fig. 343

Figs. 343 and 344: Hematoma of the proximal part of the thigh.
343: Arteriography showing the displacement of the superficial and deep femoral system
344: Phlebogram of the left lower limb showing the displacement of the upper part of the superficial femoral vein at the level of the thigh.

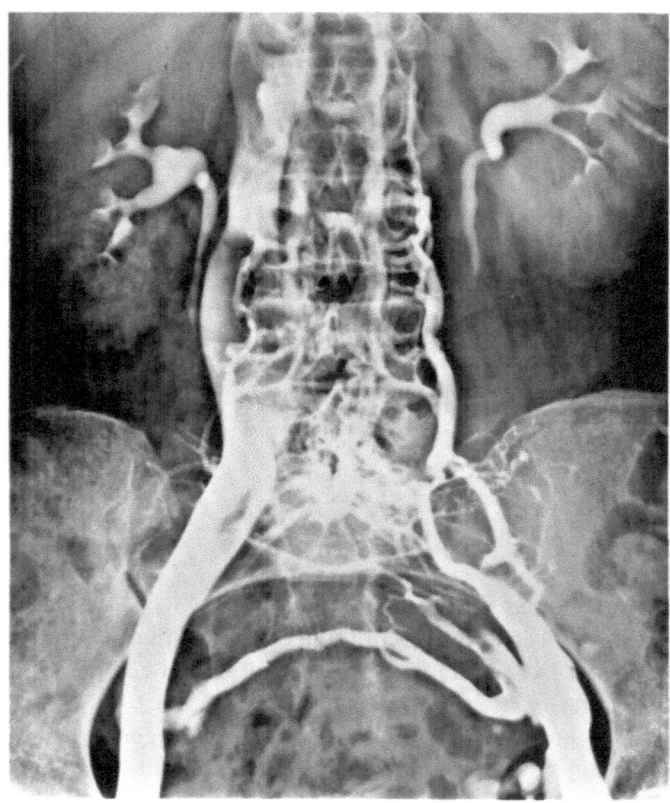

Fig. 345: Obliteration of the left common iliac vein and extrinsic compression of the infrarenal segment of the inferior vena cava by a paraganglioma of the organ of Zuckerkandl.

244

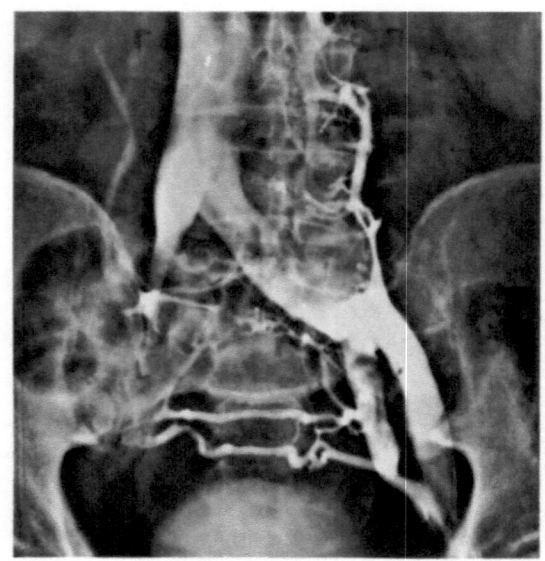

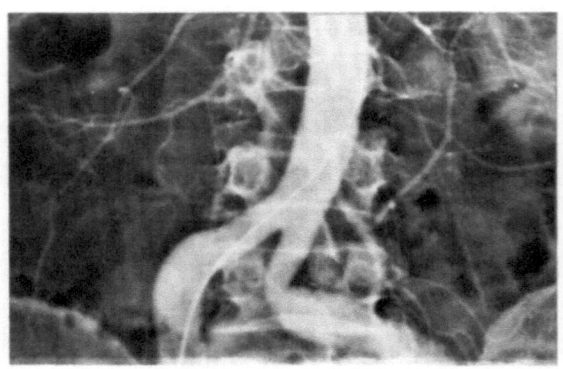

Fig. 347

Fig. 346

Figs. 346 and 347: Extrinsic compression by sinuous iliac arteries.
346: Left unifemoral cavography. Extended extrinsic impression on the entire length of the left common iliac vein. This imprint is very different from the normal imprint caused by the right common iliac artery crossing the vein at this level. It is not a matter of a Cockett's syndrome.
347: Aortogram of the same patient, showing sinuosities of the iliac arteries perfectly corresponding to the extrinsic imprints on the veins.

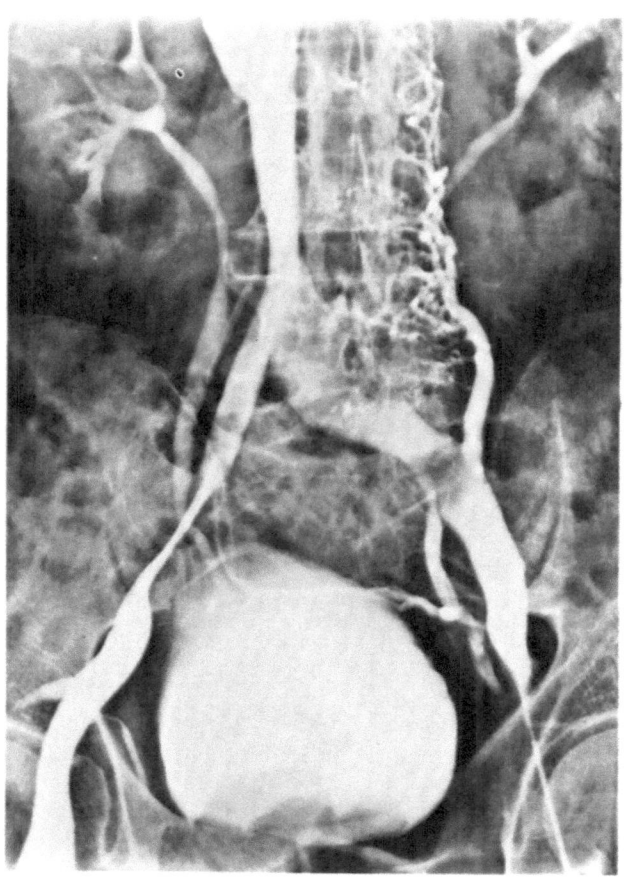

Fig. 348: Patient examined for bilateral thick leg. Bifemoral percutaneous cavography showing the ensheathed right and left iliac veins and concentric stenosis by ensheathing of the infrarenal segment of the inferior vena cava. Note the polylobate lacunar images at the base of the urinary bladder, consistent with carcinoma of the bladder responsible for adenopathies and neoplastic retroperitoneal fibrosis.

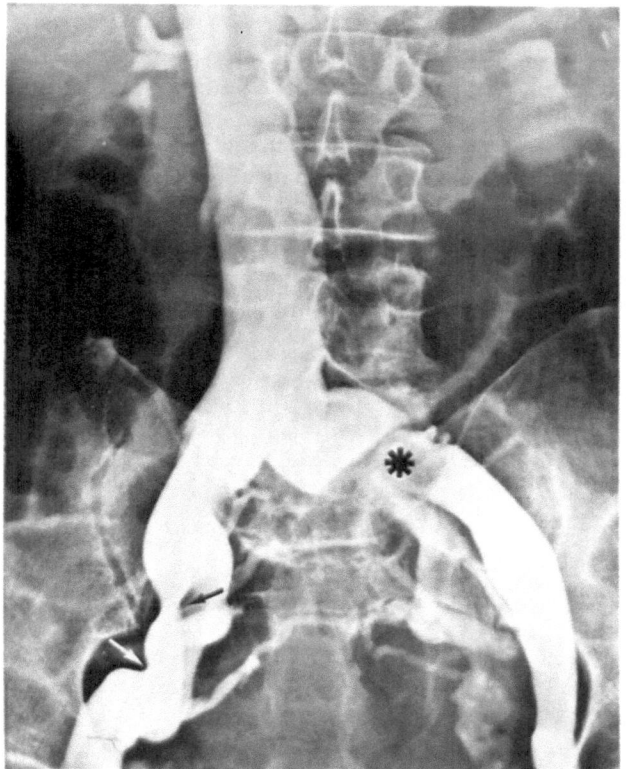

Fig. 349: Bifemoral percutaneous cavography. Voluminous * extrinsic imprints on the left iliac system, and marked extrinsic impression across the right common iliac vein † caused by dolichomegailiac arteries (aortogram not represented).

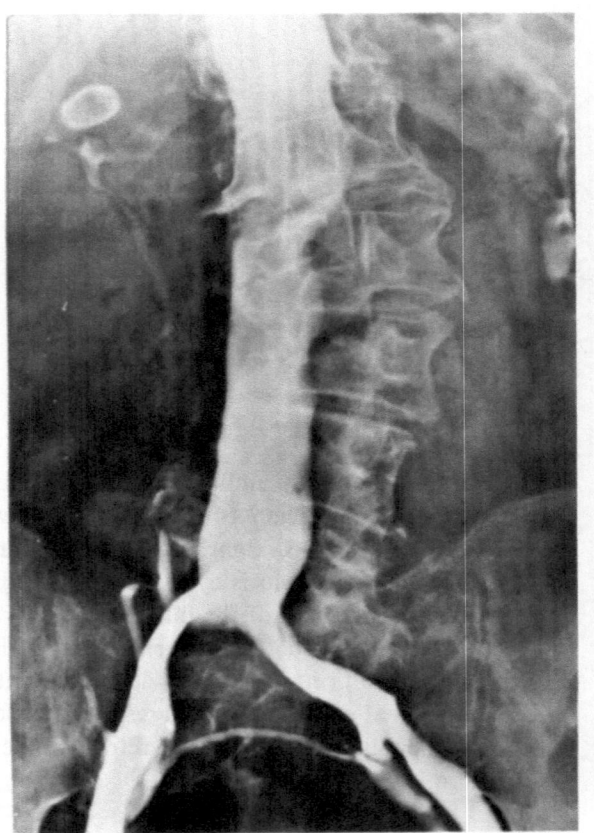 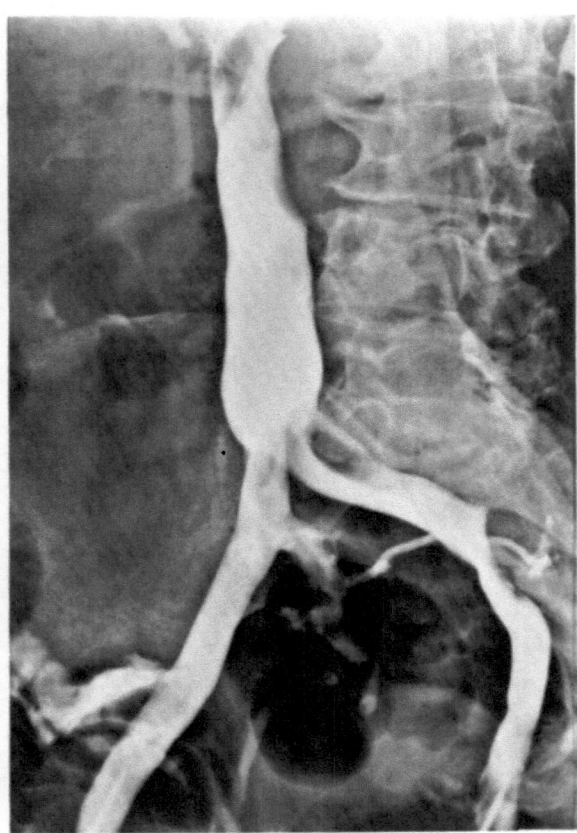

Fig. 350   *Fig. 351*

Figs. 350 and 351: Bifemoral percutaneous cavography. Frontal projection (350) and left anterior oblique projection (351). Malignant lumbar and pelvic lymph node involvements in a patient with lymphosarcoma. The pelvic features are rather signs of ensheathing and extrinsic compression: The sheathing signs are very obvious on the frontal projections (350) and the extrinsic compression signs on the left anterior oblique projections (351). Contrariwise, the retroperitoneal adenopathies are well displayed only in the left anterior oblique projection which clears the inferior vena cava from the spine and shows wide arciform imprints compressing the posterior aspect of the inferior vena cava.

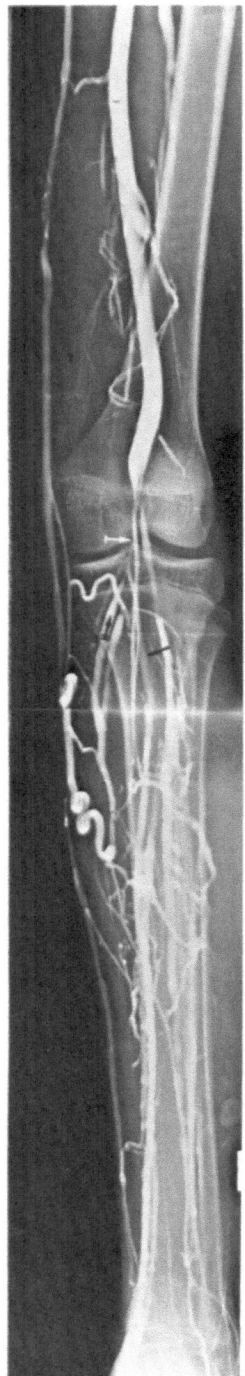

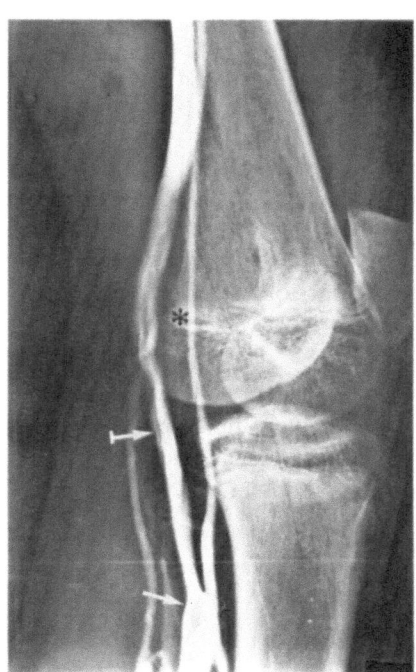

Fig. 352   *Fig. 353*

Figs. 352 and 353: Soleus muscle syndrome.

352: Phlebogram of the left lower limb, frontal projection. Stenosis of the tibio-peroneal trunk ↑ and of the lower part of the popliteal vein ↑. Collateral circulation with marked development of the internal gastrocnemial veins ↑. Stenosis due to hyperextension of the knee would be visualized at a higher level.

353: Lateral phlebography in hyperextension of the knee and dorsal flexion of the foot to exert tension on the soleus muscle. Compression and flattening involves the lower part of the popliteal vein ↑ and the tibio-peroneal trunk ↑. Filling is very laminar and opacification very faint, due to the stenosis. Note the absence of extrinsic compression of the posterior aspect of the femoral condyles. Surgery confirms the presence of a very narrow and tough aponeurosis enclosing the soleus muscle. Opacification of the internal saphenous vein ∗.

248

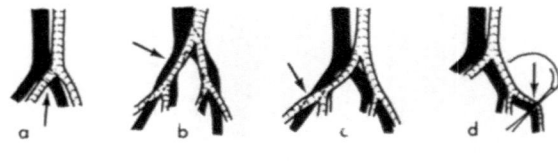

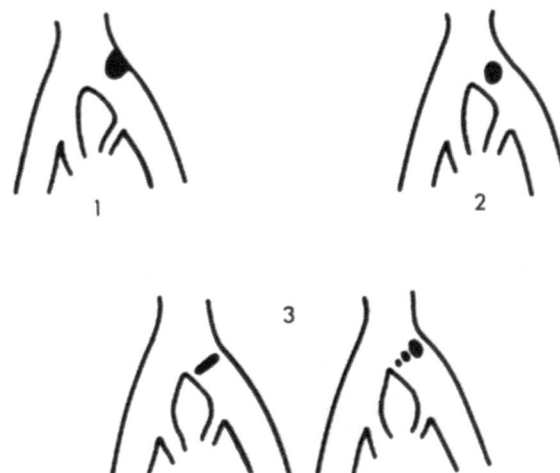

Fig. 354: Drawing demonstrating the different variations of the iliac venous compression syndrome.

a. Usual site compression (80%).

b. Complete overriding of vena caval bifurcation by aorta.

c. Compression of right external iliac vein in bifurcation of right common iliac artery.

d. Compression at inguinal ligament.

(Redrawn from H. Dodd and F.B. Cockett, p. 232, fig. 16.9.)

Fig. 355: Different types of endovenous synechia in the left iliac venous compression syndrome.

1. Lateral flap.
2. Central band.
3. Almost complete occlusion.

(Redrawn from H. Dodd and F.B. Cockett, p. 47, fig. 3.37C.)

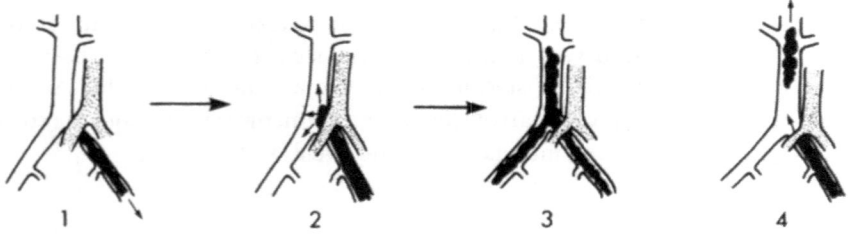

Fig. 356: Possible ways of spread of thrombosis due to iliac compression.

1–2. Spread of thrombosis.
  3. Caval thrombosis.
  4. Embolism.

(Redrawn from H. Dodd and F.B. Cockett, p. 236, fig. 16.13.)

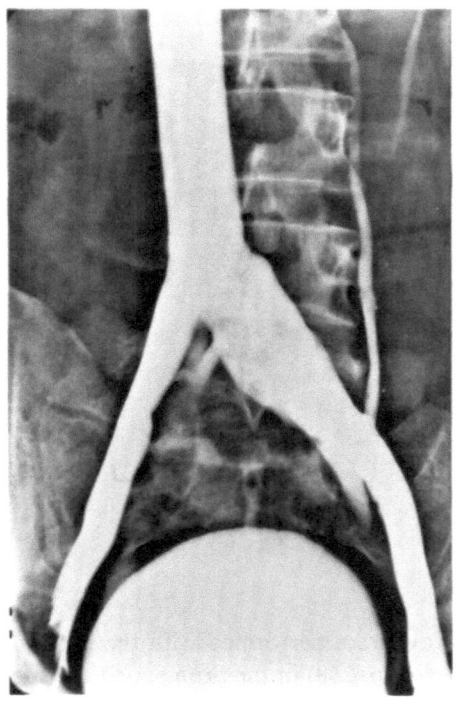

Fig. 357: Appearance of very slight left iliac vein compression with a pseudo-enlargement of the left common iliac vein. In fact there is a very significant reduction in the diameter of the lumen of the vein which is flattened in the frontal plane, producing a false enlargement image.

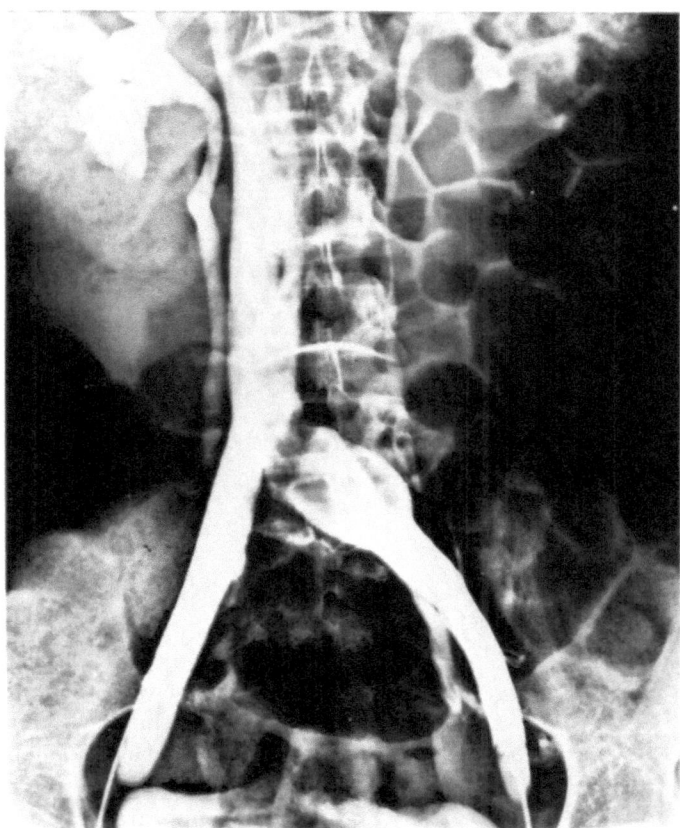

Fig. 358

Figs. 358 and 359: Left iliac venous compression syndrome. Importance of the position of the patient.

358: Cavography performed in the supine position. There is a marked extrinsic imprint.

359 (see p. 250): Cavogram performed with the patient in the prone position showing a clear diminution of the extrinsic imprint.

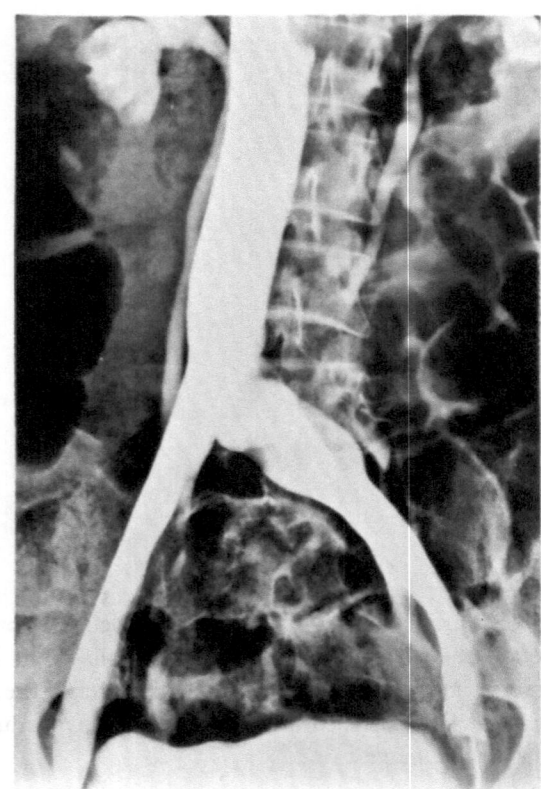

Fig. 359: Cavogram performed with the patient shown in Fig. 358 (see p. 249) in the prone position, showing a clear diminution of the extrinsic imprint.

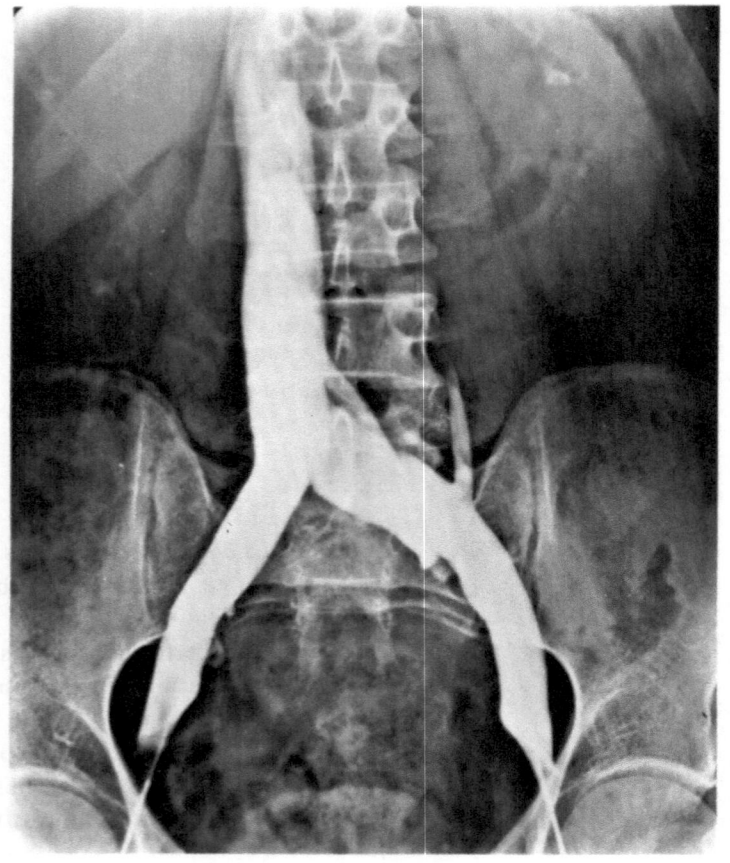

Fig. 360: Left iliac venous compression syndrome with a small synechia in the termination of the left common iliac vein which septates this vessel, producing a lamellar appearance.

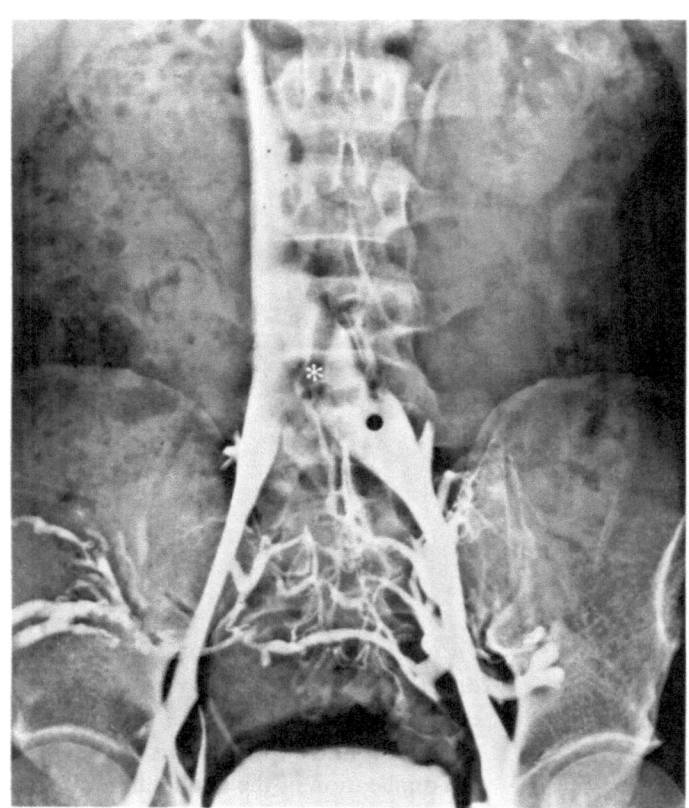

Fig. 361

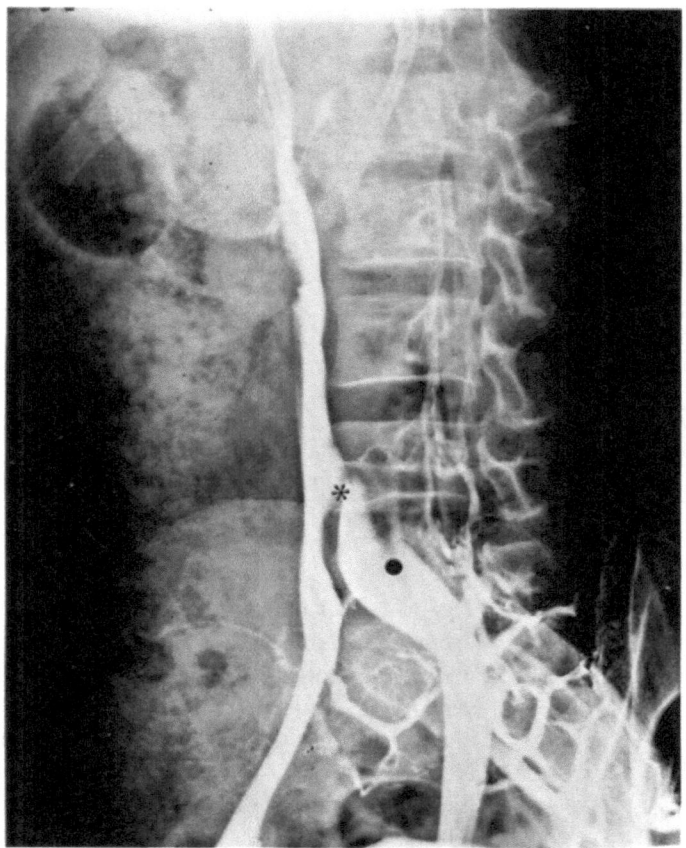

Fig. 362

Figs. 361 and 362: Frontal and left anterior oblique projection of cavography in a double left iliac venous compression syndrome. There is, in fact, a double extrinsic imprint, on the inferior vena caval origin *, and another, 2 cm below on the left common iliac vein •. This double left venous compression is well demonstrated on the left anterior oblique projection (362).

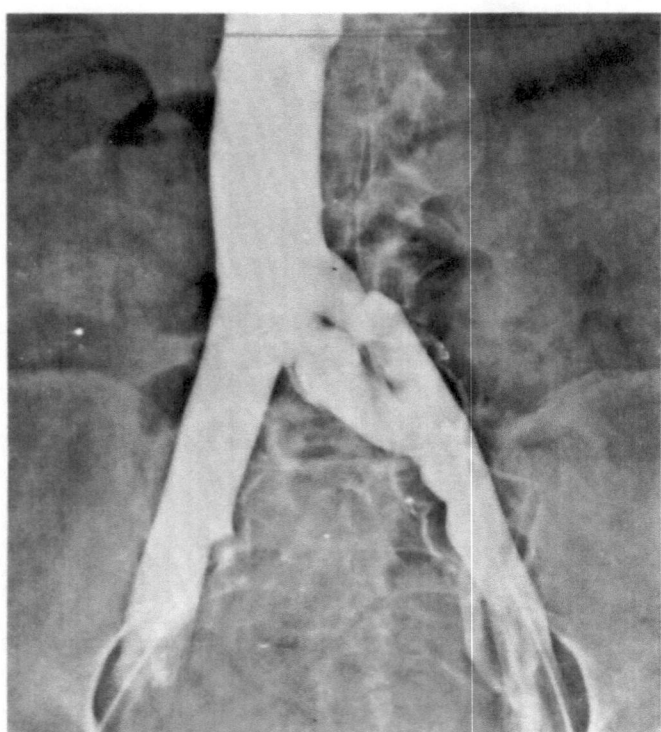

Fig. 363: Left iliac venous compression syndrome associated with a very extended synechia of the left common iliac vein. The radioanatomic appearance is similar to partial duplication of the left common iliac vein.

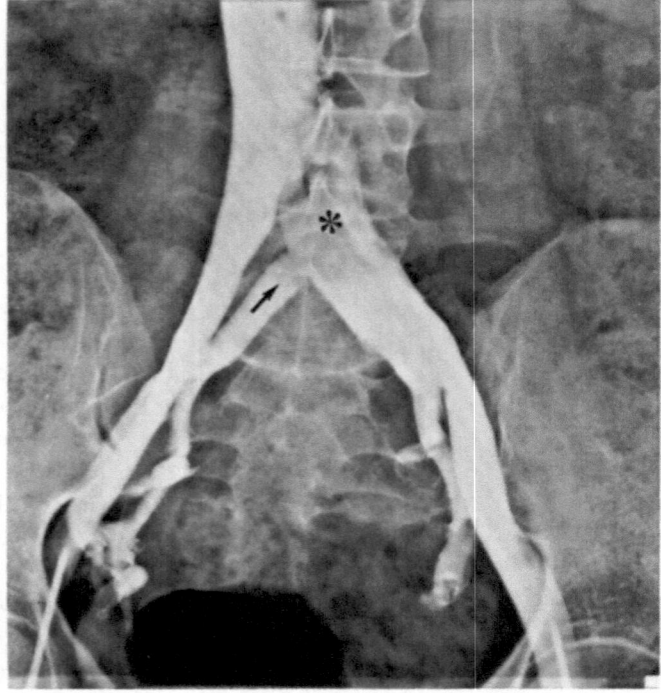

Fig. 364: Left iliac venous compression syndrome associated with a congenital anomaly of the common iliac and right internal iliac vein. As a matter of fact the right internal iliac vein ⬆ joins the left common iliac vein ✳. Note the synechia producing fenestration of the left common iliac vein which is also clearly compressed.

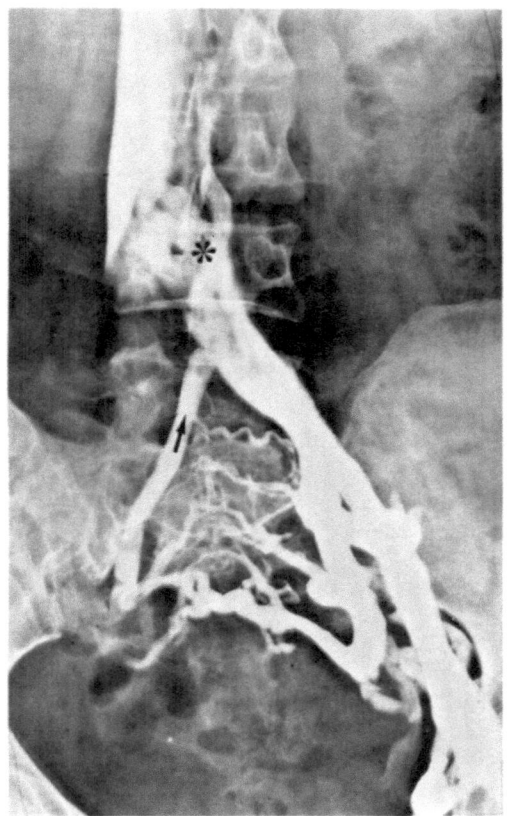

Fig. 365: Cockett's syndrome with a very significant synechia on the termination of the left common iliac vein∗. Note the congenital anomaly: the right internal iliac vein ↑ joins the left common iliac vein. Note the degree and extent of the extrinsic compression.

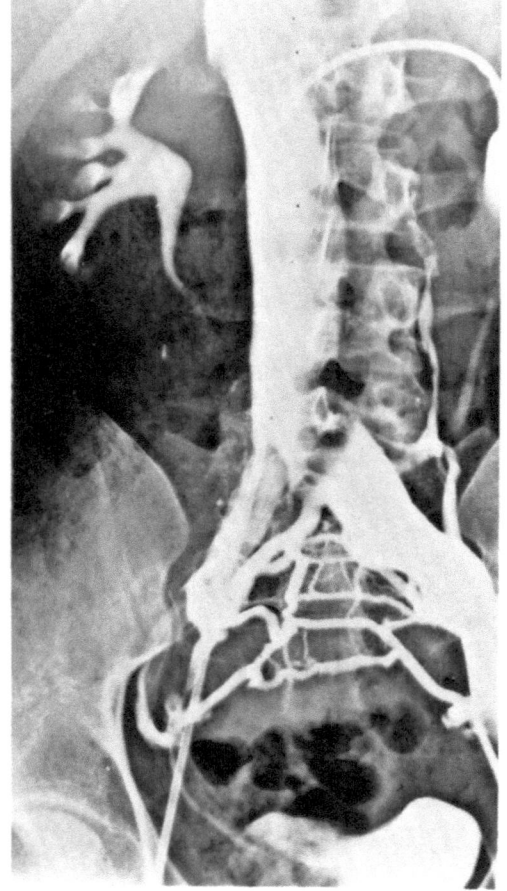

Fig. 366

Figs. 366 and 367: Association of left iliac venous compression syndrome (366) and of a left varicocele (367 — see p. 254). Figure 367 illustrates a left selective spermatic venography. Some authors have suggested the hypothesis that the genital vein could undergo varicose dilatation, in so far as it ensures decompression of the iliac venous system by means of the communication between the epigastric vein, branch of the iliac system, and the spermatic vein at the level of the inguinal ligament.

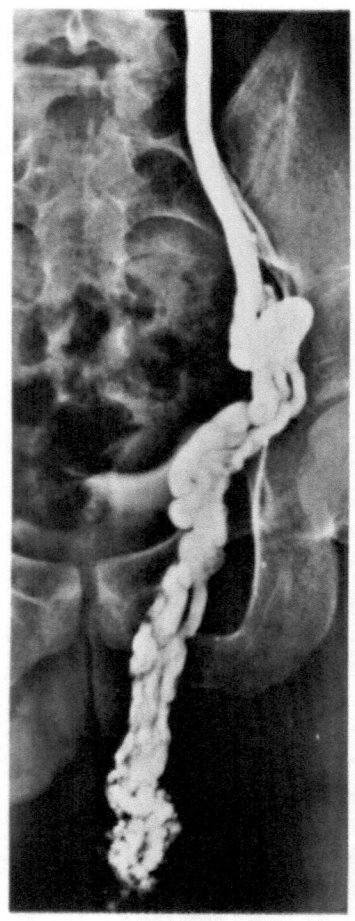

Fig. 367

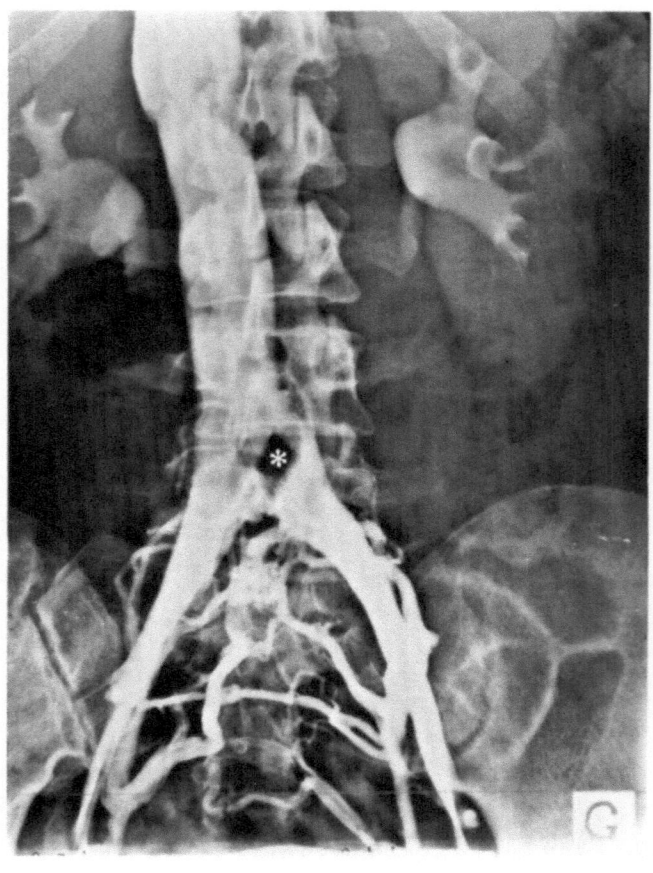

Fig. 368: Cockett's syndrome with a voluminous central ∗ synechia of the termination of the left common iliac vein.

Figs. 366 and 367: Association of left iliac venous compression syndrome (366 — see p. 253) and of a left varicocele (367). Figure 367 illustrates a left selective spermatic venography. Some authors have suggested the hypothesis that the genital vein could undergo varicose dilatation, in so far as it ensures decompression of the iliac venous system by Means of the communication between the epigastric vein, branch of the iliac system, and the spermatic vein at the level of the inguinal ligament.

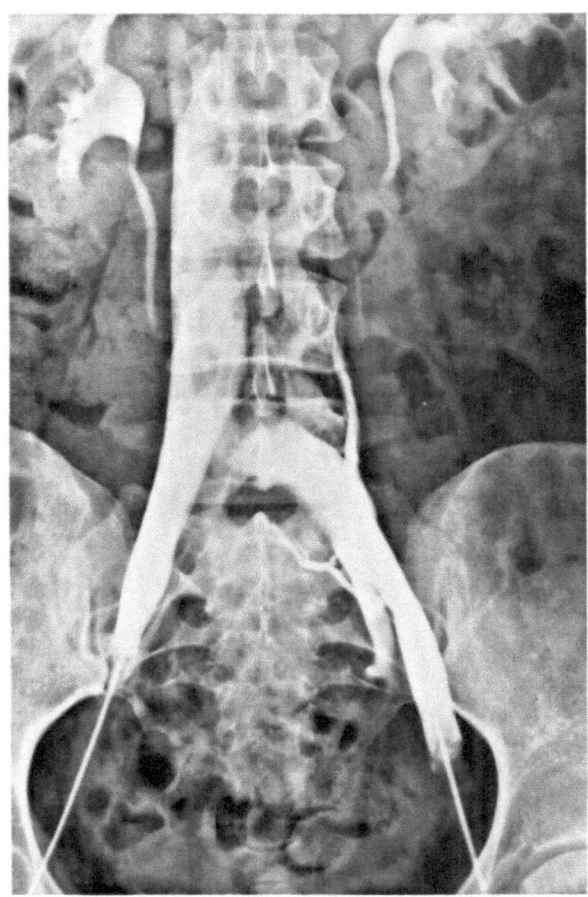

Fig. 369

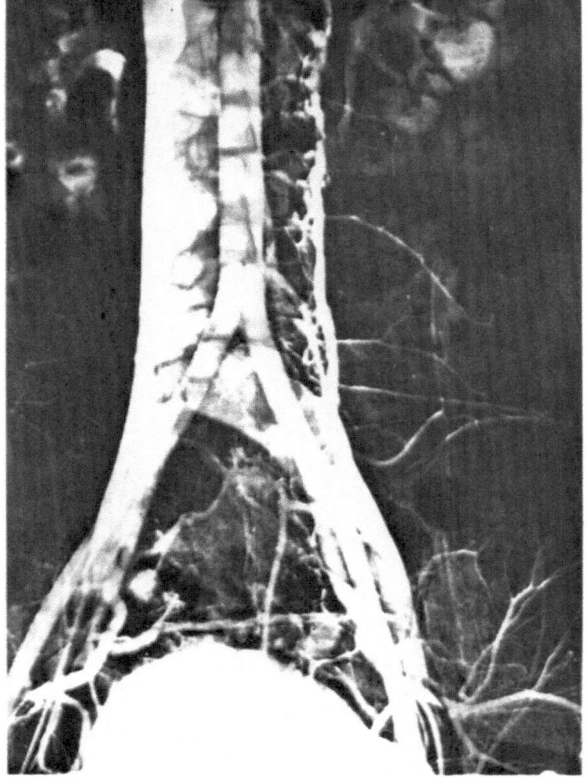

Fig. 370

Figs. 369 and 370: Moderate Cockett's syndrome in a young woman with a history of pulmonary embolisms. No other thromboembolic localization on the veins of the lower limb.

369: Bilateral cavography shows a moderate Cockett's syndrome. No synechia was demonstrable. There is only an extrinsic compression imprint on the termination of the left common iliac vein.

370: Cavography coupled with aortography demonstrating clearly the extrinsic compression of the termination of the left common iliac vein by the right common iliac artery.

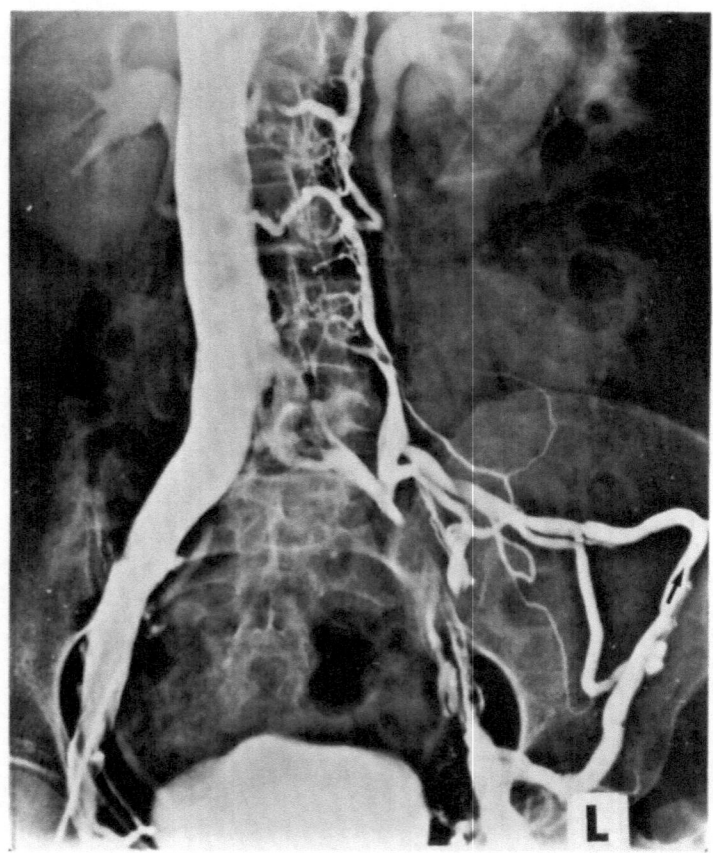

Fig. 371: Left ilio-femoral phlebitis. Bifemoral percutaneous cavography. Left iliac collateral circle faintly reopacifying the terminal segment of the left common iliac vein which is poly-fenestrated and shows multiple synechia. Cockett's syndrome with underlying phlebitis.

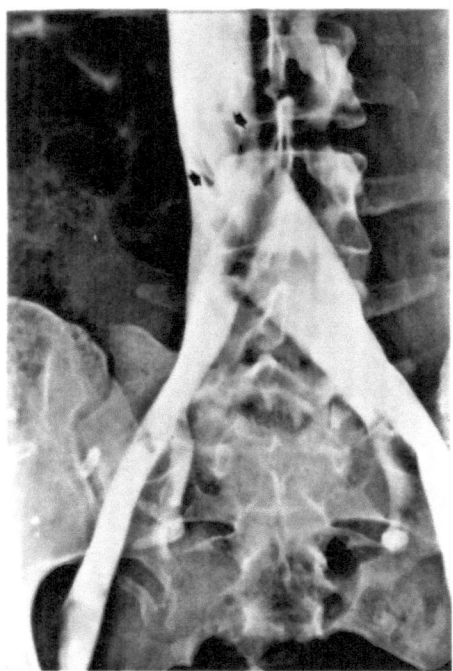

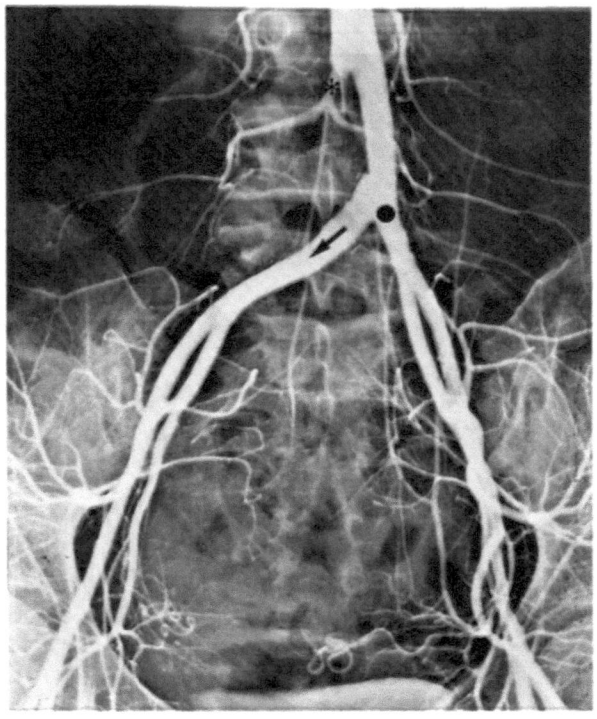

Fig. 373

Fig. 372: Bifemoral percutaneous cavography. Cockett's syndrome with "snake-head" ▲ image of phlebothrombosis proximal to the extrinsic compression. This patient has presented several successive pulmonary embolisms. No changes in the veins of the lower limbs distally. It is a case of a rather uncommon appearance of thrombosis above the Cockett's syndrome without thrombosis below.

Figs. 373 and 374: Operated-upon Cockett's syndrome.

373: Aorto-arteriography (centered onto the lesser pelvis) Uncrossing of the right common iliac artery ↑ to suppress the left iliac venous compression. Ligation of the right common iliac artery at its origin on the aorta✳ , and transposition 3 cm below onto the left common iliac artery ● .

374 (see p. 258): Left femoral percutaneous phlebography in the same patient. In spite of the patch of venous enlargement, there is still an obliteration of the left common iliac vein with contralateral derivation via the presacral plexuses.

Failure of the preventive treatment of a Cockett's syndrome in a young woman who presented pulmonary embolisms without any other sign of phlebitis of the lower limbs.

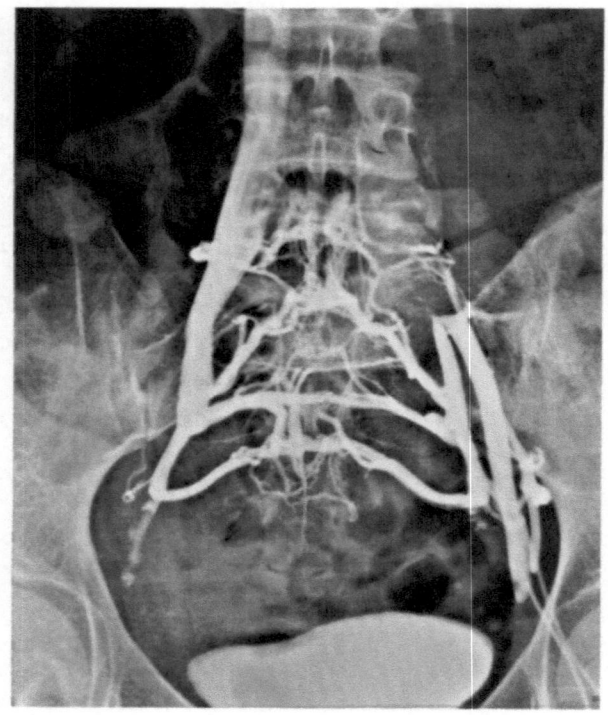

Fig. 374

374: Left femoral percutaneous phlebography in the same patient shown in Fig. 373 (see p. 257). In spite of the patch of venous enlargement, there is still an obliteration of the left common iliac vein with contralateral derivation via the presacral plexuses.

Chapter 12

VENOUS DYSPLASIAE

Figures 375–397

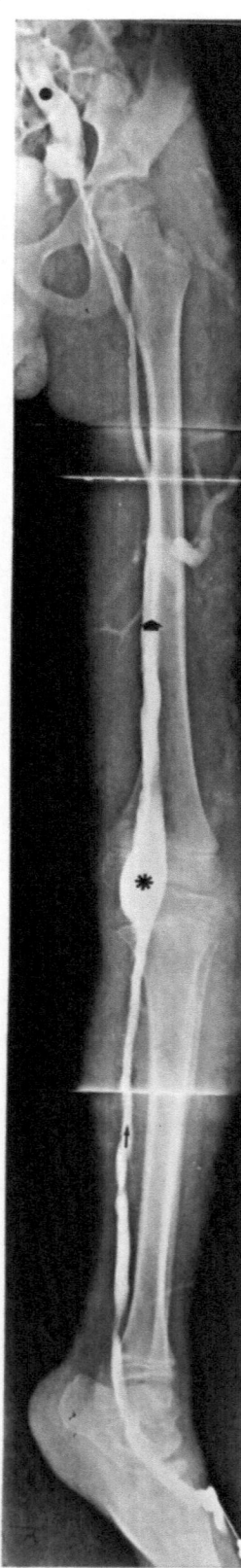

Fig. 375

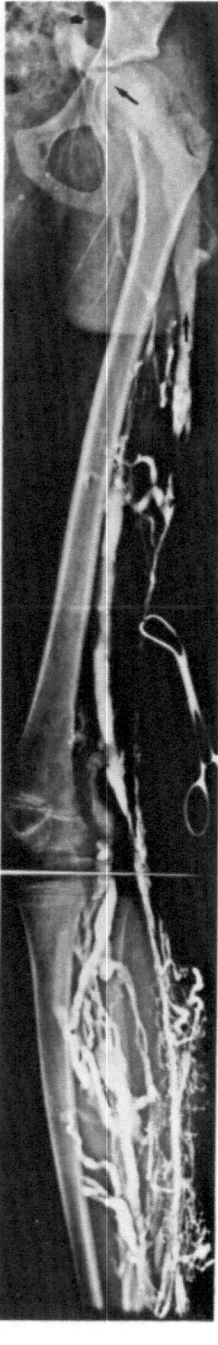

Fig. 376

Figs. 375 and 376:

375: Preoperative venography. Injection into a very voluminous vein of the dorsum of the left foot. Opacification of a single venous trunk of the leg ↑, which seems valveless. Then, filling of a gross venous ampula in the popliteal space ✳ which drains always into a unique vein at the median part of the thigh ◂, projecting onto the femoral shaft (and thus not consistent with the usual femoro-popliteal axis). Reopacification of an iliac axis of large caliber ●. Since there is no lateral projection, it is very difficult to know whether the pelvic course occurs in the buttock or in the Scarpa's triangle.

376: Phlebography performed during operation in the same patient, after cut down onto the external saphenous vein. The opacification is different (due to the fact that it is not the same vein which is punctured): the venous network is quite anarchic and never does opacify the femoro-popliteal system. But, due to the injection into the external saphenous vein, a voluminous vein on the lateral part of the thigh ↑ is demonstrated which reopacifies the hypogastric system ◂. This is a rather common drainage route seen in the Klippel-Trenaunay syndromes, i.e., a vein on the lateral aspect of the thigh which drains via the inferior gluteal venous system.

In conclusion: Klippel-Trenaunay syndrome with femoro-popliteal agenesia.

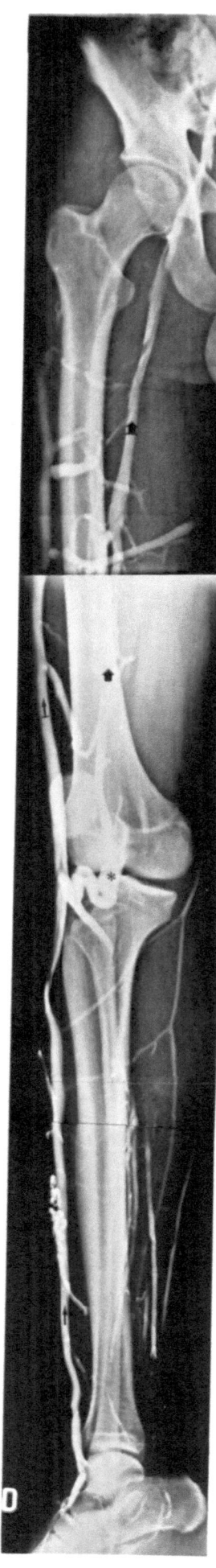

Fig. 377: Phlebography of the right lower limb from an injection into a dorsal vein of the foot. Drainage via an abnormal gross vein on the anterior aspect of the right leg ⇂. There is almost no opacification of the deep leg veins. The drainage is continued in the thigh by a large anterolateral external vein ↿ with partial opacification through a bayonet-shaped * ampullar dilatation of a deep pathway in the thigh ♠ which will give off the ilio-femoral axis. This latter vein probably corresponds to a retro-adducting vein which is drained by the profunda femoris vein ♣. Nevertheless venous return occurs clearly preferentially at the level of the thigh through a voluminous anterolateral vein ⇂. Conclusion: Klippel-Trenaunay syndrome with a deep venous malformation corresponding to probable agenesia of the deep leg veins and to unquestionable femoro-popliteal agenesia.

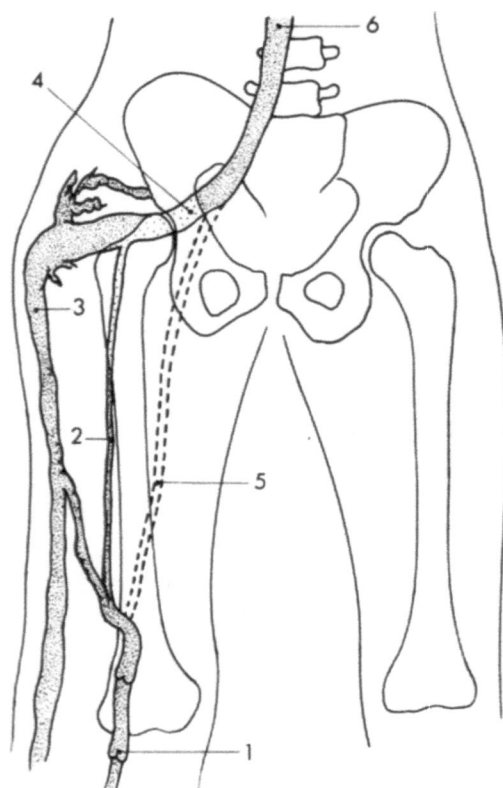

Fig. 378: Diagram of agenesia of both superficial and common femoral veins.

1. Popliteal vein.
2. Profunda femoris vein.
3. Voluminous vein at the superolateral aspect of the right thigh.
4. Ischiatic vein.
5. Agenesia of superficial femoral vein.
6. Common iliac vein.

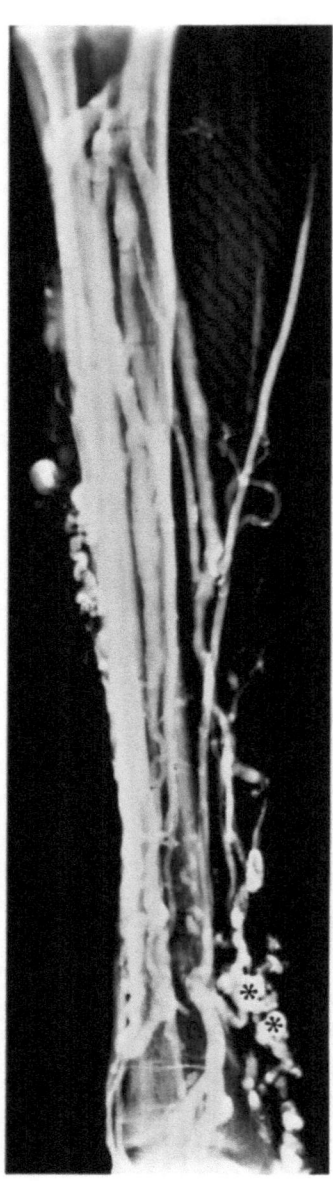

Fig. 379

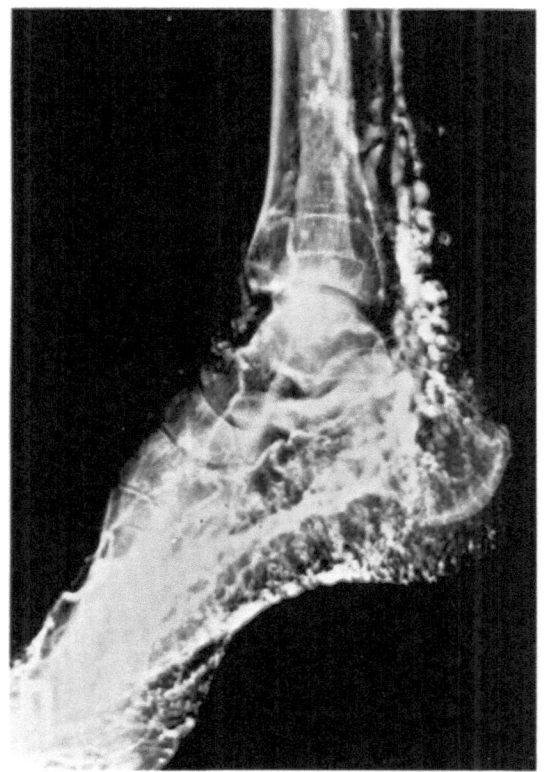 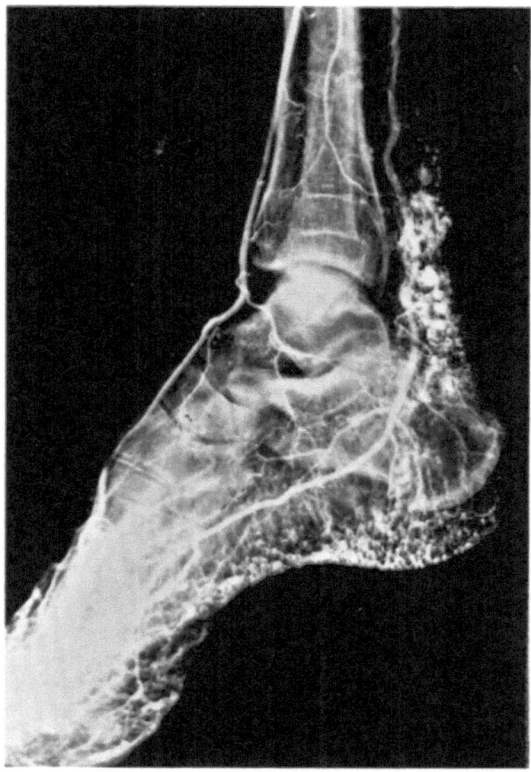

Fig. 380

Figs. 379 and 380: The right lower limb is 5 cm longer than the left. Varices. Angioma.

379: Phlebography: No malformation of the deep venous trunks in the leg. Small varices∗ in the lower part of the leg.

380: Arteriography: Arteriovenous fistula at the level of the sole and of the posterior aspect of the lower third of the leg. These images are thus superposable to the varices demonstrated by the phlebogram.

In conclusion: Congenital arteriovenous fistula with a clinical syndrome suggestive of a Klippel-Trenaunay syndrome. There is no malformation of the deep venous system

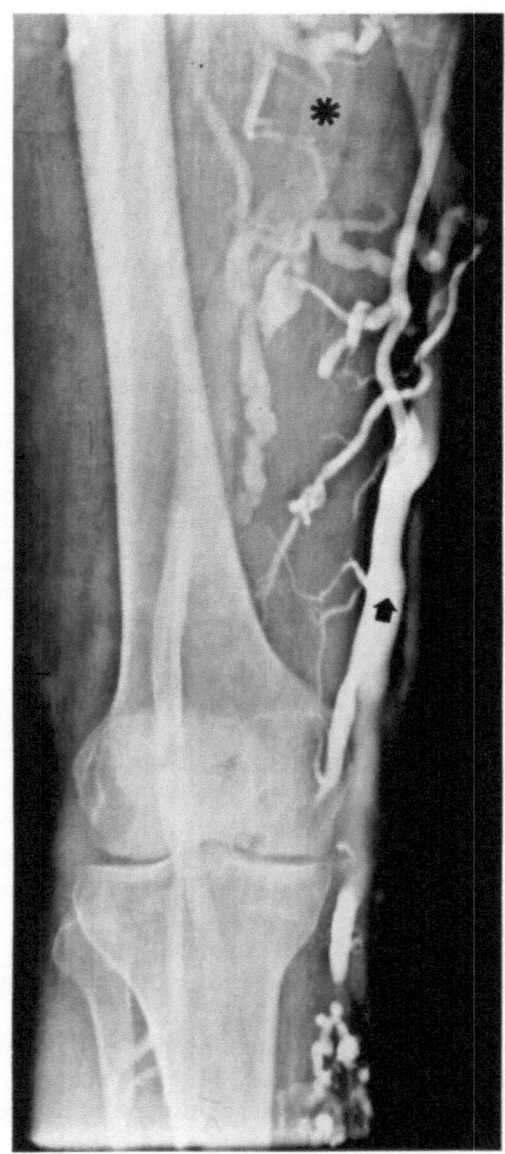

Fig. 381

Figs. 381, 382 and 383: Unilateral varices since childhood. Varicose veins of the thigh with angioma of the thigh and lengthening of the right lower limb by 4 cm.

381: Phlebography of the right lower limb demonstrating opacification of a very voluminous vein on the medial part of the leg and of the thigh, which could correspond to the very dilated internal saphenous vein ♠. The femoro-popliteal deep axis is almost not opacified, although it also seems to be significantly dilated, namely in the upper part of the film ✱. The phlebogram was performed with the patient in the supine position, so that it is difficult to affirm or disprove the valvelessness of the deep venous system.

382 and 383: Arteriography demonstrating a huge arteriovenous fistula on the thigh and upper part of the leg.

In conclusion: Congenital arteriovenous dysplasia most probably associated with a malformation of the deep system, although the latter has not been positively demonstrated.

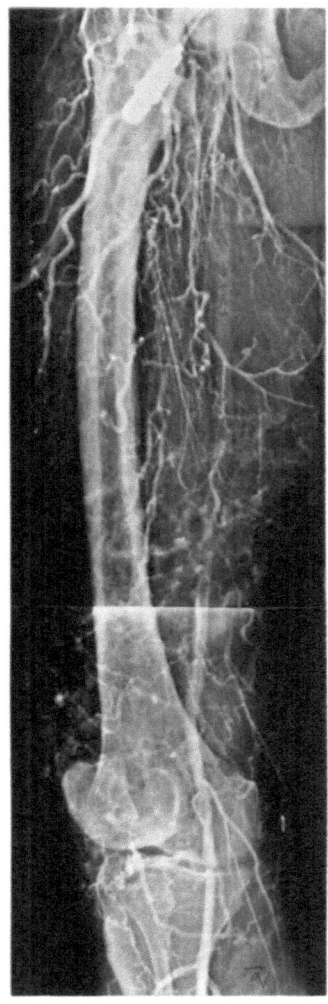

Fig. 382

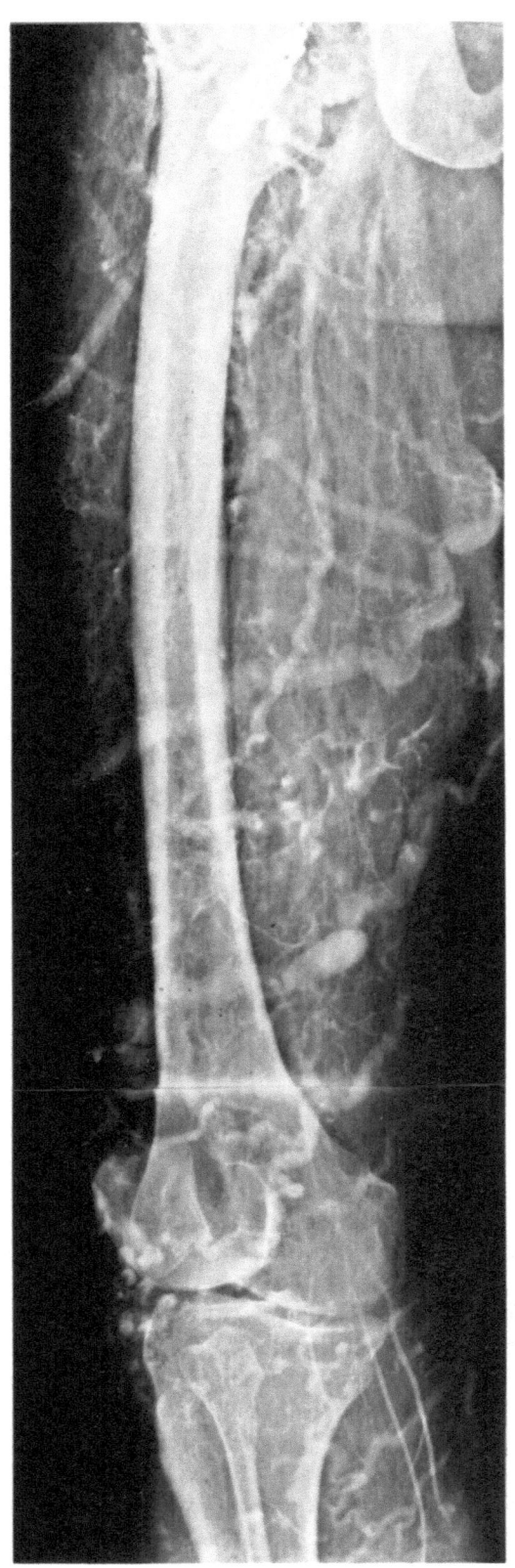

Fig. 383

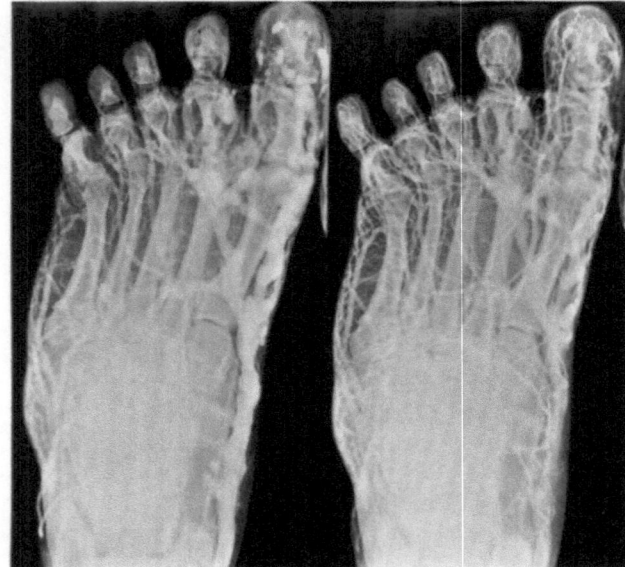

Fig. 384   Fig. 385

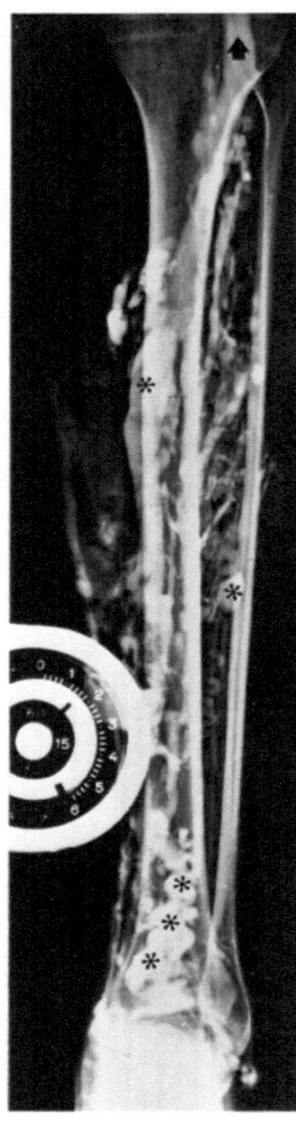

Fig. 386

Figs. 384, 385 and 386: Girl, aged 18 presenting a discrete lengthening of the left lower limb, varicose veins and an angioma on the medial aspect of the leg.

384 and 385: Arteriography of the left foot (according to Cecile's technique, with screenless films). There are arteriovenous shunts at the level of the first three toes, which are drained by a superficial venous system of large caliber, corresponding by the site to the internal saphenous vein. Note the very distal arteriovenous shunts, namely on the big toe. No other arteriovenous shunt on the arteries of the left lower limb. This shows the importance of performing arteriography when searching for arteriovenous dysplasiae, namely in association with certain Klippel-Trenaunay syndromes.

386: Phlebography of the left lower limb in the same patient. Films centered on the leg. Superficial varices * . No filling of the deep trunks. The reopacification at the knee-joint line occurs at the level of the femoro-popliteal vein ♠ which is patent. Therefore, it is a matter of agenesia of the deep veins of the leg.

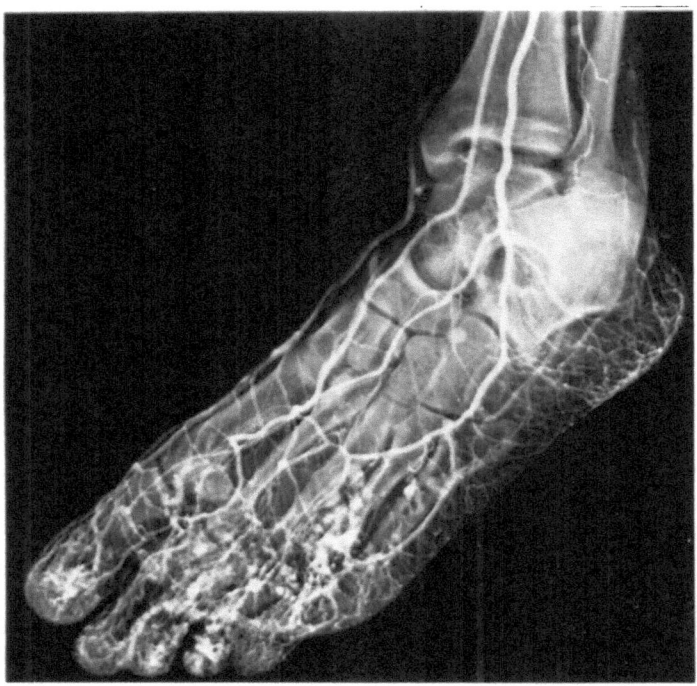

Fig. 387

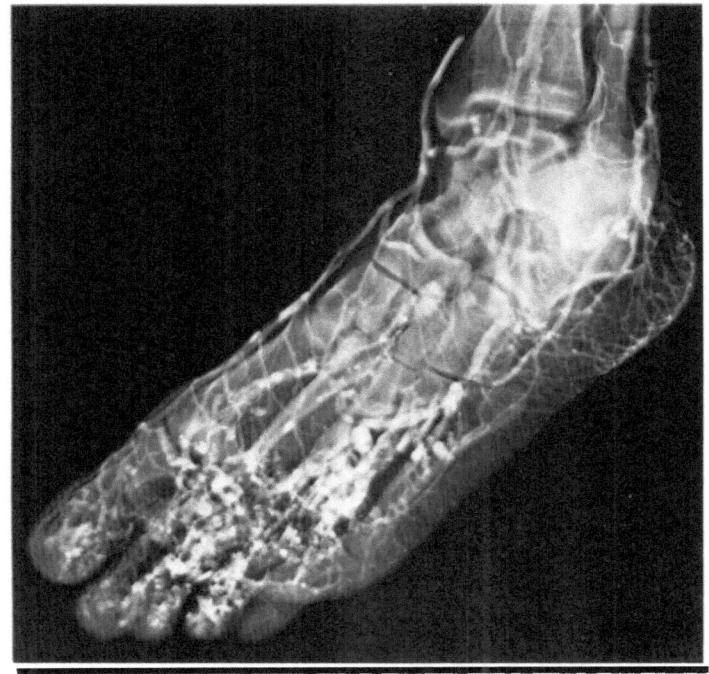

Fig. 388

Figs. 387 and 388: Arteriography of the foot. Oblique projection. Angiomatous dysplasia with multiple arteriovenous fistulae at the sole of the foot.
387: Arterial phase.
388: Venous phase.
Patient presenting all the signs of a Klippel-Trenaunay syndrome. The venogram was normal and demonstrated no obstacle or agenesia in the deep venous system.

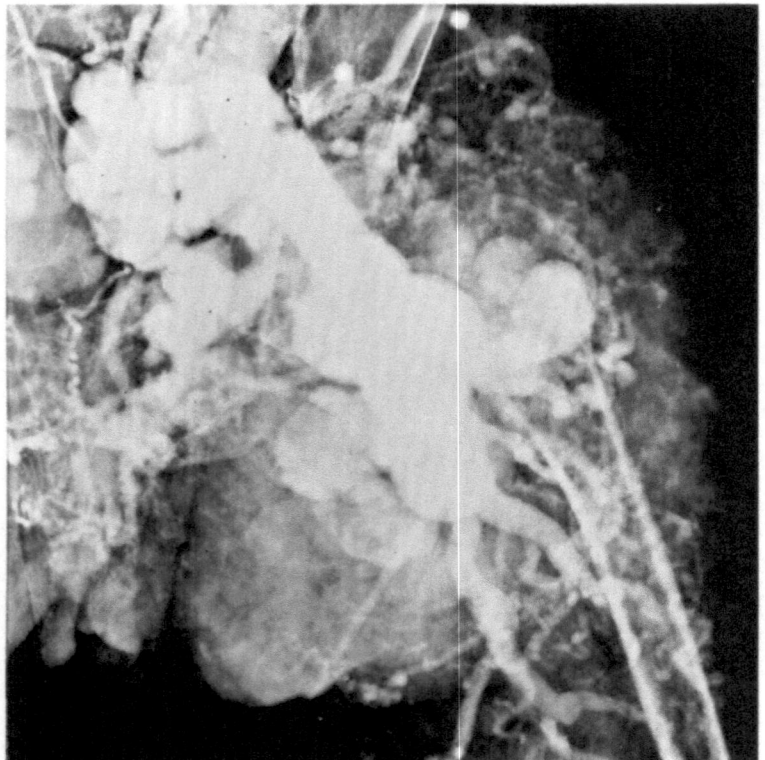

Fig. 389

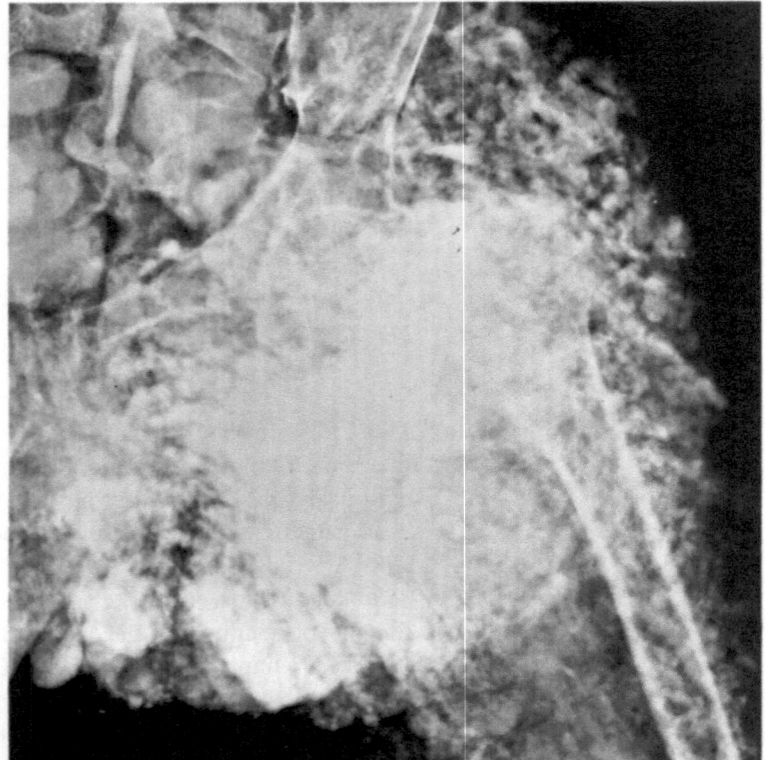

Fig. 390

Figs. 389 and 390: Klippel-Trenaunay and Weber syndrome.
389: Arterial phase.
390: Venous phase.
Huge arteriovenous dysplasia localized to the upper part of thigh, triangle of Scarpa and lesser pelvis. The patient had already undergone amputation on the thigh because of the importance of arteriovenous fistulae in the lower limb.

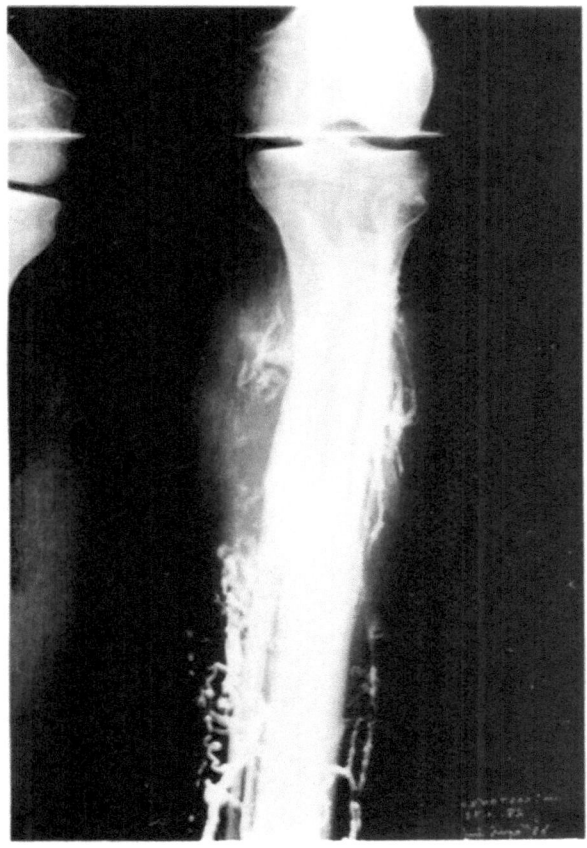

Fig. 391

Figs. 391, 392 and 393: Young man, aged 19, presenting all signs of a Klippel-Trenaunay syndrome.
391: Phlebography of the right lower limb; frontal projection. Varicose veins of the leg. Very marked stenosis of the popliteal vein. This finding could correspond (in the absence of clinical signs of Klippel-Trenaunay syndrome) to an artefact due to hyperextension of the knee as described in chapter 2.
392 and 393 (see p. 270): Right femoral arteriography. Same patient.
392: Early sequence already showing arteriovenous fistulae above the knee∗, and especially micro-fistulae in the muscular tissue of the quadriceps at the lateral aspect of the upper part of thigh ◄.
393: Venous phase of the femoral arteriography, also displaying a voluminous vein in the anterior part of the leg ↿, draining toward the upper and external thigh ⇡, as well as a greater number of muscular arteriovenous dysplasiae on the superolateral aspect of the right thigh ◄. Note that the phlebographic phase of the arteriography fails to demonstrate the stenosis of the popliteal vein. This is, in fact, totally invisible on Fig. 393.
Post-arteriographic phlebography of the lower limb is not an adequate technique for studying the deep venous system; it demonstrates mainly the superficial veins (even when a tourniquet is utilized).

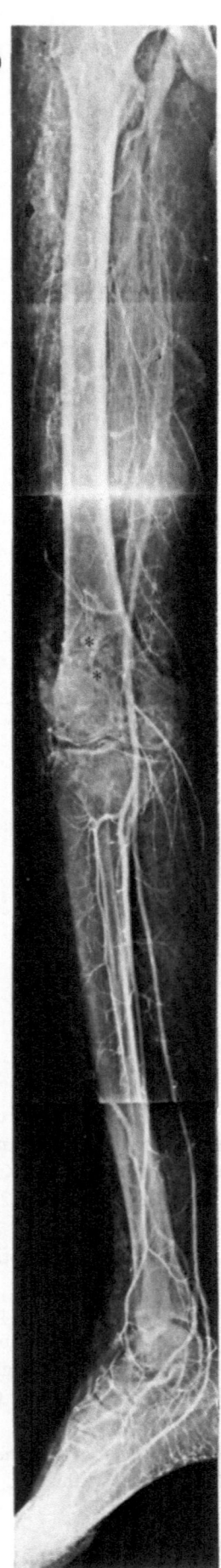

Fig. 392

(For legends to Figs. 392 and 393, see previous page.)

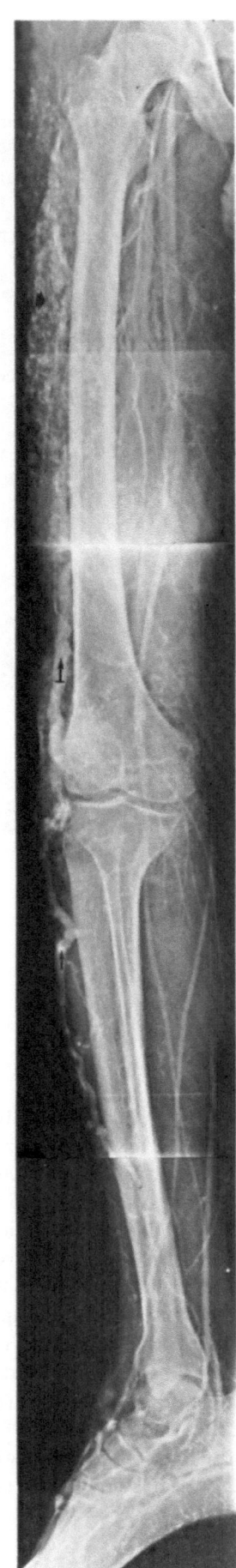

Fig. 393

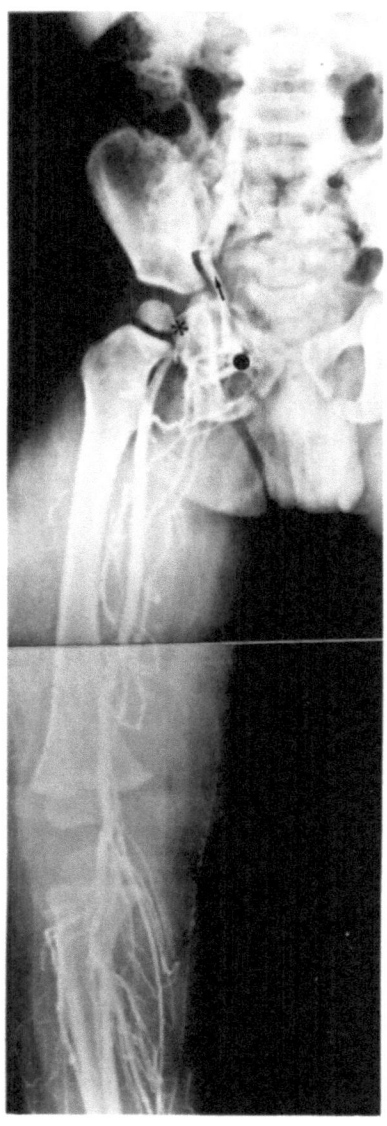

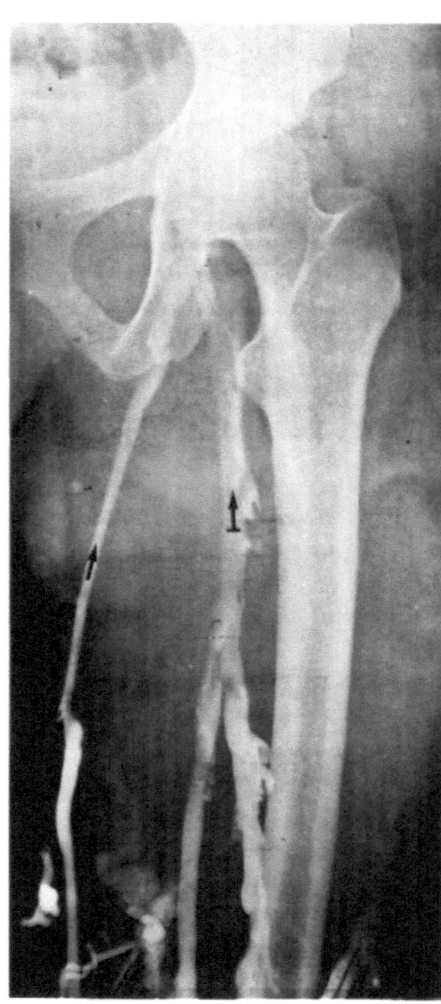

Fig. 394: Klippel-Trenaunay syndrome in a 4-year-old child. Phlebography of the right lower limb, from cut down of the vein. Agenesia of the common femoral vein and of the external iliac vein ∗, confirmed later by surgery. Note the collateral circulation through the obturator foramen ● toward the internal iliac vein ↑, and then the right common iliac vein and the inferior vena cava.

Fig. 395: Klippel-Trenaunay syndrome with a longer left leg. Phlebography. Centering on the thigh. complete agenesia of the superficial femoral vein supplied by the internal saphenous ↑ and the profunda femoris vein ↥. (Confirmed by surgery.)

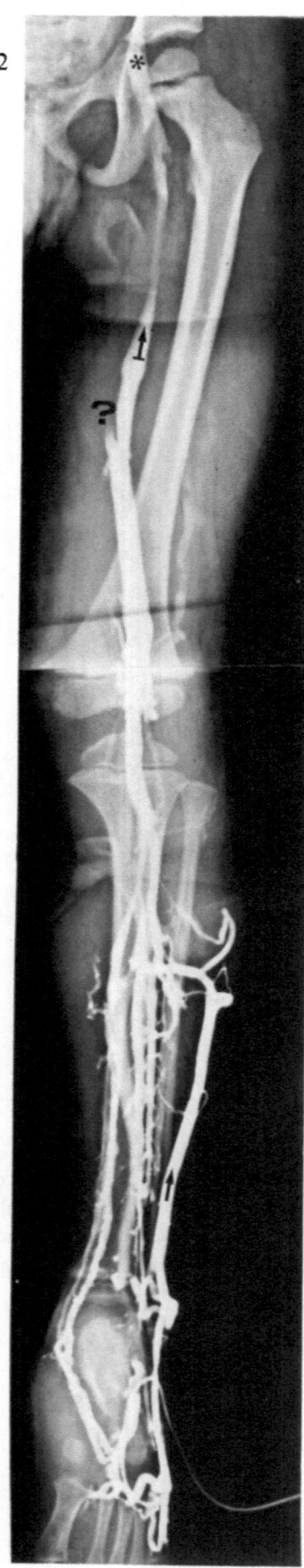

Fig. 396: Lengthening of the left leg in a child of 4. Superficial angiomatosis of the left lower limb. Phlebogram of the left lower limb demonstrates a huge vein on the anterolateral part of the leg ↿, originating at the level of the external malleolus and ascending along the lateral aspect of the leg. The deep leg veins and the popliteal vein seem to be normal. Contrariwise, there is no superficial femoral opacification **?**; venous opacification in the upper thigh corresponds to the topography of the profunda femoris vein ↿, which reopacifies the common femoral vein **∗**. Surgery confirms the presence of superficial femoral agenesia.

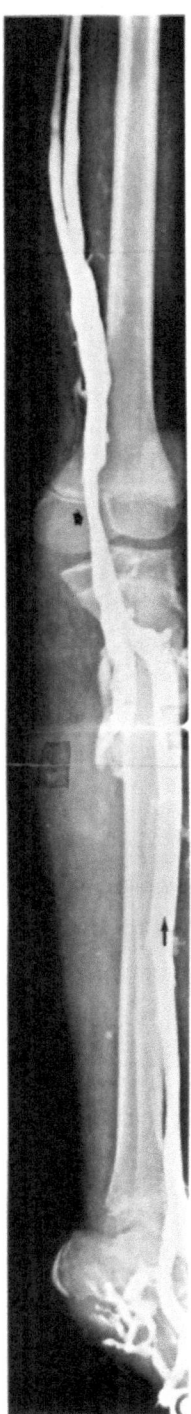

Fig. 397: Klippel-Trenaunay syndrome. Phlebography of the left lower limb. Opacification of a huge valveless vein in the anterior part of the leg ↑, without any opacification of the deep leg veins. Stenosis of the lower part of the popliteal vein ●.

Chapter 13

TRAUMATISM TO THE VEINS

Figures 398–404

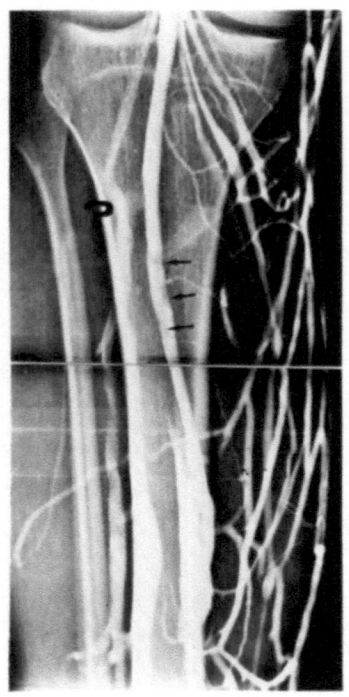

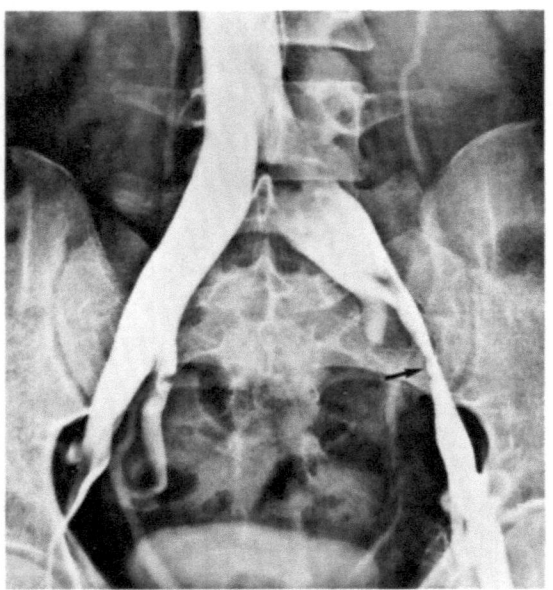

Fig. 398: Traumatism by direct blow to the leg (the patient was kicked by a horse). Phlebogram demonstrating defects in the upper part of the posterior tibial vein ↑↑ and poor filling of the peroneal veins in the upper part of the leg ?. Possible traumatism to the veins without thrombosis or onset of thrombosis.

Fig. 399: Cavography. This patient had left iliac phlebitis and had undergone thrombectomy on hand of a Fogarty's balloon catheter. Diabolo-shaped stenosis of the iliac vein ↑ due to traumatic dissection by the Fogarty catheter.

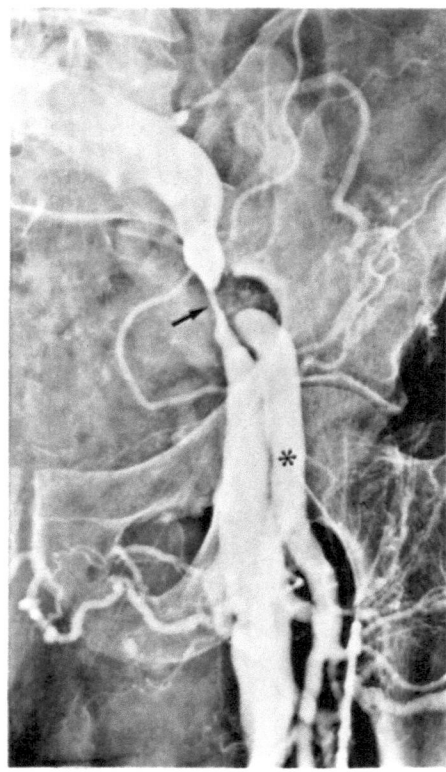

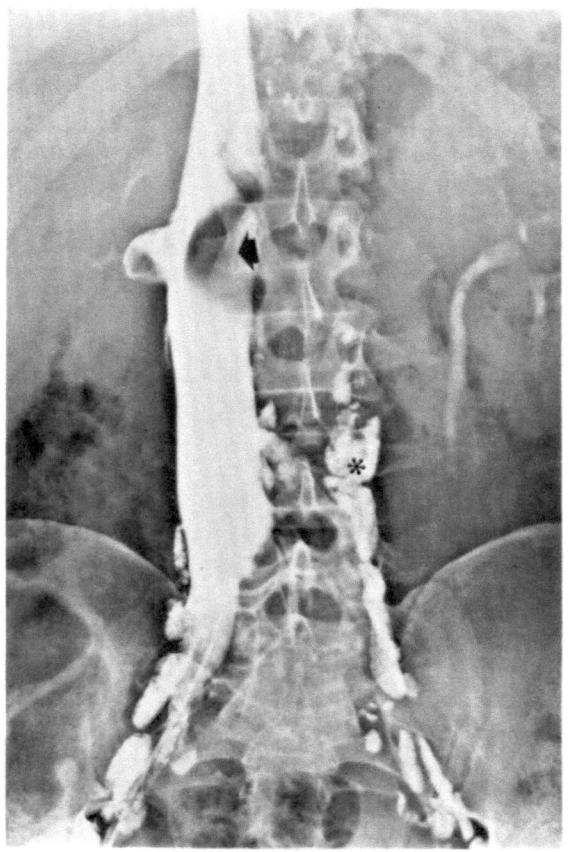

Fig. 401

Fig. 400: This patient had left iliac phlebitis and underwent thrombectomy with the Fogarty catheter and arterialization in the Scarpa's triangle. Left femoral arteriography performed with a small catheter ∗. Opacification of the arteriovenous fistula and of the iliac venous system which shows a stenosis by 90° due to dissection by the Fogarty balloon cather ↑.

Figs. 401, 402 and 403: Danger of prolonged venous catheterization in patients with sarcomatous retroperitoneal adenopathies.

401: Cavography showing a huge compression defect ◄ at the level of the left renal pedicle. Residual contrast material from a lymphography∗.

402 (see p. 278): Selective left renal venography to assert patency of the left renal vein. Global duration of the examination: 1 h 30 min.

403 (see p. 278): Edema of the left lower limbs occurring within five days following the investigation: complete ilioinferior caval thrombosis. Thrombosis of the left renal vein, confirmed by the post-mortem report. Risk involved by venous catheterization in patients with lymphosarcoma.

278

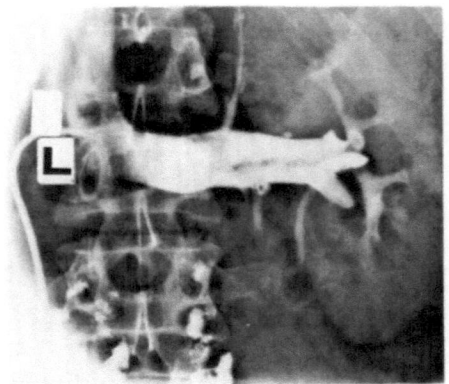

Fig. 402

Fig. 403

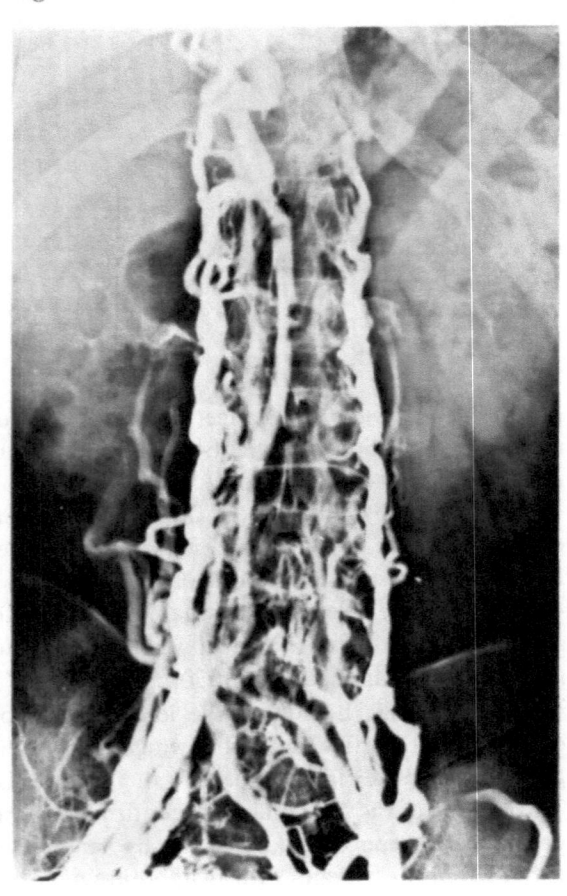

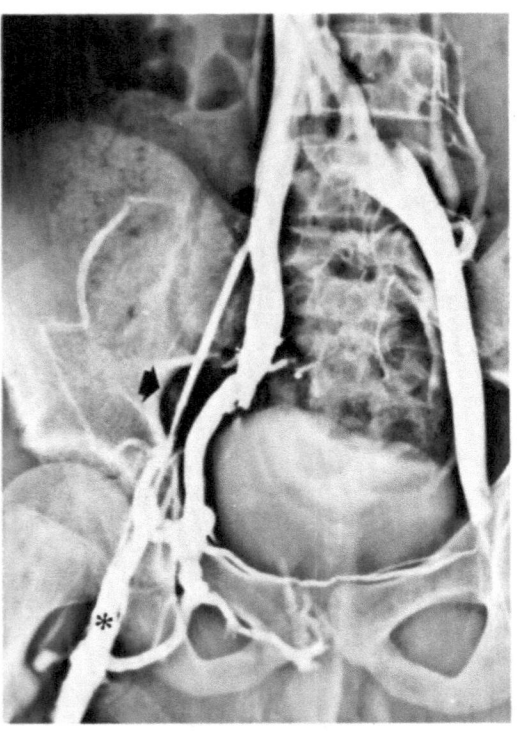

Fig. 404: Operative treatment of a right inguinal herniation in a child aged 14. Traumatism to the veins with a wound during surgery. Follow-up cavography shows the irregular appearance of the common femoral vein ∗ with almost complete stenosis of the external iliac vein ◂.

402: Selective left renal venography to assert patency of the left renal vein. Global duration of the examination: 1 h 30 min.

403: Edema of the left lower limbs occurring within five days following the investigation: complete ilio-inferior caval thrombosis. Thrombosis of the left renal vein, confirmed by the post-mortem report. Risk involved by venous catheterization in patients with lymphosarcoma.

(See also Fig. 401 on p. 277.)

Chapter 14

VARIOUS PATHOLOGIC CONDITIONS OF THE VEINS OF THE LOWER LIMB

Figures 405–409

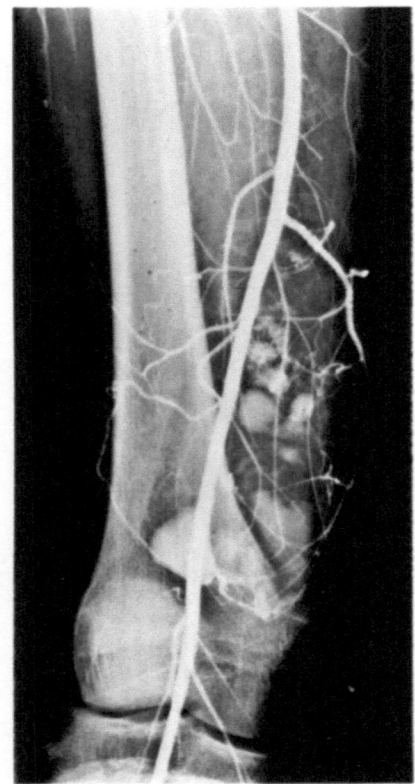

Fig. 405

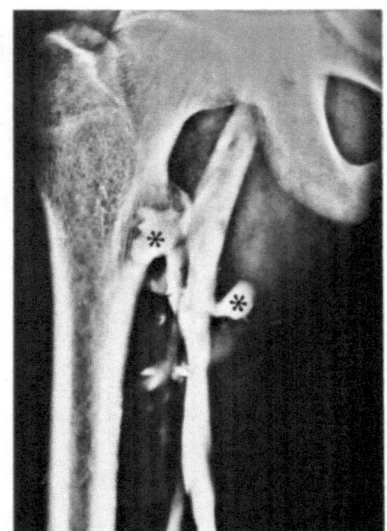

Fig. 407

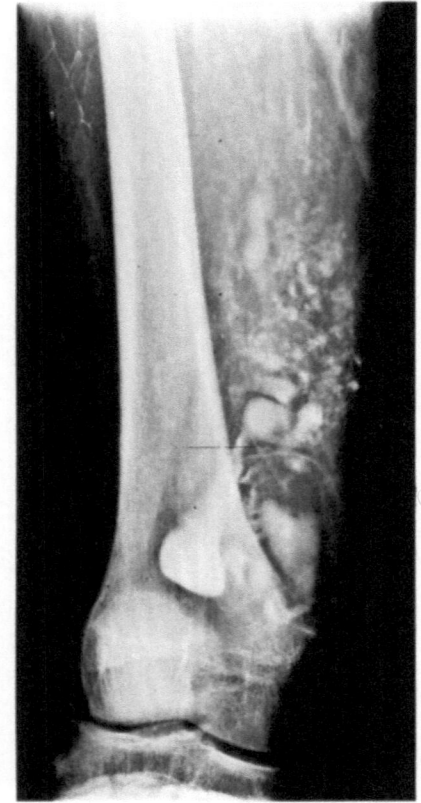

Fig. 406

Figs. 405, 406 and 407: Cystic lymphangioma in a child.
405: Femoral arteriography. Early phase.
406: Later phase of the femoral arteriography showing opacification from the arterial route of a cystic lymphangioma in the lower part of thigh.
407: Phlebography of the lower limb in the same patient showing in the upper part of the thigh, a lympho-venous communication between the cystic lymphangioma and branches of the profunda femoris vein. One of the cysts is displayed on the lesser trochanter *, the other is located more medially* and seems to be communicating with the superficial femoral vein.

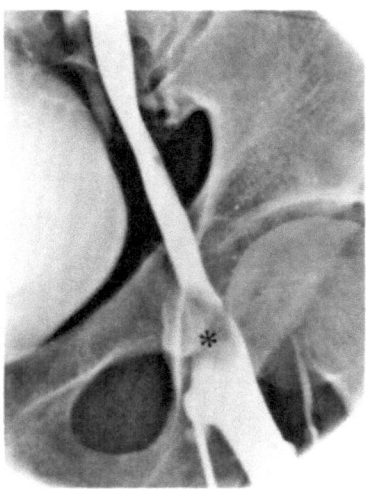

Fig. 408: Patient aged 26, athletic, presenting a thick leg and a thick thigh. Filling defect, occluding * almost completely the common femoral vein. Cyst on the posterior wall of the femoral vein. No communication between the cyst and the coxofemoral joint; it is thus not a matter of a synovial cyst but of a primary tumor of the vein.

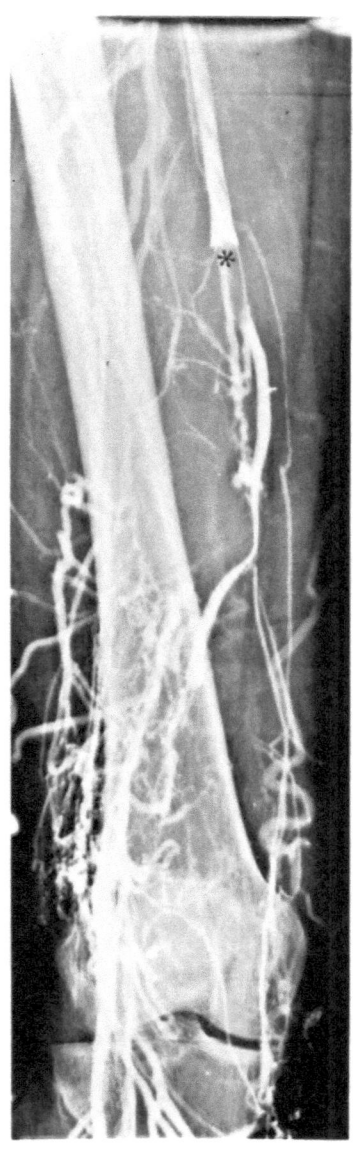

Fig. 409: Thick right leg in a woman aged 50. Suspicion of phlebitis. The venogram of the right lower limb shows partial femoro-popliteal obliteration with a downward concave cupuliform image in the superficial femoral vein * . Femoral phlebitis is diagnosed and the patient is given anticoagulant treatment. No improvement. Worsening of the thick leg. Surgery shows a primary fibrosarcoma of the femoral vein.

Chapter 15

RADIOISOTOPE PHLEBOGRAPHY

Figures 410–418

by Aslam Siddiqui, M.D.

The concept of utilizing radioisotopes in the detection of venous thrombosis is not new; however, there has been a recent flurry of research activity in this area. Table 1 lists most of the radiotracers which have been tried with varying degrees of success in humans and experimental animals. The most simple and convenient method of performing isotope phlebography is by using technetium-99m labeled albumin particles (macroaggregates or microspheres). These are readily available and are in routine use for pulmonary perfusion scintigraphy. These radiolabeled particles adhere to newly formed clots in vivo and appears as hot spots. Other findings on technetium-99m labeled albumin particle phlebography which suggest thrombophlebitis include non-visualization of a venous segment or system, collateral vessels and stasis of the radiotracer distal to the clot. When isotope phlebography, using ^{99m}Tc macroaggregates or microspheres, is performed and interpreted properly, the accuracy is over 90% when compared to contrast phlebography. Although the contrast phlebography is still the most reliable technique for detection of deep venous thrombosis, complications such as thrombophlebitis due to contrast material, local trauma and sepsis at injection site, etc., are not rare. It also can not be used in patients who are allergic to contrast medium or in those who have edematous legs or have small veins unsuitable for large volume injection. For isotope phlebography a very small volume injection is required; therefore, very thin needles can be used and allergic reaction is not a problem. Furthermore, the isotope phlebography can be combined with pulmonary perfusion scintigraphy without any extra discomfort or radiation dose to the patient.

The technique of technetium-99m macroaggregate or microsphere phlebography is very simple but exacting. Large field of view gamma camera is the instrument of choice; however, standard gamma cameras equipped with diverging collimators can also be used. No patient preparation is necessary. It is preferable that there is an interval of 24 hours between contrast and isotope phlebography since endothelial damage from contrast medium injection can give false positive scan results. Briefly the technique of isotope phlebography is as follows:

A. Four syringes are prepared, two with 2.5 mCi of technetium-99m macroaggregate or microsphere diluted with 1–2 ml of saline in each, and each of other two syringes, containing about 3 ml of sterile saline. Gamma camera should be set for 10 000-count images and the intensity should be set accordingly.

B. A radioactive marker is taped between patient's legs at knee level and another one at symphysis pubis. The marker should not be too "hot".

C. Tourniquets are applied firmly just above the ankles and immediately below the knees and the patient lies supine with the detector of the gamma camera over the calves with radioactive knee marker just on the top of the field of view.

D. Slow injection of radiotracer is made in dorsal pedal veins of each foot simultaneously, followed by saline flush. Use of a three-way stopcock system is optional. During intravenous injection, blood should not be withdrawn into the syringe and held there for any length of time, since radioactive clots will form, giving false positive results.

E. As soon as radioactivity is seen in calves, the ankle tourniquets only are released and an image is made over the calves.

F. Next image is over the thighs with knee marker at the lower edge of the field of view and symphysis marker at the top.

G. Following that an image over the upper thigh

and pelvis is made with pubis marker at lower edge of the field.

H. After repositioning the patient as in F, the knee tourniquets are released and another image over the thighs is obtained (knee marker just at the lower edge of the film).

I. Another image over the pelvis is obtained as in G.

J. The patient is repositioned with detector over the calves and the knee marker just at the top of the field of view. In this position an image is obtained accumulating about 10 000 counts (depending on residual radioactivity), but for not more than 2 min. Intensity is set accordingly.

K. The patient then actively exercises lower extremities for about 2 min, by, for example, flexing and extending ankles against resistance (technicians pushing against the soles of the feet of the patient) or flexion and extension of the knees with the legs elevated on two pillows under the heels.

L. Another image is obtained as in J.

M. If after exercise persistent radioactivity is seen in the calves, lateral views should be obtained, right lateral for right calf and left lateral for left calf.

N. If pulmonary perfusion study is not requested, one anterior view lung image should probably be obtained anyway if the isotope phlebography is abnormal.

O. When a particular image takes a long time, imaging should be stopped at 2 min.

Table 1: Radiotracers used for isotope phlebography

Macroaggregates and microspheres of albumin	Labeled with technetium-99m
Fibrinogen	Labeled with iodine-123,125, 131, technetium-99m, indium-111, mercury-197, bromine-77
Streptokinase, urokinase	Labeled with iodine-123,125,131, technetium-99m
Plasminogen, plasmin	Labeled with iodine-123,131
Fibrin	Labeled with iodine-123
Antihuman fibrinogen antibody	Labeled with iodine-131
Platelets	Labeled with indium-111, chromium-51, technetium-99m
White blood cells	Labeled with chromium-51, indium-111, iodine-131, technetium-99m–sulfur colloid
Technetium-99m pertechnetate infusion venography	
Fibrinogen turnover test	Iodine-125 label
Regional clearance of xenon-133	

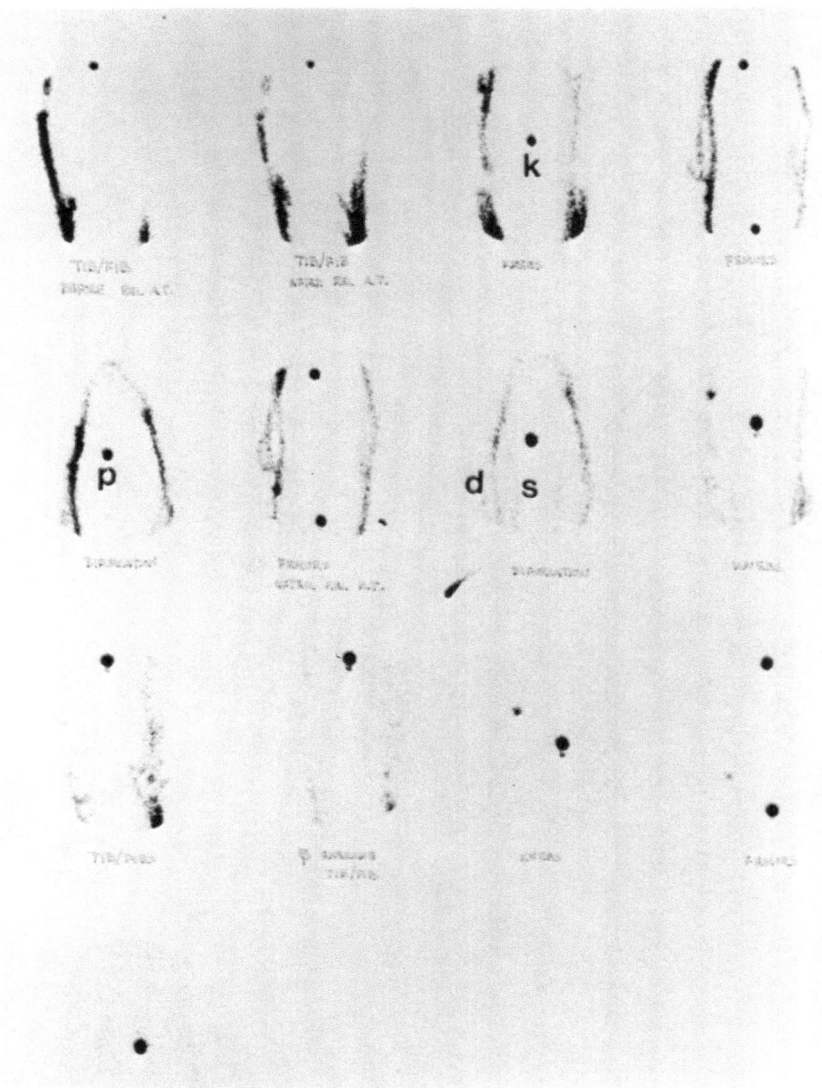

Fig. 410: Images over the calves (Tib/Fib) are obtained immediately after injection of technetium-99m MAA into the pedal veins of each foot — before and after release of ankle tourniquet. Subsequently 10 000-count images are obtained over knees, thighs (femur) and pelvis (bifurcation). The knee and symphysis pubis are marked by letters k and p respectively. The knee tourniquets cause the radiotracer to go into the deep venous channels (d). Removal of knee tourniquets causes the residual radioactivity in the calves to be emptied through the superficial venous system (s). The superficial system is always seen medial to the deep. After exercise there is usually no residual radiotracer in the lower extremities. Incidentally, it is not unusual to see some degree of collaterization in the deep venous system in thighs in normal individuals. Overall, this is a normal isotope phlebogram.

286

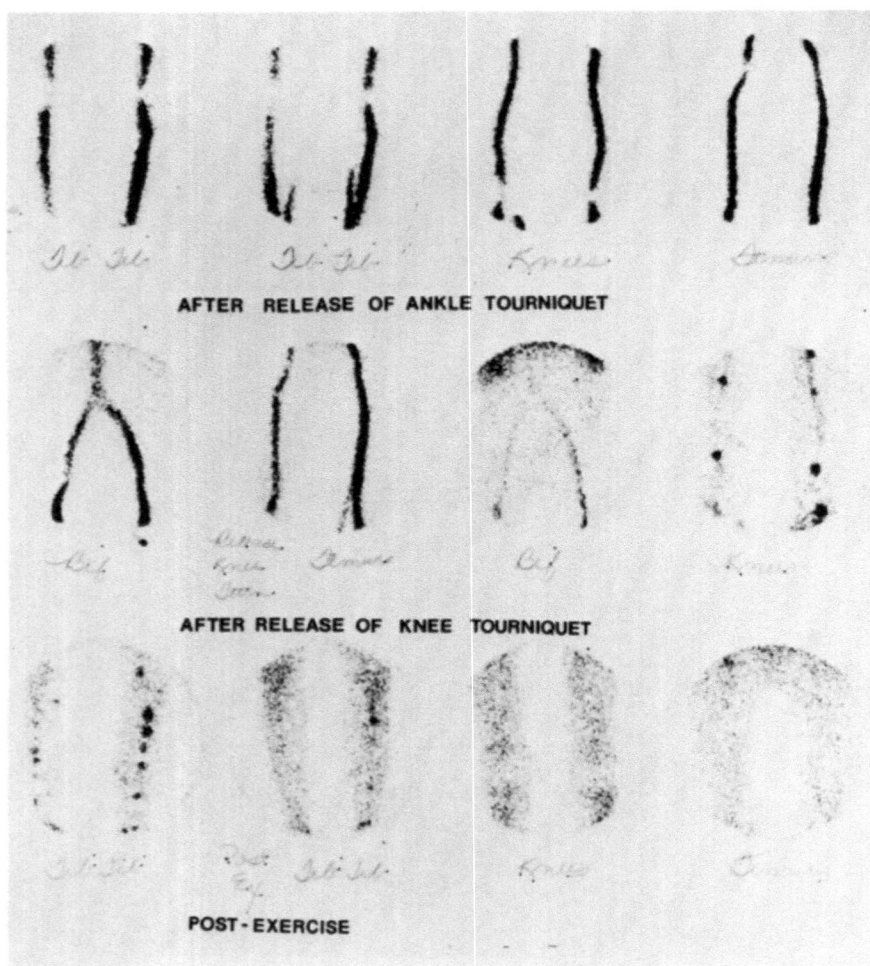

AFTER RELEASE OF ANKLE TOURNIQUET

AFTER RELEASE OF KNEE TOURNIQUET

POST - EXERCISE

Fig. 411: Another normal isotope phlebogram. The superficial venous system in the thighs in not visualized, despite a technically adequate study. This finding is not unusual. Multiple punctate areas of hang-up of radiotracer are noted in the calves in the late part of the phlebogram. These probably represent radioactivity around the venous valves — normal or hypertrophied. As in this case, the exercise usually clears this hang-up.

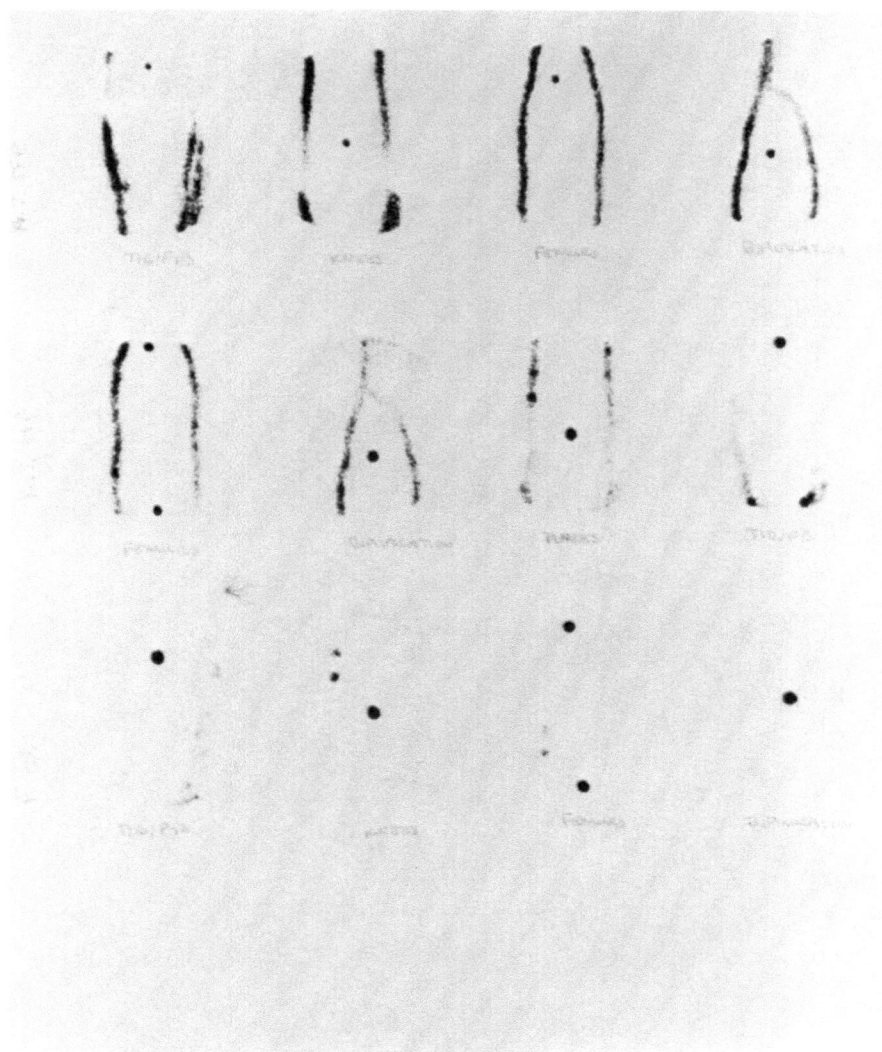

Fig. 412: Another normal study showing very rapid clearance of the radiotracer from the lower extremities. Two small punctate areas of radioactivity persist in the lower portion of the right thigh. The shape and size of this hang-up is suggestive of retention of technetium-99m MAA at venous valves.

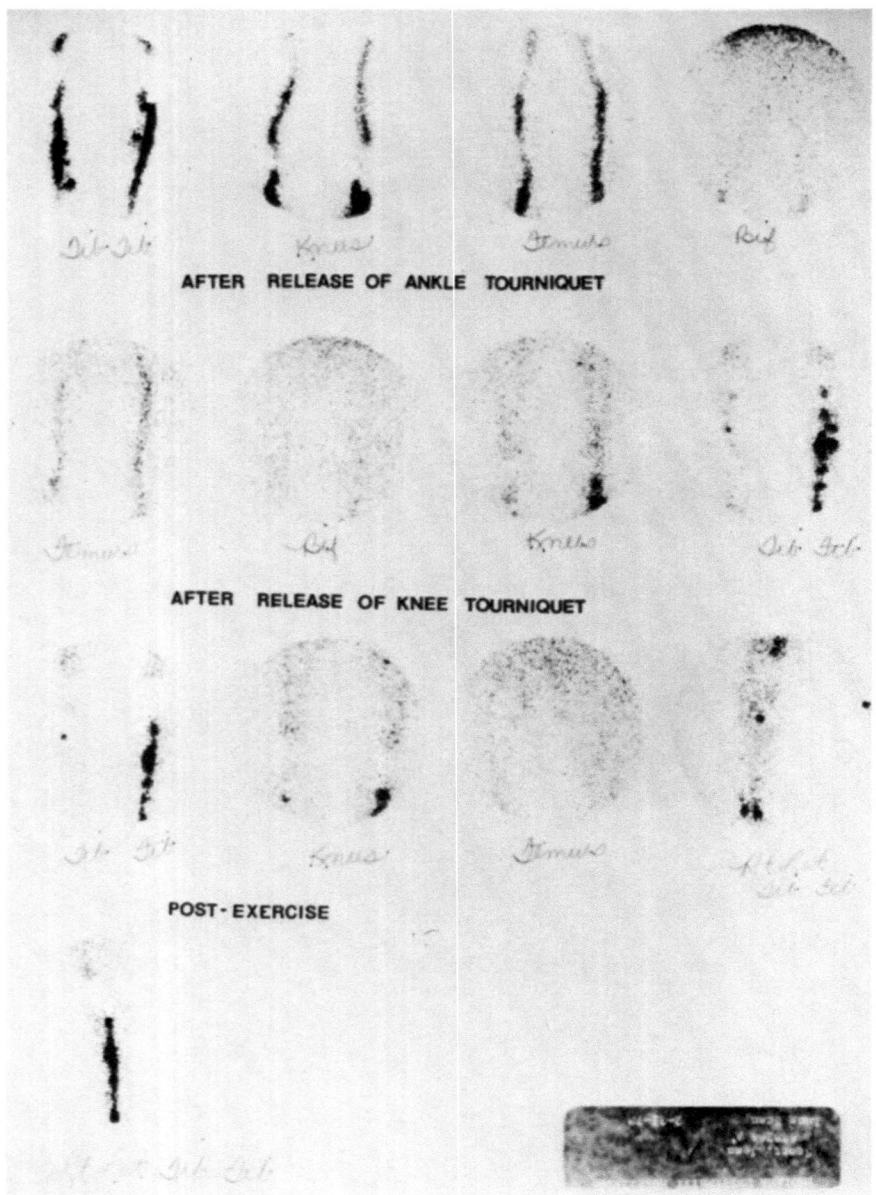

AFTER RELEASE OF ANKLE TOURNIQUET

AFTER RELEASE OF KNEE TOURNIQUET

POST-EXERCISE

Fig. 413: In this isotope phlebogram, there is quick clearance of radiotracer from the lower extremities; however, there is hang-up in the left calf. This appears somewhat irregular and linear and the exercise has no definite effect on it. This is technetium-99m MAA adhering to a fresh thrombus. Contrast phlebogram confirmed this finding.

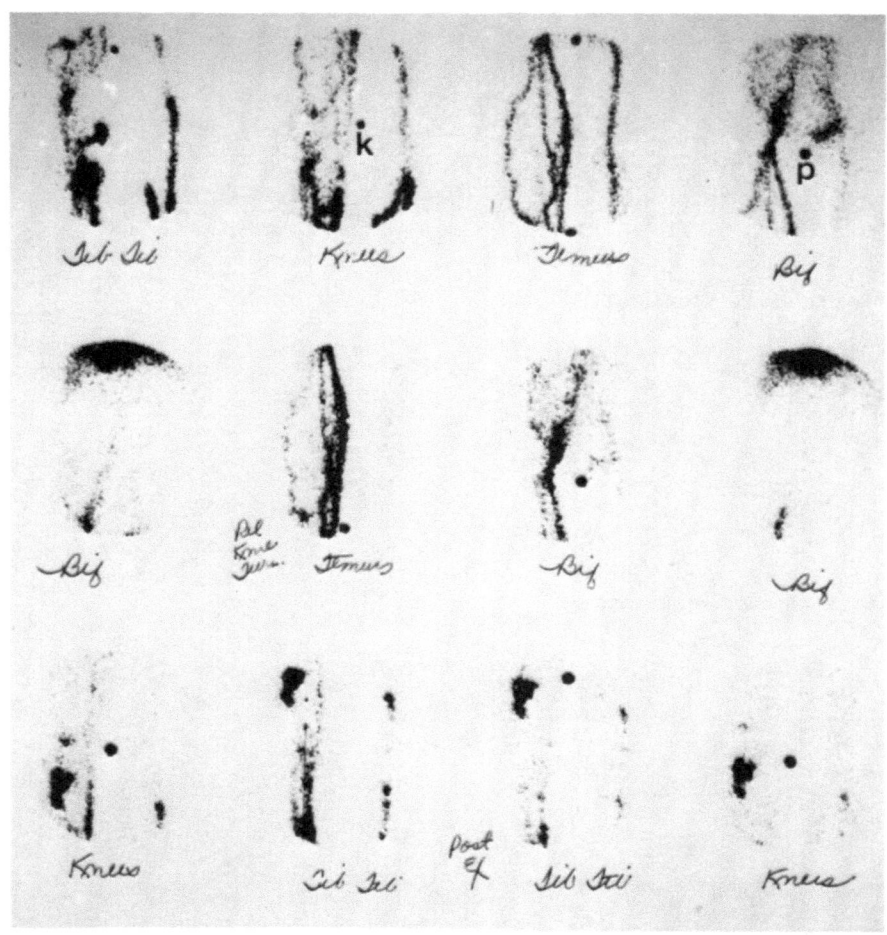

Fig. 414: This isotope phlebogram was performed in a man who was clinically suspected to have pulmonary embolism and had minimal symptoms to suggest thrombophlebitis of right lower extremity. The phlebogram on left is within normal limits. There is extensive collaterization in right calf, thigh and pelvis. The deep system in the right thigh is not visualized. The vein on the medial aspect of the right thigh represents the superficial venous system which is filling despite the knee tourniquet. This finding in combination with two irregular-looking collateral veins is highly suggestive of deep venous thrombosis in right thigh. Transpelvic and other collateral are also seen in this area. Persistent area of hang-up is also noted around the right. Diagnosis in this patient is acute and chronic thrombophlebitis in right lower extremities.

290

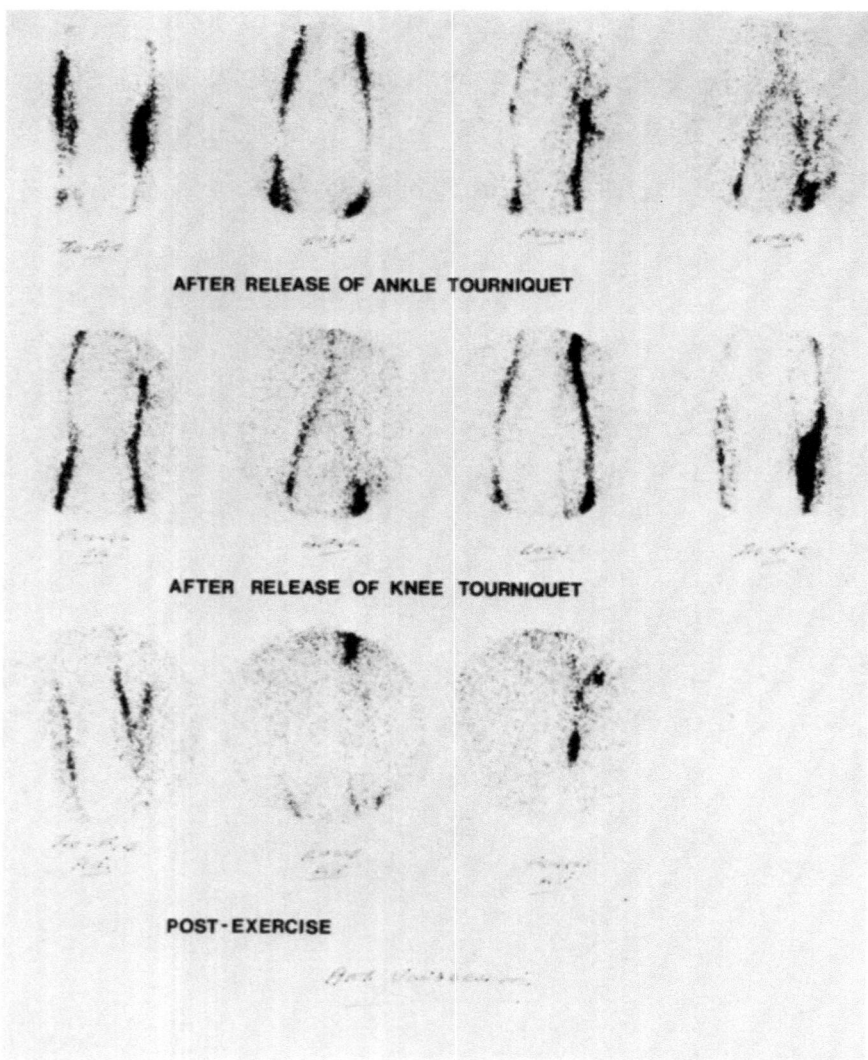

AFTER RELEASE OF ANKLE TOURNIQUET

AFTER RELEASE OF KNEE TOURNIQUET

POST-EXERCISE

Fig. 415: In this isotope phlebogram, the deep venous system in the left thigh is well visualized; however, in the upper 1/3 of the thigh there is an abrupt cut-off and evidence of collateral circulation. In this patient with pulmonary embolism this was considered to be the source of emboli. The findings of this isotopic study were confirmed by contrast phlebogram. The areas of increased radioactivity around the area of phlebitis represent stasis of blood in the veins distal to the clot and in the collateral vein.

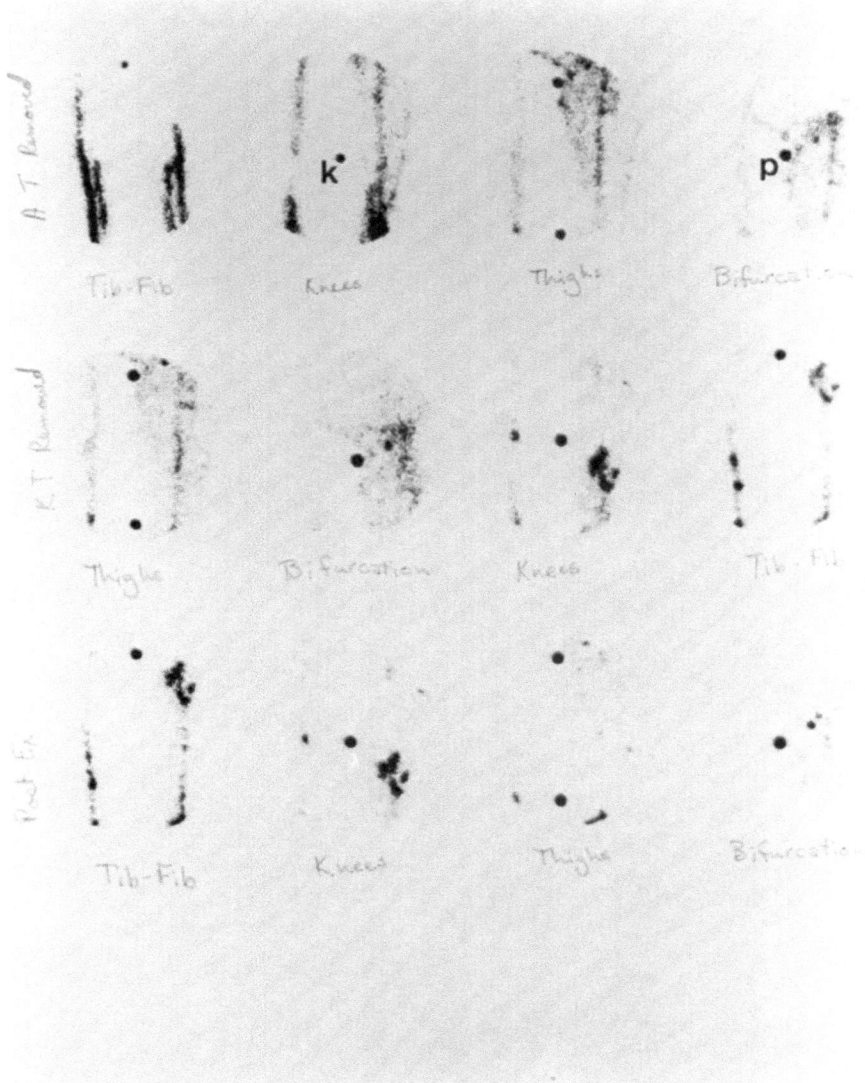

Fig. 416: This is a study in a patient with old thrombophlebitis in the region of left thigh. The deep venous system in the thigh appears to have recanalized; however, left iliac vein still shows no activity and there are transpelvic and other collaterals. There appears to be vague diffuse type of distribution of the radioactivity in the thigh. This is due to multiple small collaterals and perforators. There is probably some acute thrombophlebitis around left knee as evidenced by post-exercise hang-up. This study demonstrates the difficulty of differentiating acute thrombophlebitis from chronic using isotope phlebography. If definite abnormal areas of hang-up are seen after exercise, this would be suggestive of acute phlebitis. Otherwise, collateral circulation and absence of filling of a venous system is seen in both acute and old thrombophlebitis.

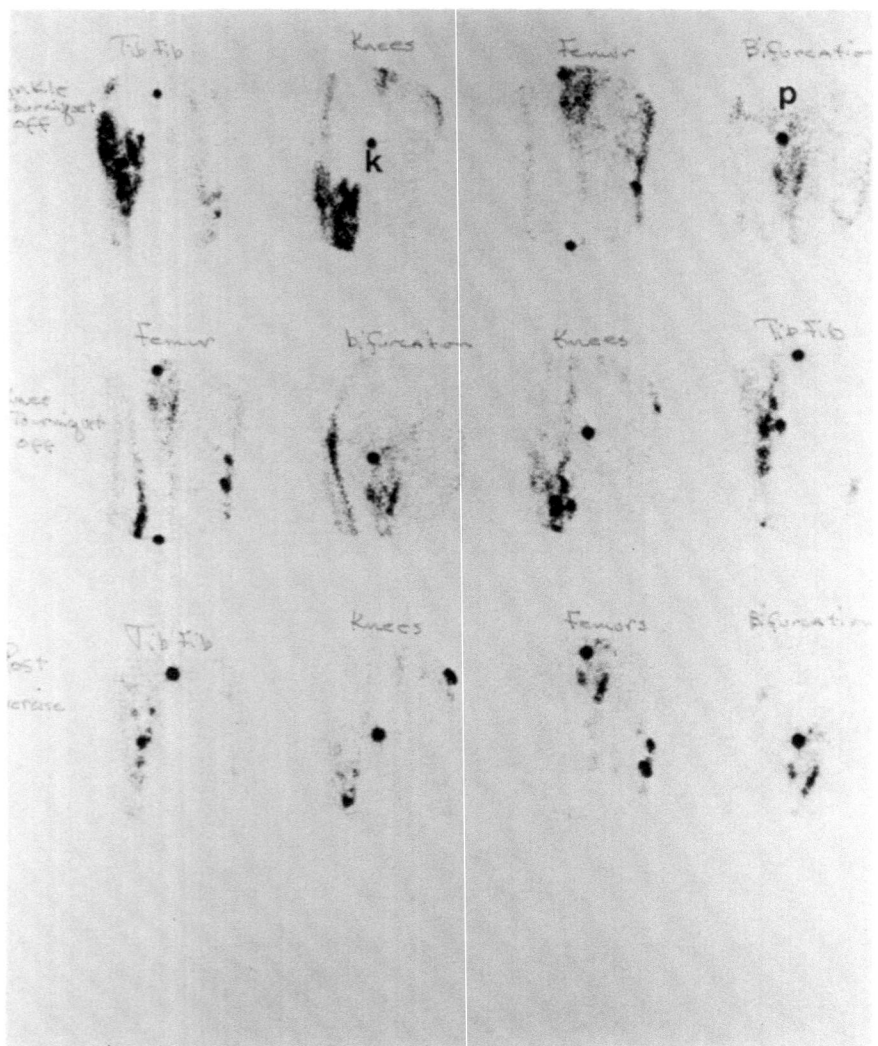

(a)

Fig. 417: (a) This patient had multiple episodes pulmonary emboli and thrombophlebitis in past resulting in interruption of inferior vena cava. This study was performed approximately 6 months later. Except for some stasis in varicosity due to chronic venous insufficiency, the right lower extremity phlebogram is essentially normal. On the left the deep venous system is not visualized and there are numerous collaterals. Iliac veins are not well visualized on either side. Findings are consistent with thrombophlebitis. (b) Anterior view of perfusion lung scan on the same patient shows normal lungs without any defects to suggest

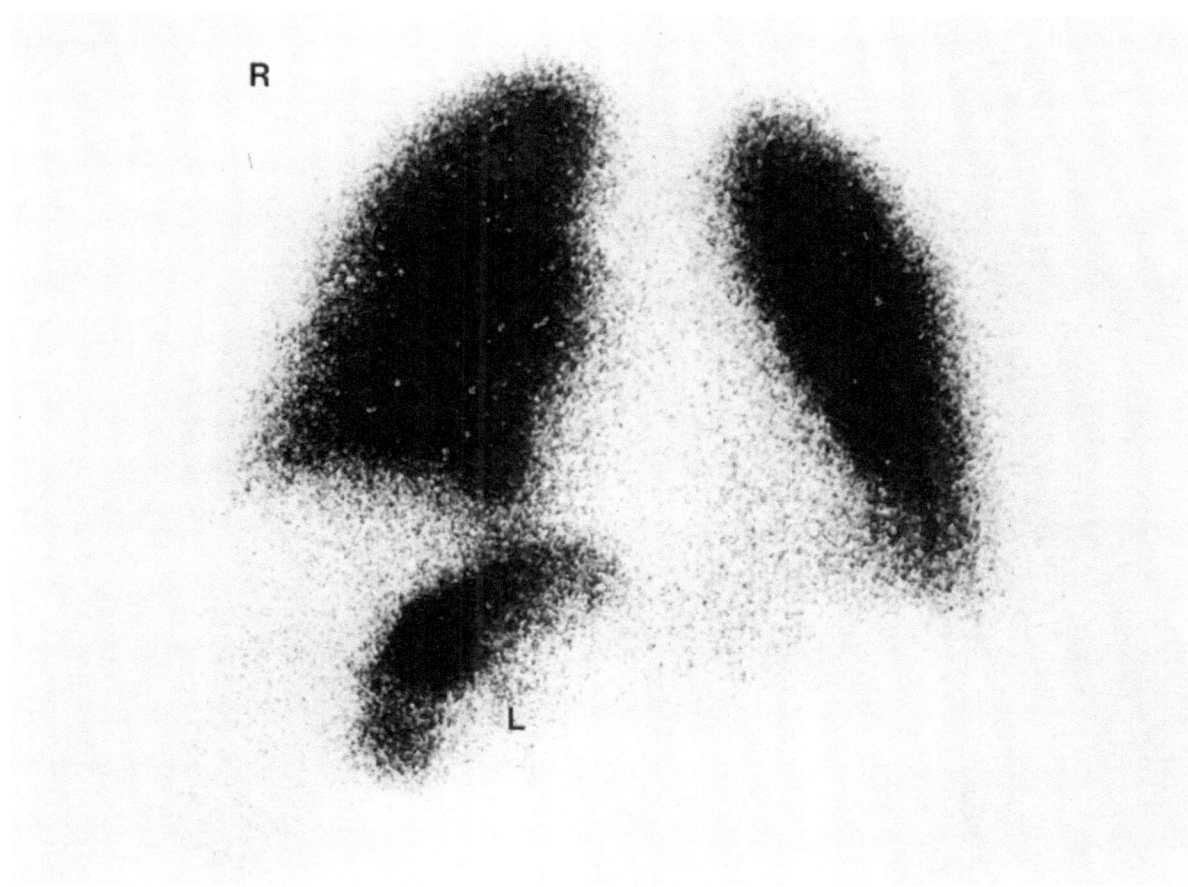

(b)

pulmonary emboli. Also seen is the entrapment of the technetium-99m labeled MAA in a portion of liver. When inferior vena cava flow is interrupted, numerous collateral venous channels open up, including veins in the anterior abdominal wall and umbilical vein. The umbilical vein drains into the quadrate and caudate lobes of the liver. In this patient some of this radiotracer was being drained from the lower extremities through the umbilical vein and thus got trapped in the region of caudate and quadrate lobes of the liver.

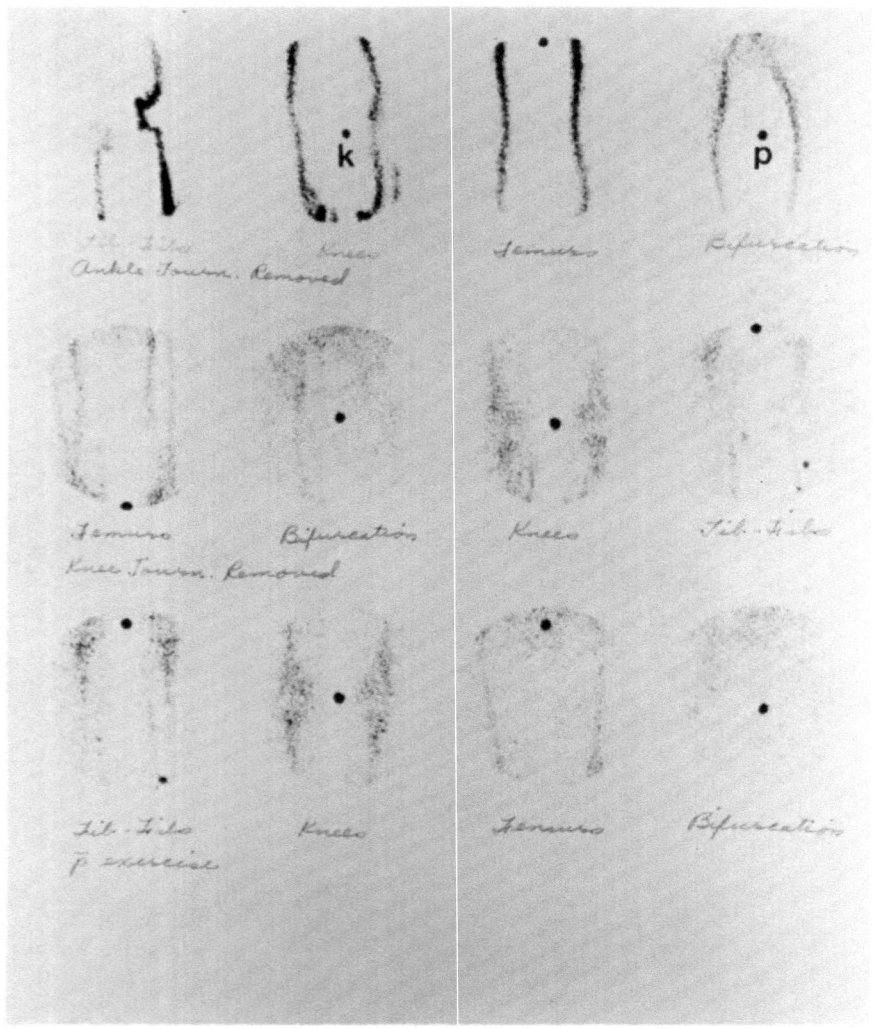

Fig. 418: In this isotope phlebogram, the initial flow appears to be within normal limits; however, in later phase of the study, there is visualization of the skeleton in the lower extremities. This patient had an intracardiac right to left shunt and the technetium-99m MAA particles were able to get into the systemic circulation. Besides the skeleton, these particles were also trapped in various organs, including kidneys and brain.